WHEN YOUR DOCTOR DOESN'T KNOW BEST

Medical Mistakes That Even the Best Doctors Make— And How to Protect Yourself

Richard N. Podell, M.D., and William Proctor

Simon & Schuster

New York London Toronto Sydney Tokyo Singapore

SIMON & SCHUSTER
Rockefeller Center
1230 Avenue of the Americas
New York, New York 10020

Designed by Irving Perkins Associates
Manufactured in the United States of America

1   3   5   7   9   10   8   6   4   2

Library of Congress Cataloging-in-Publication Data
Podell, Richard N., date.
    When your doctor doesn't know best: medical mistakes that even
the best doctors make—and how to protect yourself / Richard N.
Podell and William Proctor.
        p.   cm.
    Includes index.
    1. Medical errors.   I. Proctor, William.   II. Title.
R729.8.P63   1995
610—dc20   94-33561
                            CIP

ISBN: 0-671-87112-9

To my parents, Lawrence J. Podell and Florence Podell, and to three professionals who taught me to respect the patient's perspective: Anne R. Somers; Kurt Deuschle, M.D.; and Donald Kent, M.D.

A Note to the Reader

To ensure that every section of this text is medically accurate and relevant to patients' needs, I have asked knowledgeable and caring physicians in a wide variety of specialties and backgrounds to read and comment on the successive drafts of this book.

Each section has been reviewed by two or more primary care physicians—family physicians or internists—and by two or more board-certified physicians from the following specialties: allergy and immunology, cardiology, clinical nutrition, endocrinology, gastroenterology, general surgery, gynecology, neurology, oncology, orthopedics, psychiatry, pulmonary disease, and urology.

Although I take complete responsibility for the final text, I am profoundly grateful for the contributions that these medical experts have made in helping me produce as useful a tool as possible for patients who want to secure the best-available medical care.

As this is a book about medical error, it is doubly important for you to keep in mind that *you should not alter the dosages of your medicine or any other aspect of your medical treatment without first consulting your doctor.* Each reader's medical situation is unique. It is impossible for a book such as this, written for a wide audience, to anticipate all the factors that should enter into making your personal health care decisions.

Your personal physician is the adviser best able to help you adapt what you learn from this book to your specific health needs. What I hope the book will do is teach you how to ask the right questions and obtain the right answers, so you can become a more effective partner with your doctor in caring for your health.

Contents

Errors:

TREATMENT OF CANCER

Foreword

Despite this century's brilliant medical advances, a feeling of genuine well-being continues to elude most Americans. From all sides, we are bombarded with health advice and health warnings. Ironically, this heightened health consciousness tends to make us more aware of our personal vulnerability. In fact, we appear to be increasingly beset by forces that are inimical to our well-being. What were once presumed to be innocuous activities—such as basking in the sun, drinking a glass of tap water, or enjoying a juicy steak— now seem fraught with potential hazard. Even when our life is apparently safe and healthy, it often feels precarious and uncertain.

Traditionally, we have assuaged this insecurity by turning to medicine, religion, social-service institutions, or some other source of wisdom and comfort. Whether our help comes from a physician, minister, teacher, or other professional, much of its effectiveness depends upon our ability to trust its source. Throughout history, physicians have been held in particularly high trust because of their apparent power over life and death. This apotheosis of the physician may have culminated in the late 1960s with the advent of cardiac transplantation. For a brief period, cardiac transplant surgeons had near-godlike status in the public eye. Before long, however, the wheel had turned full circle, and public opinion seized upon the mistaken prophecies that often mark the early stages of any new medical treatment. Although we had been ready to transplant the human heart, we were unable to manage the rejection and infection that inevitably followed. Most centers abandoned the procedure until better drugs that would control or eliminate these dreaded complications became available.

This temporary suspension of heart transplantation by most centers symbolized a more general, widespread disillusionment that began during the early 1970s. Probably the greatest change in the

American health care system since that time has involved the transfer of power and authority from physicians to patients and third parties. Despite the erosion of doctor-patient relationships, we continue to have high expectations of medical treatment. We want to believe that, in a world perceived as increasingly dangerous, physicians are still among our greatest allies.

Unfortunately, a trip to the doctor's office or the hospital may provide one more good reason for worry. Because our health care system has become so complex and depersonalized, there is increasing leeway for medical mistakes. This does not mean that medical personnel are incompetent but, rather, that they are human. Like other human beings, physicians are frequently overstressed. Today's physicians are also subject to a variety of pressures that have been imposed by the increasing complexity of the medical system and of health care reform. Under these circumstances, medical errors can occur and include not only over- or undertesting, misdiagnosing, and prescribing medications carelessly, but also overlooking subtle signals of disease, failing to give important information, and recommending unnecessary procedures (or failing to recommend needed ones).

All of these possible errors and more are covered by *When Your Doctor* Doesn't *Know Best*, an invaluable guide for helping patients communicate assertively with their physicians and assume ultimate responsibility for their own health care. The book covers a wide spectrum of medical and surgical conditions, ranging from cancer and cardiac disorders to Lyme disease, estrogen replacement therapy, and senility. In a clear, congenial style, the authors outline a comprehensive program for preventing or rectifying physician and hospital error. Their message is sobering but never unduly alarming. *When Your Doctor* Doesn't *Know Best* is a valuable and potentially life-saving guide that is highly recommended to all patients and their families. In our precarious and uncertain world, this is one guide that can be trusted.

Denton A. Cooley, M.D.
Surgeon-in-Chief
Texas Heart Institute
Houston, Texas

Introduction

A Program to Protect Yourself from Medical Error

When I, as a practicing physician, become a patient, I have a better shot at protecting myself than you do. But that's only partially because I'm a doctor. The truth is that when a doctor is a patient, he or she usually isn't treated any differently from anyone else. That's why I don't hesitate to be assertive in my own defense. Because most of my successes while on the receiving end of the stethoscope have *not* been due to my professional credentials, I feel quite comfortable speaking to you from your point of view.

The kind of assertiveness I'm talking about is something I've learned the hard way through years of trial and error. Increasingly, I've been impressed by the need *all* patients have for a practical program to prevent medical mistakes, especially when I hear so often complaints about misdiagnosis, physician insensitivity, unnecessary tests and procedures, not answering questions, and oversights and mistakes that can be traced back to medical offices overwhelmed by administrative complexities and paperwork.

The nagging sense of worry you frequently have when you enter your doctor's office or a hospital is, unfortunately, often warranted, even in the best medical settings. With every day that passes, the chances increase that you or I will fall victim to error. What exactly is provoking this?

What's Causing the Mistakes?

Whatever happens under the Clinton plan or in the years to follow, the problems *and* the remedies discussed in this book will not change. For one thing, your doctor's office sessions—those intimate face-to-face chats when he or she is able to hear your complaints and prescribe treatment—will continue to be cut to the bone. Instead of focusing mainly on caring for you, the typical doctor will increasingly spend her time focusing on high-tech procedures, tunneling out from under a blizzard of insurance forms and government-mandated paperwork, or scrambling to meet productivity quotas designed by the managers of your health plan.

The more sophisticated and, therefore, more costly medical tests and procedures become, the more likely it is that care will be fragmented by a bottom-line consideration: Who will pay for it? As you're shunted from internist to specialist to technician, you will find out whether you belong to the top tier of medical care, to the middle, or to the bottom. You can't take it for granted anymore that your personal physician's decisions will be determined solely by his understanding of your health needs. He will inevitably have to classify you as belonging to the medical "haves" or the "have-nots."

This impersonal atmosphere, with no firm hand on the medical tiller, fosters situations that are ripe for error. But it's important to recognize that the medical errors you face aren't primarily a result of bad or greedy doctors, though such physicians are sometimes the problem. In fact, most medical error is embedded in a complex and defective system, and so to a large degree, it's inevitable. Certainly, it's essential to identify and root out the incompetent or dishonest doctors. But good physicians also make mistakes, and they make them every day—and I include myself in this group.

Even in well-organized offices, lab work, letters from specialists, and other patient data get misplaced or misread a minimum of 2 percent of the time. A Harvard Medical School study of 30,000 hospitalized patients found that injuries caused by flaws in medical management occurred in 3.7 percent of all hospitalizations—and one in seven of these led to death. In poorly run clinics, the incidence of such error is much higher still.

Also, doctors with excessive patient loads and administrative responsibilities (and that includes *most* physicians) can experience lapses in concentration, even with patients who have been coming to them for years. A rushed or distracted doctor may even fail to take an adequate medical history. As a result, he may overlook the fact that you have a particular illness that makes you vulnerable to the side effects of a particular drug or procedure that he prescribes.

For example, your physician may give you erythromycin for your bronchitis even though his records show you are taking Seldane, an antihistamine, for your allergies. In the back of his mind, the doctor knows that Seldane and erythromycin are potentially a deadly combination, which may trigger heart rhythm irregularities or worse. But at the instant of decision, the fact that you're on Seldane just doesn't click in.

Other errors can be traced to the way doctors and health administrators function in the different medical care systems that now exist. The stresses and strains of a high-pressure practice can trigger mistakes no matter what the setting—whether it's the traditional office of an independent physician or a clinic run by a health maintenance organization (HMO).

Are There More Mistakes in an HMO?

The main issue is not which type of health care system produces more mistakes, but, rather, the *kinds* or *categories* of errors that are likely to characterize different medical settings. Traditional fee-for-service medicine, administered by a private practice doctor, tends to err on the side of doing *too much* for the patient. A major reason is that private physicians have no upper limit on the services they can offer, and their payment depends on what the patient's insurance or pocketbook will bear.

Managed care organizations, such as the HMO, which are fast becoming a dominant form of care in the United States, tend to err on the side of doing *too little* for the patient. A source of this problem is that these groups have a fixed, nonexpandable budget, and if one patient is given more, another patient may have to make do with less. HMO managers and administrators, who may not have medical degrees, set the cost-cutting tone, and practicing physicians have to respond accordingly.

The doctors in these two systems don't come to different conclusions about the same medical problem because they are dishonest. Instead, because many health conditions lie in a gray area that requires the doctor to make a judgment call, a doctor's decision may tend to conform to the bias of the system.

For example, it's often not easy to decide the following:

- Should this child be delivered by cesarean section or the natural way?

- Does this bleeding fibroid really need to come out, or can we stall until menopause?

- Should we replace your hip to relieve your arthritis pain, or will physical therapy be good enough?

When the answers to such questions are clear-cut, only a criminally minded doctor or health plan administrator will give the wrong answer just to make or save a buck. But when the answer can go either way, you shouldn't be surprised to hear different responses. The fee-for-service private physician may say, "Let's give this treatment or procedure a try!" Yet the people with the fixed-budget plan, such as an HMO, may answer, "Let's wait and see if we really need to do anything else."

Even though the first thing a doctor thinks about may not be the amount she'll receive, financial considerations can come into play, either consciously or subconsciously. It's obvious, for instance, that the more care you're given by a private physician, the more money that physician will make. A kind of reverse phenomenon is at work in managed health plans. There, you may not be aware of this twist: Your primary care doctor—also called your "gatekeeper"—may have funds *deducted* from her own income each time she refers you for a consultation with a specialist! So the pressure is on her to limit your care to what *she* can provide, not to take advantage of the expertise of other physicians.

Clearly, there are strong dollars-and-cents reasons that may cause doctors to give you more or less care, depending on the system in which they are operating. This situation came home to me in a very personal way recently when both an uncle and a cousin of mine were diagnosed with a similar early stage of prostate cancer.

My uncle, who had been cared for in an HMO for many years, was seen there by an internist, who in turn sent him to a urologist. The urologist advised him nothing should be done except to recheck certain blood tests after one year. The odds were better than fifty–fifty, the urologist said, that my uncle would live out his life before the cancer spread. Besides, he noted, despite the popularity of surgery or radiation in dealing with cancer of the prostate, there was no solid proof that these measures actually save lives. On the other hand, he said, there was a good chance that either of these procedures could cause impotence, urinary incontinence, or other unpleasant side effects.

My cousin, who had basically the same prostate problem as my uncle, carried traditional medical insurance—a circumstance that put him on quite a different path of treatment. He went first to his personal doctor, a private fee-for-service internist, who then referred him to a urologist as well as an oncologist (cancer specialist).

The urologist recommended surgery to remove the cancer. As for the cancer specialist, he felt it was necessary for my cousin to have a consultation with a radiotherapist, who was qualified to treat the cancer with radiation.

With all the specialists' recommendations before him, the cancer specialist (oncologist) ultimately decided that my cousin's chances of being alive and well five years or more in the future were best with surgery. He felt radiation should be a second choice. My cousin decided to go with the surgery option.

In these two scenarios no one is the "bad guy." It's just that when the facts and outlook for a certain health condition are fuzzy, there's a predisposition for doctors in different systems to lean toward those strategies that butter their own bread. So on the one hand, it's understandable that there would be fewer referrals with the HMO and that a wait-and-see attitude would be taken toward further treatment. On the other hand, it's *also* understandable that the private fee-for-service physicians would come down on the side of more aggressive, extensive—and expensive—treatments.

The important thing for you, as a patient, to understand is that there are peculiar biases and weaknesses in whatever system is providing your health care. If you're unaware of these tendencies, you're much more likely to be sold a bill of goods or to be blinded to the fact that you might be better served by some other option.

Throughout the book, I'll arm you with questions to ask in different medical situations so that you can elicit the facts you need to know about the treatment options that are available. Fortunately, most medical mistakes are predictable and preventable once you know what to look for.

The main problem plaguing too many patients is that they are so respectful toward—or intimidated by—their doctors that they don't realize they have a *right* and an *obligation* to be assertive in gathering facts about their situation. In the impersonal and harried environment that now exists in many doctors' offices and hospitals, you, as a patient, must become an activist in the best interests of your own health.

Once you know the kinds of questions that should be raised, you'll be in a much stronger position to prevent errors that could threaten your health and even your life. You don't have to try to become an amateur doctor. But you do need to educate yourself so that you can understand the basics about the symptoms and treatment of your own disease or condition. You must become alert to possible weak points in your particular medical system that may make you the victim of error. Such preparation will place you in the strongest possible position to monitor your own health and to work hand in hand with your physician to prevent error in a wide variety of circumstances.

Done smartly and diplomatically, being alert as a patient should improve, not harm, your relationship with your doctor. One colleague put it well: "I hope all my patients read this book. It teaches the skills that they need to do their job as patients. That helps me to do a better job as their doctor!"

What Types of Errors Might You Face?

With this book in hand, you'll be able to ask the right questions and make the best decisions when you're in situations like these:

- You're a 38-year-old woman whose doctor tells you that a lump that you can feel in your breast doesn't require further treatment because the lump has failed to show up on a mammogram. Should you accept his evaluation?

- Your doctor feels you need a kidney X ray, but when you go in for the procedure, you learn that you'll have to receive an injection of a dye into your blood—a prospect that worries you because you suffer from a number of serious allergies. Neither the radiologist nor any other physician is there to explain whether there could be an allergic reaction to the dye. To make the situation even more frustrating, the X-ray technician won't give a definite answer when you ask if there's a safer way to do the kidney test. Do you have the right to insist on an answer? Should you demand to see a qualified doctor? Should you refuse the dye injection?

- You're a 37-year-old woman with recent irregularities in your menstrual cycle. While you're undergoing a routine gynecological exam, your doctor recommends a costly and invasive biopsy of the lining of the endometrium (uterus), which she says can eliminate any question of cancer. How should you respond?

- You're admitted to a hospital for surgery, but the anesthesiologist fails to ask you if you snore. Is this an important omission?

- Your husband can't maintain his erection long enough to satisfy you. You wonder if his high blood pressure pill might be the problem, even though the doctor didn't say anything about sex problems being a side effect. Your husband is too embarrassed to bring up the topic with the physician. Should you pursue the issue? Is there any literature you can turn to for advice?

- As a female patient, you've become aware that the drug your doctor has prescribed for you, though tested on men, has never been tested on women. Should you be concerned that your doctor brushes aside your concerns with a glib "Oh, don't worry about that"?

- You're rushed to the emergency room with abdominal pain and are examined there by an intern or resident but not by a senior emergency room physician. Is that all right?

- You're given a large dose of antibiotics because you've been bitten by a deer tick, but there's no indication that you have Lyme disease. Is this a good idea?

- You've been unusually tired for a few months, but your blood tests come out normal. Your doctor concludes that you must be depressed. Should you accept this opinion? What are the alternatives?

- Your doctor refuses to help you design a program of vitamin therapy as part of your cardiac or cancer treatment. Is she being unreasonable?

- Although you're only in your late thirties, your doctors says you should have an exercise stress test every year. How should you respond to him?

- You must undergo a serious operation, but your doctor discourages you from checking into a large city hospital known for treating your particular condition. Instead, she insists that you use a nearby local hospital. What should you do?

- The doctor you often use for your medical exams schedules a chest X ray, even though you've had one within the previous twelve months. Should you go along with him?

If you've been plagued by such questions, don't feel alone—and don't feel paranoid. The reality is that far too many mistakes are made in doctor's offices and hospitals. Yet most patients don't know how to protect themselves, their relatives, or their close friends who may be facing a personal health crisis. What you need is a practical program to help you deal with medical error—the kind of program I've created in the following pages.

How Error Slips Through the Door

How may error enter, and how can you overcome it through the principles and techniques described in this book? To answer this question, let me tell you about Emma, Hal, Steve, Trudy, and Linda, each of whom had to deal with health-menacing and sometimes life-endangering medical mistakes.

TWO ERRORS THREATEN EMMA. Emma, a 38-year-old secretary, was always haunted by her memories of her mother, who had a small breast cancer removed when she was 49 years of age. Although the mother was doing well at age 65, Emma knew that her family medical history doubled her chances of developing breast cancer. But she contained her anxieties by telling herself that *her* high-risk period, like her mother's, would be at least ten years away.

Emma's family doctor, Dr. Caldwell, examined her breasts about every two years when she came in for a Pap smear. Unfortunately, he left it to her to schedule these visits, and he didn't remind her that the American Cancer Society and other expert panels have recommended that a breast exam be done yearly, not every two years. Nor had he ever asked Emma to demonstrate her self-examination technique to him, so that he could determine if she did it correctly. Had he done so, he might have learned that she wasn't being thorough.

Emma didn't examine her breasts very often because she wasn't confident about the procedure. Instead of pressing systematically with the pads of her four fingers throughout the entire area of each breast, she pinched a few places and left large sections unexamined. This was probably the reason that she didn't notice a one-inch-wide lump in her right breast until her husband called it to her attention.

Emma went quickly to her doctor, who said that although he wasn't sure, he didn't think it was a cancer. He asked her to get a mammogram at a clinic in which he owned a part interest. Despite the doctor's financial connection, the mammography unit was perfectly respectable, not the nonaccredited fly-by-night type you sometimes find in a shopping center. So what happened next wasn't the unit's fault.

Emma's mammogram results were normal. There was no evidence of cancer in the breast even though both Emma and her doctor could still feel a definite lump. Reassured by the negative report, her doctor told Emma that it was safe to wait awhile before she underwent tests. He asked her to return for another exam and mammogram in about six months.

That was a mistake. As is the case with many premenopausal

women, Emma's thick, dense breast tissue made reading a mammogram difficult. At least 15 percent of breast cancers that can be felt by hand can't be seen on a mammogram.

Fortunately, Emma became nervous after about two months had passed, and so she made an appointment with Dr. Arnold, a respected older surgeon who had operated on her mother. Alarmed that Emma had waited so long to take action, Dr. Arnold scheduled an immediate biopsy. He asked Emma to sign a paper stating that if cancer was found on the *frozen section* of the biopsy, then she would remain under anesthesia, and the doctor would proceed to remove the tumor and the breast. This is a standard operation known as a *radical mastectomy.*

That's exactly what happened. When Emma woke up, her right breast was gone. Once she realized what had happened, her first reaction was gratitude, especially when Dr. Arnold emphasized how lucky she was. He said the cancer had been confined to the breast, and all the lymph nodes he had extracted from the area near her shoulder tested negative for cancer. Losing a breast was a small price to pay for this assurance, he said.

Maybe yes, and maybe no. It took Emma about six weeks to learn from her outside reading that most modern breast cancer experts now believe that a much smaller operation, called a *lumpectomy*, could have given her as great a chance of cure. At the same time, this procedure would have allowed her to preserve almost all of her breast.

When she questioned Dr. Arnold about her findings, she found out that he was well aware that expert opinion had changed since his professors had taught him to remove all of the breast. He just didn't believe the new approach was valid.

"Fads come and go," Dr. Arnold told her. "But I'm not taking a chance with any of my patients."

Emma realized immediately that there was no point in arguing with him. She didn't even feel it would be worthwhile to express her growing anger that he had taken her choice away from her without informing her about other surgical alternatives. Dr. Arnold may have meant well, but Emma had paid a high price.

As a result of this bitter lesson, Emma transformed herself into a better-educated and more assertive patient. Although Dr. Arnold had told her she was "cured," Emma sought out a second opinion from an oncologist, a physician trained in both internal medicine and cancer. From this specialist, she learned that even though her chances of being cured were quite good without any further treatment, the risk could be reduced by another 25 to 30 percent if she began to take tamoxifen, a hormone-related chemotherapy drug.

It's now been five years since Emma's breast was removed. She's off chemotherapy and still doing well. She regrets not having had the chance to save her breast, but she's also thankful because she managed to survive two major medical errors.

When she reflects on the first error, she shudders to think what might have happened if she had accepted her family doctor's verdict that her "normal" mammogram meant she could safely delay having a biopsy done on her breast lump. The second error cost her a breast, but at least now she's more in control of her health and much less likely to be victimized by the kinds of mistakes that confronted her in the past.

Sometimes, an error may at first seem much less threatening than those that confronted Emma. But as a man named Hal learned, when it comes to your health, there's often no such thing as a minor mistake.

THE MYSTERY SURROUNDING HAL'S HIGH BLOOD PRESSURE. Hal's doctor diagnosed him as being hypertensive. In other words, like an estimated 40 to 60 million other Americans, he had high blood pressure. Hal's average blood pressure reading at the medical clinic was 162/98, while normal pressure is below 140/90. But for some reason, the doctor failed to tailor his treatment to Hal's individual body rhythms and daily health habits. The results came perilously close to disaster. Check the following facts, and see for yourself.

After making his diagnosis, the physician prescribed a common medication, an angiotensin-converting enzyme (ACE) inhibitor, to bring Hal's blood pressure readings down to normal. He was told to take the drug twice a day, at breakfast and with dinner.

Unfortunately, the physician failed to take a couple of key factors into account in his treatment. First of all, he apparently forgot that Hal was also taking an antidepressant in the evening. Or if he was aware of the other medication, it didn't register with him that there might be an interaction between the ACE inhibitor and the antidepressant, both of which tend to drive the blood pressure down.

Second, the doctor didn't bother to check the fluctuations in Hal's blood pressure at different times during the day just to be certain that the drug was being used to the best effect. He could have done this by recommending that Hal take his own readings with a generally available and easy-to-use home blood pressure monitoring device.

Hal suspected that there might be a problem related to his antihypertensive medication when he began to feel unusually tired, weak, and dizzy as bedtime approached. On one occasion, he almost fell down when he got up in the early morning hours to urinate. He had to steady himself against a wall for a minute or two before he could proceed to the bathroom.

Although he trusted his doctor, Hal was a great believer in doing his own homework, especially in matters relating to his health. So he began to read extensively in the vast body of lay literature that is available on hypertension. Before long, he discovered that many people with high blood pressure take their own readings at home. This way, their doctors have more information to work with in directing treatment.

Hal went right out and bought a home monitoring device at a local medical supply store. Within a few days, he noted that his blood pressure consistently dropped quite steeply as the evening wore on. By the time he went to bed, his readings averaged only 115/75, well within normal range. And on two occasions, when he measured his pressure just after midnight after taking both his ACE inhibitor and his antidepressant, he discovered that the readings were only 99/61!

When he reported his symptoms and also his home-monitored readings to his doctor, the physician immediately understood the problem. Hal was experiencing *hypo*tension, or excessively low blood pressure, as a result of the two medications he was taking. The doctor adjusted Hal's drug schedule by giving the blood pressure pill in a single morning dose, which produced a stronger effect during the day and a lesser effect at night.

The final result of all this monitoring and investigation was a better form of medical treatment and a healthier life for Hal. But it's likely that without the actions of an alert patient, this doctor's error would gone undetected until Hal experienced a serious fall or worse from hypotension.

HOW STEVE'S DOCTOR STUMBLED OVER SNORING. Do you often snore? If so, you'll be interested in the situation faced by Steve, who was admitted to a hospital for a surgical procedure. Because the procedure required general anesthesia, Steve met with his anesthesiologist the night before the operation to go over his medical history.

During the discussion, the specialist seemed tired and distracted. At one point, he complained that he was just finishing one of his longest and most demanding days in memory. He then proceeded in a rather perfunctory way to ask Steve a series of questions attached to a clipboard on his lap. He rushed through the questions so quickly that he seemed to be assuming the answers before Steve even responded.

The next day, Steve went in for what was supposed to be a routine operation. But when the surgeon had completed his work and Steve was transferred to the recovery room to allow his anesthesia to wear off, the nurse in charge of his case was horrified to find that Steve would stop breathing entirely for as long as a minute at a stretch. Finally, a full medical team managed to bring Steve back to consciousness, and fortunately, later tests showed that he hadn't suffered any brain damage or other injury. But it had been a close call.

The problem? The anesthesiologist had failed to probe deeply enough in his preoperative interview to see if Steve's personal health history contained any signals that anesthesia might be dangerous. Although Steve was a chronic snorer, the doctor had never asked him about this habit. A small percentage of people who snore have a breathing disorder known as *obstructive sleep apnea.* While they are asleep, their breathing may stop for a minute or more, and the levels of oxygen in the blood plummet.

Although this condition is usually not an immediate danger in normal circumstances, the application of anesthesia slows the working of the respiration centers of the brain and may aggravate the impact of sleep apnea. The result may be a serious cutoff of blood flow, with the patient possibly suffering a stroke or heart attack.

Steve was lucky. He escaped unscathed from the potentially devastating effects of this serious medical mistake. Furthermore, he knew that if he ever had another operation that required anesthesia, it would be essential for him to bring up his snoring at the outset of the interview with the anesthesiologist. This way, the doctor would be alerted to warn the postoperative staff to watch for a potential problem.

It's always important to assume leadership over your own health care whenever you suspect there may be a problem with the treatment you're receiving—even if you can't quite put your finger on what that problem is. That's what Trudy did when she finally decided her doctor couldn't figure out how to treat her headaches.

WHY TRUDY'S HEADACHES GOT WORSE BEFORE THEY GOT BETTER. Throughout her adult life, Trudy had been struck periodically by one of the most common health complaints: severe headaches. They became so painful and debilitating that it eventually became evident that she was suffering from chronic migraines.

The cause of the headaches was uncertain, but Trudy was able to get some relief for a while from a migraine medicine, Cafergot, which her doctor directed her to take. But within a month or two, the pains returned with a vengeance. They were more frequent than ever before, even after the doctor increased the dosage of the Cafergot.

The doctor seemed at a loss about what to do. He suggested that there might be some sort of psychological connection to the headaches and that Trudy should see a psychiatrist. Instead, she decided to seek out another internist, a known headache specialist, for a second opinion.

The second doctor's response was quite different from what you might expect. He quickly identified Trudy's problem as the medicine itself! He told her that ergot-type migraine medicines, such as Cafergot, can actually *cause* headaches or increase their intensity for some patients. Among other things, they have an addictive quality that makes it necessary for certain patients to take larger and larger doses to get the same level of relief. The more of the medicine you take, the more pain you may experience later, especially if you miss a dose or are late taking it.

This doctor put Trudy on a nonaddictive calcium channel blocker, which can help relieve headaches without increasing their intensity. Monitoring her daily, he tapered off the Cafergot while moderating her "withdrawal" headaches by using injections of a powerful antimigraine medicine, dihydroergotamine. Trudy had a hard time during the first week of withdrawal, but it was worth it. As a result of the adjustment, her daily headaches vanished, and her occasional serious attacks were much easier to control.

Although most doctors are honest and ethical, some are not. A patient by the name of Linda ran into one of these "bad apples."

LINDA'S HIGH-PRESSURE GYNECOLOGIST. Linda had experienced one irregular menstrual period and mentioned the concern to her gynecologist during one of her routine checkups. He immediately displayed a worried look and suggested that she might be in danger of developing cancer. Understandably Linda became upset. The doctor continued to press her to undergo an immediate biopsy of her endometrium, the membrane that lines the uterus. Although the test was expensive, he said that if he performed it during this visit, he could give her a discount.

"Of course, I don't know that anything is actually wrong with you," he said. "But this procedure will make us all rest easier if the results are negative."

Feeling extremely pressured by her physician, Linda agreed reluctantly to go ahead with the biopsy, which turned out to be much more uncomfortable and invasive than she had expected. She continued to have doubts about the necessity of the procedure, but she decided she had no choice but to trust her doctor.

The results, which the doctor forwarded to her later, were negative. But Linda wasn't particularly relieved. In fact, she was *furious* with her physician because after checking with other patients and also with a doctor friend, she had learned that the procedure had almost certainly been unnecessary. Apparently, the test had become rather fashionable among gynecologists in her area because it was easy to perform and carried a high price tag. Also, she had gone through many anxious moments while waiting more than a week for the results to arrive.

What can you do if you find yourself in Linda's position in your doctor's office? First of all, don't be intimidated or rushed into a test or procedure unless your doctor assures you that a genuine emergency is involved. Increasingly, sophisticated and costly diagnostic tests are being used inappropriately as screening procedures. The doctor's rationale that he was testing for cancer was equally inappropriate.

Also, remember that making decisions about your health care is similar to making any consumer decision. So evaluate the services and tests that are being offered, compare prices, and, whenever possible, check your physician's qualifications and track record in handling other patients with your particular condition. You may know other patients who have dealt with this physician, or you may even be friendly with another physician or nurse who can give you some advice about the kind of medical expertise you need. Any information you can gather will pay off by enabling you to protect your health better and save money on medical costs.

Such mistakes as those just described can turn your life into a living hell—and for no good reason. *Most* errors are avoidable if you are knowledgeable about the facts and alert to your avenues of recourse. The fundamental strategy in identifying and countering a medical error is to get an idea about what to look for and to understand how to employ the most effective antidote against the mistake.

The Four Basic Antidotes to Error

As we've seen, when I refer to medical error, I'm not just talking about the rare instance of incompetence or malpractice, such as amputating a right leg when the operation calls for removal of the left one. Certainly, this book contains strategies for protecting yourself from such gross mistakes. But there are also many routine glitches that occur thousands of times every day in hospitals, clinics, and doctors' offices across the country. These mistakes may not pose an immediate threat to your life or limb. Unattended over a period of time, however, they can cause unnecessary discomfort or even danger.

Error emerges in many guises, with each mistake having its own peculiar characteristics and demanding its own special responses. If you're dealing with an error related to a respiratory disease, for instance, your specific tactics will differ from those who are facing an orthopedic problem. The particular approaches to such errors are covered in succeeding chapters.

In addition to these specific responses, there is also a *general* strategy of protection that underlies all the special tactics that I've summed up in terms of the following four "antidotes" to medical error.

Error Antidote 1: Courage. To be able to operate effectively as a patient in the current health care environment, you must have the guts to stand up to your doctor and to ask him pointed questions. The alert—and safe—patient is the one who is able to be assertive, even aggressive, with her physician.

I'm not suggesting that you pick a fight with your doctor, but it is important to work hard toward an active collaboration with him. Your relationship with your physician should be a partnership, not a contest. At the same time, you must see yourself as an equal partner who participates in the big decisions. All the information in the world won't help you if you're too timid or cowed by the professional status of your doctor to speak out on your own behalf. I'll provide you with the questions to ask, but it's up to you to do the asking.

Error Antidote 2: Facts. To be your own best advocate with the health care establishment, you have to acquire a basic understanding of your condition, including the various medications and procedures that may be available for treatment. Effective self-education, including a knowledge of relevant medical terms and buzz words, will provide you with important armor to protect yourself from mistakes.

How do you get this information? Under the discussion of each error, I've included the key facts and terms you need to know to defend yourself against misdiagnosis, physician insensitivity, and unnecessary procedures and tests. In addition, you should get into the habit of conducting your own research into your condition.

Suppose your problem is high cholesterol. You might clip all newspaper articles on new breakthroughs or warnings on blood lipids. Find books in your local bookstore and library on cholesterol and look them over. Take notes on points that you feel you should raise with your doctor.

If you're unusually inclined to do independent research, you may even want to go to your library and check out copies of leading medical journals, such as *The New England Journal of Medicine* and *The Journal of the American Medical Association,* which contain landmark articles on your condition. Your librarian can help you find these studies through the *Index Medicus* or another medical index. You certainly won't understand everything you read. But the more you expose yourself to these specialized reports, the better educated you'll become about your condition.

Although this idea of doing amateur research into your medical problems may seem a bit of overkill, there's nothing wrong with becoming as well informed as you can about medical challenges you face. Again, I'm not suggesting that you "play doctor" and try to treat yourself. But patients who do their homework are patients who are likely to protect themselves most effectively against serious medical mistakes.

Error Antidote 3: Tips. Keep your ears open. If you encounter another patient with a problem similar to yours, share war stories. Explore in detail the problems that person has faced with doctors and hospitals. You can learn a great deal from other people's experiences.

Error Antidote 4: Second opinions. If you're not satisfied with what you're hearing from your doctor, find another physician who can double-check the first. But be careful that you don't fall into what I call the "second opinion trap."

Avoiding the Second Opinion Trap

As valuable as second opinions can be, some are definitely not worth the effort. A common reason is that many doctors absolutely refuse to criticize or contradict one another. To make the situation worse, a patient will often end up seeing a second doctor who has been recommended by the *first* doctor.

Put yourself in the second physician's shoes: Would you criticize a friend or colleague who probably plays tennis with you, knows your spouse, belongs to the same club, and is referring business to you? Of course you wouldn't, and neither will that doctor rendering the second opinion.

The only way to secure a reasonably valid second opinion is to go to a doctor who has nothing to do with the first one, and that may mean traveling to another part of town or even to another city. Of course, you'll probably have to pay a first-visit premium to the second doctor, but the extra cost will be worth it if you're facing a serious health crisis.

Whatever approach you take with a second opinion, however, you must remain careful and alert. Even an independent second doctor might not criticize the first opinion too severely, even if that first opinion was diametrically opposite. Doctors are conditioned from their days in medical school to be wary of stepping on their fellow physicians' toes. That's just the way the medical profession works.

To help you wend your way successfully through the second opinion maze, the description of various medical errors in this book will provide you with illustrations of subtle signals that will help you identify disagreements that the second doctor may have with the first. For example, if the second doctor indicates *any* reservations, qualifications, or differences of opinion, you must seize on this signal and press the doctor for more information. Even if he just says, "I wonder . . ." or "That's unusual . . . ," your medical-consumer antennae should go up.

Finally, you'll be armed with means to protect yourself against the "entrepreneurial" second opinion doctor, who may try to line her own pockets by pulling your business away from the original physician. Competition is fierce out there in the real medical world. So a physician may say, "Yes, you need an operation. But your doctor is proposing the wrong one. Now, let me show you what *I* can do for you."

Clearly, medical error may don many masks.

In the following pages you'll learn to identify and defend yourself against the major mistakes that are being made again and again in the treatment of hundreds of major and minor health problems. You'll learn how to ask the right questions and push for satisfactory answers, even if your doctor seems pressed for time or reluctant to go into detail. The presentation of information in this book has been designed to put you, the patient, in charge of your health. Just turn the page and prepare to be empowered!

PART ONE

Danger in the Heart Zone

SPECIAL ALERTS: CARDIOVASCULAR CONDITIONS

- If you're an asthmatic taking a beta-blocker for high blood pressure, the medication may aggravate asthmatic symptoms, such as wheezing and shortness of breath, and you could face sudden death. (See error, p. 60.)

- If you're taking a beta-blocker drug for high blood pressure, a reaction from allergy injections, bee stings, or food allergies can be much more severe. (See pages 65 and 66.)

- If you are a diabetic taking a beta-blocker for high blood pressure, the drug may be masking sudden drops in your blood sugar level, which could result in a stroke. (See error, p. 66.)

- If you're simultaneously taking a blood-thinning medication for clogged arteries *and* an antibiotic for an infection, you're at serious risk for bleeding in the brain. (See error, p. 72.)

- If you suffer a stroke, it's essential that your doctor immediately consider two often neglected tests: a computed tomography (CT) scan and an echocardiogram. Otherwise, you are at high risk for a second stroke. (See errors, pp. 81 and 83.)

- You increase your risk of sudden death from a heart attack unless your doctor helps you *rehearse* an attack before you have one. (See error, p. 103.)

- You increase your risk of sudden death from a heart attack in the emergency room unless you know how to move to the head of the patient line. (See error, p. 107.)

- If you agree to a coronary arteriogram (an invasive procedure involving injection of a dye and then observing the state of the vessels of the heart) and if the procedure is really not justified, you could suffer an unnecessary stroke or heart attack. (See error, p. 111.)

Blood Pressure

Your Doctor Says You Have Hypertension, but You Don't

You've had your blood pressure checked by your doctor on two visits to her office in the last six months, and in both cases, the readings were high. The first time, an average of two measurements was 150/94. The second time, a single measurement showed your pressure was even higher—154/95. In explaining her diagnosis that you have hypertension, she informs you that normal pressure should be below 140 for the first, or upper, number and below 90 for the second, or lower, number. Now, she's recommending that you go on low doses of an antihypertensive drug.

But you have some questions. From everything you've read, you understand that temporary, variable factors, such as the level of stress in your life, can be important in affecting blood pressure. You know that you don't handle stress very well in many situations. Also, you always feel extremely nervous when you go in for a medical checkup.

"I've heard that something called 'white coat' hypertension can occur when some people get tense in the doctor's office," you say. "In other words, their pressure goes up only when they see a doctor."

"Do I really scare you?" the doctor replies with a laugh. "There are very few people who have this white coat problem, and I'm sure you're not one of them. I've taken measurements of your blood pressure on two different occasions, and you can assume that if it's too high in here, it's too high at other times during the day. I think medications are the only answer for you.''

FACTS: Blood pressure is not a constant set of numbers that will be the same on every occasion a measurement is taken. Readings may bounce up or down dramatically, from minute to minute, or hour to hour.

The numbers may indeed be raised by temporary influences, such as the amount of stress you're under, the fact that you have a full bladder, a wrong-size arm cuff for measuring pressure, or a variety of other factors—including your worry or discomfort about going to see the doctor. In other words, there *is* such a thing as "white coat" hypertension, and contrary to the views of your doctor, it's not at all rare. Even some people who are not aware of becoming nervous at the doctor's might find that their blood pressure rises in this setting.

The most accurate reading is an *average* of *two* measurements taken on three separate occasions, several weeks apart. Your doctor made her diagnosis after too few measurements. The best physicians will also recommend out-of-office or at-home monitoring for patients who are suspected of having white coat hypertension.

WHAT TO DO: Don't accept a diagnosis of hypertension unless your blood pressure has been abnormal on three separate visits to your doctor, with two readings at each visit. Check the readings taken on each occasion, and ask the doctor about variations. Usually, your blood pressure will decrease after the first reading taken on each visit. As I've already said, an average of the readings should be the basis of any diagnosis.

Also, before you accept a diagnosis of hypertension, you should have your pressure checked *outside* the doctor's office just to be sure you're not a victim of the white coat syndrome. You can go to another lower-stress site away from your doctor's office, such as the local pharmacy or the medical department at your place of employment.

Even better, you can take the measurements yourself at home with an electronic digital device that can be purchased at most local pharmacies or medical supply stores.

The most sophisticated way to see if you really have high blood pressure is for your doctor to monitor it over a twenty-four-hour period with a portable, computerized blood pressure device attached to your arm. This test is usually available only from high blood pressure specialists or from a hospital. The procedure costs perhaps $250 and is certainly not needed by everyone, but if there's any doubt about the diagnosis, your doctor may recommend this approach.

If your high blood pressure does turn out to be of the "white coat" form, it's still wise to keep an eye on your blood pressure. A fair proportion of people with "white coat" reactions will later go on to develop more general high blood pressure.

Here are some other steps you can take to avoid an erroneous blood pressure reading:

- Be sure that if you're exceptionally heavy or muscular, the readings are taken with a large-size cuff. Point out your large arm size to the doctor or technician taking your pressure. Most cuffs have markings that indicate whether or not their size matches your arm. All your doctor has to do is measure the circumference of your biceps with a tape measure to see what size cuff is appropriate.

- Empty your bladder before the measurement.

- Avoid talking during the measurement.

- Don't smoke or eat anything for at least an hour before the checkup.

- Avoid exercise, including fast walking, just before the measurement.

- Obey the doctor's instructions to sit quietly for four or five minutes before the reading is taken, to avoid tensing your muscles during the exam, and to place the arm being measured on a firm support at heart level. (The doctor's desk or examining table may be an appropriate place to prop your arm as you sit in a chair.)

Caution: The foregoing suggestions apply to borderline to low-moderate elevations of blood pressure. If a first measurement of your blood pressure is in the high-moderate range or higher, say, a diastolic pressure of over 105, you should expect immediate treatment. (Consult the accompany charts to get an idea about your status.)

The Meaning of the Blood Pressure Numbers

The first, or upper, number in a blood pressure reading is the *systolic* pressure. This is the pressure the blood exerts against the arteries when the heart is actively contracting during a beat. The second, or lower, number is the *diastolic* pressure, or the force of the blood against the arteries between heartbeats. All blood pressure is measured in terms of millimeters of mercury, or mm Hg.

Blood pressure is considered normal when the readings are below 140/90 mm Hg and high when the measurement is 140/90 mm Hg or above. If *either* the systolic or diastolic numbers are in the high or hypertensive range after an adequate set of readings have been taken, then you are considered to have high blood pressure.

The following table lists a more specific breakdown of classifications of blood pressure readings as reported in the 1993 Fifth Report of the Joint National Committee on Detection, Evaluation, and Treatment of High Blood Pressure.

CLASSIFICATION OF BLOOD PRESSURE
FOR ADULTS 18 YEARS OLD AND OLDER

Category	Systolic Blood Pressure (mm Hg)	Diastolic Blood Pressure (mm Hg)
Normal	< 130	< 85
High normal	130–139	85–89
Hypertension		
Mild (Class I)	140–159	90–99
Moderate (Class II)	160–179	100–109
Severe (Class III)	180–209	110–119
Very severe (Class IV)	210 +	120 +

ERROR:

Your Doctor Doesn't Warn You About Possible Interactions Between High Blood Pressure Medications and Other Drugs

You're taking another drug—even an over-the-counter product like aspirin—but your doctor fails to ask you about your other medications. Or if he knows about the other medications, he neglects to inform you about possible interactions with your antihypertensive drug.

FACTS: Many drugs may interact with different high blood pressure medications in ways that can put your health at risk. Here are some of the possibilities:

- Certain aspirinlike medicines and related nonsteroidal antiinflammatory agents (e.g., Advil and Motrin) promote fluid retention in the body and blunt the effect of blood pressure medicines. Nasal decongestants, diet pills, and certain female hormones may also raise blood pressure.

- Other drugs may lower blood pressure and aggravate dizziness or weakness, especially after exercise or standing up suddenly. These include antidepressants, antipsychotic or strong tranquilizer drugs (e.g., Mellaril and Thorazine), and certain heart medicines, such as nitroglycerin.

- Diuretics, which are among the most commonly used high blood pressure drugs, may increase the risk of being poisoned (toxicity) by lithium or digitalis. They may also make it more difficult to control diabetes and high cholesterol.

- The blood levels and impact of beta-blockers, which limit the heart rate, may be *increased* by cimetidine (Tagamet), which slows the metabolism. Quinidine, a heart medicine, can also increase the risk of beta-blocker-caused side effects.

- The blood level and effect of beta-blockers may be *decreased* by rifampin (an antituberculosis medicine), cigarette smoking, and phenobarbital.

- Beta-blockers can increase the blood levels of theophylline (an asthma medicine), lidocaine (an anesthetic also used to treat heart rhythm problems), and phenothiazines (a class of anti-psychotic drugs or strong tranquilizers).

- Angiotensin-converting enzyme (ACE) inhibitors may increase the potassium-raising effect of potassium supplements (including over-the-counter salt substitutes), potassium-sparing diuretics, and aspirin/ibuprofen-type medicines.

- ACE inhibitors may increase lithium blood levels and the risk of lithium toxicity.

- The blood level and effect of calcium channel blockers may be reduced by rifampin, barbiturates, and carbamazepine (Tegretol).

- The side effect of calcium channel blockers may be increased by cimetidine (Tagamet) and beta-blocker drugs. Calcium channel blockers and beta-blockers are often used together, but this combination should be approached cautiously. Both drugs have similar potential side effects, including weakening the force of the heart muscle's contractions. This is especially likely to be a problem for people over age 50 who take a specific calcium channel blocker, verapamil (Calan, Isoptin), together with a beta-blocker.

- Calcium channel blockers may increase the risk of toxicity from beta-blockers, digoxin, digitalis, carbamazepine (Tegretol), prazosin (Minipress), quinidine, theophylline, and cyclosporine (an immune system suppressant).

- Aldomet may increase the risk of toxic reactions from lithium, L-dopa (used to treat Parkinson's disease), and certain oral diabetic drugs.

WHAT TO DO: Ask your doctor this question: Are there any drug interactions I should be aware of with this high blood pressure medicine I'm taking? To help him answer the question accurately, give him a list of *all* the drugs you're taking, whether prescribed or over-the-counter.

It's also wise to check with your pharmacist. She should be able to help you review all your medicines and check them against her computerized drug interaction list when you purchase an over-the-counter medication or pick up a prescription.

Finally, ask your pharmacist for the drug package insert for each of your medications and look for the section dealing with drug interactions.

If all three of these sources agree, you can be fairly certain that you have identified the most important dangers and discomforts that may arise from the interplay of your drugs.

ERROR:

Undertreatment of Older People with High Blood Pressure

You're over 70 years of age, and your blood pressure is 160/80. Yet your doctor says something to the effect that "this level is normal for your age, so don't worry about it."

FACTS: An old, now disproven notion is that as long as your systolic pressure (the upper, or first, number) is no higher than 100 plus your age, there's no need to be concerned. Also, doctors have traditionally been reluctant to treat those over age 70 with high blood pressure medications because they tend to be more vulnerable to the medication's side effects. In addition, in the past there was some doubt whether keeping the blood pressure at a lower level would really help older people live longer.

More recent research has shown that men and women over 70 who have high blood pressure will benefit from treatment and be at lower risk for serious conditions like stroke and congestive heart failure.

WHAT TO DO: Many people well up into their seventies and eighties can enjoy relatively low systolic pressures if they pay close attention to pursuing a healthy lifestyle, such as maintaining a low level of body fat, limiting alcohol consumption, and exercising regularly. Those who can't lower their high systolic pressure by these nondrug means may be candidates for low doses of a high blood pressure medication. Your physician or a hypertension specialist should be consulted to see if you should receive such treatment.

All classes of blood pressure medicine work well to lower readings in older patients. But thus far, scientific research has proven only that diuretics and beta-blockers definitely reduce the incidence of cardiovascular illness and death. Certainly other antihypertensive medicines *may* reduce this health risk; it's just right now, scientific proof is lacking on this point.

Finally, a word on the threat of excessively *low* blood pressure: Older people on blood pressure medicines should be monitored very closely because they are more sensitive to these drugs than those who are younger. It's easy to "overshoot" with older people by giving them too large a dose of a medication. The result can be blood pressure that is too low, with such symptoms as dizziness or blacking out.

To guard against too low blood pressure, be sure that your doctor measures your blood pressure when you're in the *standing* position as well as when you're seated or lying down. Taking the reading while you're standing can provide an early tip-off of a low blood pressure problem, which can be critically dangerous for those over age 70.

ERROR:

Not Emphasizing Nondrug Treatments for Your High Blood Pressure

Your doctor correctly diagnoses you as having high blood pressure—specifically, with a reading of 158/97, which classifies you as a class I or mild hypertensive. She then prescribes a particular antihypertensive medicine, an ACE inhibitor, and she hands you several typed sheets of paper.

"Be *sure* to take your medicine as prescribed," she says. "If you do, your pressure should go down to normal. But don't miss a dose, or your pressure may rise again. Come back here for another checkup next month. And by the way, those sheets have some useful tips that may also help you control your pressure."

With that, she waves good-bye, and you're left with the task of sorting through the information on the sheets and determining how to apply it. After you've returned to your office, you read through the sheets and find there is information in them on lowering blood pressure through low-salt foods, weight loss, reduced alcohol consumption, regular exercise, and lowering stress.

For a few moments, you compare this advice to your own situation: You've never even considered lowering the salt content of your food, and you have no idea how to evaluate the amounts you're taking in each day. In any event, you don't seem to put any more salt on your food than anyone else. You know you're about 15 to 20 pounds overweight, but you've always felt you carry the extra pounds pretty well.

You regularly drink about three to four mixed drinks every evening, and sometimes you have one drink during lunch, but you never get drunk or feel you lose control. You think you exercise fairly regularly—a round of golf or maybe some tennis on the weekends and occasional weight training at your local health club.

As for stress, you know your job involves high-pressure decisions and interactions with others. Sometimes, as you think about deadlines or battles that you'll face the next day at work, you have trouble getting to sleep at night. And you do keep a roll of antacid tablets in your pocket at all times for that nervous stomach that seems to plague you fairly regularly. But again, you don't really think you're experiencing any more stress than your co-workers.

So you drop the sheets your doctor gave you into the folder labeled Personal Health in your file cabinet, and you immediately put everything out of your mind except for the need to take your blood pressure medicine regularly.

FACTS: Many doctors and patients share the misperception that a physician is really "doing something" only if she writes a prescription or performs some medical procedure. In fact, educating the patient about *how to care for himself* is one of the most important things a doctor can do, especially in combating high blood pressure.

A personalized nondrug program involving low-salt, low-fat foods; regular endurance exercise; reduced alcohol intake; and, perhaps, stress management can restore blood pressure to normal in about half of all people who have mild hypertension. This means that if you follow the suggestions on those sheets that your doctor so cavalierly tossed at you, you might very well be able to eliminate the medicine she prescribed—along with its potential side effects.

Even for those who do need medicine, appropriate lifestyle modifications can mean that less medicine is needed. The result will be a lower cost of medical care and potentially fewer side effects, such as reduced sexual performance or dangerous interactions with other drugs you may be taking.

WHAT TO DO: Here's a brief overview of the lifestyle changes you can make to control your blood pressure. Discuss these with your physician before you try to incorporate them into your life.

Eliminate those extra 15 to 20 pounds! Your extra body fat may be responsible for much if not all of the mild hypertension you're experiencing. According to the Framingham Heart Study, those who weigh in at 20 percent or more above their ideal weight are eight times as likely to become hypertensive as those who maintain their proper weight. Any doctor treating you for hypertension should emphasize this factor and should insist that you go on a low-fat, lower-calorie diet combined with regular endurance exercise to lose those extra pounds.

Excess upper body fat (around your belly and waist and on the upper part of your torso) is an especially important risk factor for hypertension. But because spot reducing isn't really possible, you should concentrate on lowering your overall weight; the upper body fat should decrease along with the excess poundage on the rest of your body.

Reduce the salt or sodium in your diet. This measure doesn't work for everyone. It has been estimated that about 50 percent of all those who have high blood pressure are salt sensitive, that is, their blood pressure readings climb as their salt intake increases. The vulnerability to salt is especially high among African-Americans and among older people of all races. If you're a salt-sensitive person, reducing your salt intake can lower your blood pressure by 5 to 10 mm Hg or even more.

To be precise in evaluating the level of salt in your diet, you should know that the main thing we're concerned about here is the *sodium content* of the salt, which comprises about 40 percent of the salt you take into your body through your diet. (See the accompanying box, How to Calculate the Sodium Content in Your Daily Diet.) *Almost everyone* should restrict sodium consumption to no more than about 4 grams daily, and those with hypertension should try to keep their daily intake at around 2 grams.

Go on a high-potassium diet. Keeping your intake of potassium high is especially important if you're on a diuretic medication that causes a depletion of potassium through urination. Potassium depletion tends to raise blood pressure even before a low level of potassium in your blood can be picked up on a blood test. To be safe, you should design your diet so that you take in at least 4,000 milligrams of potassium each day. This means emphasizing foods like bananas, grapefruit juice, tomato juice, baked or boiled potatoes, and beans, which are relatively high in potassium content.

How to Calculate the Sodium Content in Your Daily Diet

In calculating the level of sodium in your daily diet, include the following:

- Sodium content on the labels of food you eat (including prepared or packaged meats).

- Table salt you add to your meal after it's cooked (sodium content will be 40 percent of the grams of salt).

- Fast foods and snack foods, which are characteristically *very* high in sodium content.

Although a detailed listing of the sodium content of different foods is beyond the scope of this book, you should be able to get the information you need from your physician. Or you can refer to publications containing gram listings of the nutritional contents of foods as provided by the U.S. Department of Agriculture. One example is *The Handbook of the Nutritional Contents of Foods* by B. K. Watt and Annabel L. Merrill (Dover Publications, Inc., New York), 1975.

Do regular endurance exercise. Sedentary living or infrequent exercise, including weight training, won't help and may hurt those with a propensity toward high blood pressure.

What sort of program should you follow? Three to four days per week, you should pursue a medically approved program of aerobic exercise training, with an emphasis on steady endurance exercise, such as brisk walking, slow jogging, cycling, or swimming.

Caution: Violent, strenuous exercise or heavy muscle-building exercises, such as weight training, can actually raise blood pressure levels and may be dangerous for those with high blood pressure.

Reduce or eliminate alcoholic beverage consumption. For those with hypertension, the safest approach is not to drink alcoholic beverages at all. Some people are so sensitive to alcohol that any amount will affect their blood pressure. If you do drink, your absolute upper daily limit should be two mixed drinks *or* two glasses of wine *or* two beers. To put this another way, you should avoid drinking more than about one ounce of pure alcohol per day.

Consider taking mineral supplements. Ask your doctor about whether or not you should take magnesium, calcium, or potassium supplements, which are sometimes used to counter hypertension.

Also, raise a question about whether stress management or psychological counseling might be helpful for your problem. Poorly managed stress can raise blood pressure significantly. So if you can identify stress as a personal problem, you should explore possible antidotes, such as making changes in your work or family environment or incorporating relaxation techniques into your daily routine.

Still, *most* people with high blood pressure do not seem either to be under abnormal stress or to be unable to handle the stress in their lives. While some scientific studies report beneficial results from such measures as relaxation techniques, other studies do not. It will be up to you and your physician to determine whether you have the type of personality that might benefit from a special stress reduction program.

In any event, you should raise these nondrug treatments with your doctor. If she shows little or no interest in working with you to develop any sort of lifestyle management regimen, you should find another doctor. Nondrug treatments are an essential component of any blood-pressure-lowering program and must not be neglected by patient or physician.

ERROR:

A Hypertensive Asthmatic on Beta-blockers May Face Sudden Death

Henry had suffered from asthma as a child. But the problem subsided as he grew older, and at age 40, he only experienced an occasional episode of bronchitis. Also, after a bad cold, he might do some mild wheezing, and exposure to outdoor air in the winter might trigger some coughing or shortness of breath. Among other things, he attributed his improvement to excellent physical fitness and regular workouts in a gym.

During a medical exam conducted just after Henry's fortieth birthday, his doctor detected high blood pressure and placed him on a beta-blocker but without questioning him about previous respiratory problems. At first, Henry began to feel a little breathless after taking the drug, but he put these incidents out of his mind. Still, as he pursued his exercise routine, he found it was becoming less fun. He had to concentrate to get through his workout without respiratory discomfort.

In late September of that year, about three months after he had started taking the beta-blocker, Henry's seven-year-old son brought home a cold from school. Henry caught it, and within two days, he wound up in the emergency room at 3:00 A.M. with a rip-roaring asthma attack. Henry came close to death during the first hour of the attack, but his family's quick response in getting him to the hospital saved his life.

After getting Henry's symptoms under control by about 5:00 A.M., his doctor remarked, "Apparently, you're developing asthma, so we'll have to switch you to another blood pressure medicine. Beta-blockers tend to make asthma worse."

"Why didn't you tell me that before?" Henry exploded. "I've had respiratory problems off and on all my life! I had asthma when I was a kid!"

"So why didn't you tell me about your asthma?" the doctor retorted, rather miffed.

Who was right and who was wrong in this situation?

FACTS: As a matter of fact, both Henry and his doctor were at fault to some extent. Certainly, your doctor should know all about your health vulnerabilities before he starts you on a medicine. But it's common for patients to end up in a situation where their physician doesn't know their personal health story as well as he should to provide proper treatment.

For one thing, a doctor may not ask all the right questions before he prescribes a medicine. That was the mistake of Henry's physician. Or a doctor may have the right information at one point and then in a moment of distraction or fatigue, he may forget a patient's history.

On the other hand, a patient may fail to fill out completely or accurately the patient health history form his doctor gives him at the beginning of their relationship. As it turned out, Henry hadn't indicated on his form that he had suffered from asthma as a child and still had mild respiratory symptoms. He figured that his exercise program had taken care of this problem, and he didn't want to admit, even to himself, that he might still have an ongoing physical weakness.

Beta-blockers are wonderful drugs for treating high blood pressure, angina, migraine headache, glaucoma, and other conditions, even stage fright. But their main strength, which involves blocking certain actions of the hormone adrenaline, is also their main weakness as far as asthma is concerned.

High Blood Pressure Medicines and Their Main Side Effects

Class of Blood Pressure Medicine	Selected Side Effects	What to Do
diuretics (except for potassium-sparing): e.g., chlorothiazide, furosemide	low blood potassium; low blood magnesium; sexual problems for men or women; weakness; may increase blood sugar, calcium, cholesterol, triglyceride, uric acid	Monitor blood potassium, supplement potassium or add compensating medicine to keep potassium well in the normal range. Notify doctor immediately if heart rate irregular, very rapid or slow, or if weak, dizzy, or unusually fatigued.
diuretics (potassium-sparing type): e.g., Aldactone, triamterene	high blood potassium especially if also taking potassium supplements, ACE inhibitors, or aspirin type NSAIDs (nonsteroidal antiinflammatory drugs) may cause sexual problems or enlarged breasts in men	Avoid potassium supplements, ACE inhibitors. Be cautious with NSAIDs. Notify doctor immediately if heart rate irregular, very rapid or slow, or if weak, dizzy, or unusually fatigued.
beta-blockers: e.g., propranolol (Inderal), atenolol (Tenormin), nadolol (Corgard), metoprolol (Lopressor), acebutolol (Sectral), betaxolol (Kerlone), pindolol (Visken)	asthmalike symptoms (shortness of breath, wheezing, cough), fatigue, insomnia, reduced exercise tolerance; congestive heart failure; masks hypoglycemia if on insulin; slow heartbeat; may cause rebound high blood pressure or angina if stopped suddenly	Do not use if you have asthma, chronic lung disease, slow heartbeat (heart block). If you have congestive heart failure use cautiously—might provide benefit or harm. Notify doctor immediately if heart rate is irregular, very rapid or slow. Do not stop suddenly. Check electrocardiogram.

ACE inhibitors: captopril (Capoten), enalapril (Vasotec), lisinopril (Prinivil, Zestril)	throat-clearing type cough, hives or skin swelling (angioedema), high potassium, distorted taste/smell, kidney disease deterioration	Report symptoms to doctor. Check blood potassium, kidney tests, urinalysis. Note: despite potential for kidney damage, might retard kidney damage in juvenile diabetics.
alpha-blockers: doxazosin (Cardura), prazosin (Minipress), terazosin (Hytrin)	fatigue, may cause extreme low blood pressure with first dose, weakness, dizziness, palpitations, headache	Report symptoms to doctor.
calcium channel blockers: diltiazem (Cardizem), verapamil (Isoptin, Calan, Verelan), nifedipine (Procardia)	headache, dizziness, fluid retention (edema), angina, rapid heart rate, constipation, overgrowth of gums, slow heart rate	Notify doctor immediately if you have heart rate abnormalities. Use cautiously if there is congestive heart failure. Avoid if heart block. Check electrocardiogram.
central alpha stimulants: Aldomet (methyldopa), clonidine (Catapres), gaunabenz (Wytensin), guanfacine (Tenex)	sedation, dry mouth, fatigue, dizziness; stopping suddenly may cause rebound high blood pressure.	Report symptoms to doctor. Don't stop suddenly.
alpha-blockers: Ismelin, reserpine	depression, diarrhea, fatigue, nasal congestion, low blood pressure with exercise	Report symptoms to doctor.
vasodilators: hydralazine (Apresoline), minoxidil (Loniten)	abnormal antinuclear antibody (lupus) test, increased hair growth, fluid retention, inflammation of pericardium (sac around heart)	Report symptoms to doctor; blood tests.

Matching Patient Needs with Blood Pressure Medicines

Your Lifestyle Priorities or Health Vulnerabilities	Type of Blood Pressure Medicine Most Likely to Match Well	Type of Blood Pressure Medicine Most Likely to Not Match Well
Avoid sedation or fatigue	ACE inhibitors, diuretics	Central alpha-stimulants, e.g., Clonidine
Maintain active sex life	ACE inhibitors, calcium channel blockers, beta-blockers (all sometimes cause problems but not too often)	All others especially diuretics, Clonidine, reserpine, Minipress, and methyldopa
Enjoy vigorous exercise	Most okay	Beta-blockers
Sensitive to sun	Most okay	Diuretics
Frequent urination inconvenient	Most okay Hytrin (terazosin)	Diuretics
Overweight problem	Most okay	Beta-blockers may slow metabolism.
Asthma	Most okay	Beta-blockers
Diabetes	Alpha-blockers, ACE inhibitors, calcium channel blockers	Diuretics raise blood sugar; beta-blockers mask symptoms of low blood sugar if taking insulin.
Fluid retention or edema	Diuretics	Calcium blockers
Angina or coronary heart disease	Beta-blockers, calcium channel blockers help	Vasodilators
Congestive heart failure	ACE inhibitors, vasodilators, diuretics help	Beta-blockers (can worsen heart failure, but also sometimes help treat it), calcium channel blockers

Condition		
Excessively slow heart rate or heart block		Beta-blockers, calcium channel blockers
Kidney disease	ACE inhibitors may slow progression of kidney disease in diabetes (juvenile or Type I)	ACE inhibitors, potassium-sparing diuretics
Vulnerable to allergic reactions/hives/angioedema/anaphylaxis. Those taking allergy shots		Beta-blockers, ACE inhibitors
Gout, high uric acid		Diuretics except for potassium-sparing diuretics
Depression		Reserpine and Ismelin often cause depression; beta-blockers, central alpha-stimulants, e.g., Clonidine and calcium channel blockers sometimes do.
High cholesterol	Alpha-blockers pindolol (Visken)	Diuretics, beta-blockers
Osteopororsis	Diuretics	
Peripheral vascular disease (e.g., pains in legs due to partial blockage of arteries)		Beta-blockers
Liver disease		methyldopa, Labetalol
Headache	Beta-blockers and calcium channel blockers help migraine	Calcium channel blockers and vasodilators may cause headache.
Pregnancy	methyldopa	Diuretics, ACE inhibitors

Adrenaline-type chemicals help prevent asthma by keeping bronchial tubes relaxed. In fact, an infusion of adrenaline from within the body or from a shot is our most effective antidote to allergy and asthma reactions. Conversely, stopping the flow of adrenaline with a beta-blocker may aggravate asthmatic symptoms, including wheezing and shortness of breath. As with Henry, a beta-blocker may even place an asthmatic at risk of sudden death.

WHAT TO DO: Always ask your doctor these questions before you start a new blood pressure medicine: Are there any health conditions that may be aggravated by this medicine? Do I have any of these conditions? What other risks may be associated with this drug?

Next, familiarize yourself with the special strengths and weaknesses of some major medicines by glancing through the accompanying boxes, High Blood Pressure Medicines and Their Main Side Effects and Matching Patient Needs with Blood Pressure Medicines.

Finally, you should ask your doctor or pharmacist for the package insert that goes with the new medicine. This document will tell you the side effects and other characteristics of the drug.

If Henry had taken these steps, he would have learned that while beta-blockers are fine for many people, they can be inappropriate or dangerous for those with a history of bronchial problems (e.g., asthma, bronchitis, and emphysema). Also, they should not be taken by those receiving allergy shots or those who are vulnerable to serious allergic reactions (e.g., anaphylaxis, or shock, as a result of a bee sting, food allergy, or other severe allergic reaction).

ERROR:

A Hypertensive Diabetic on Beta-blockers May Be in Danger of a Stroke

Nina, who had been diagnosed as having diabetes, had started taking insulin for her condition. But her physician overlooked the fact that another doctor, a hypertension specialist, had placed her on beta-blockers for high blood pressure about a year before.

Soon after she started taking the insulin, she began to perspire profusely, had a rapid heartbeat, and in general felt agitated. Then, one morning after taking both her insulin and beta-blocker, she found she couldn't talk clearly, and her left side felt weak. A neighbor who happened to call on her knew that something serious was wrong and rushed her to the hospital. She had experienced a transient ischemic attack (TIA)—just short of a stroke.

FACTS: Beta-blockers can mask the ability of those with diabetes to recognize the early symptoms of low blood sugar reactions (hypoglycemia), such as sweating, rapid heart rates, and agitation. Without early corrective action, for example, eating something or lowering the insulin dose, blood sugar can continue to drop to very low levels. This can bring on mental confusion, epileptic seizures, or even stroke, as was the case with Nina.

Diuretics may pose some problems for diabetics because they tend to increase blood sugar and also blood cholesterol levels. But these effects are usually modest, and most experts feel that diuretics are useful and reasonable medications for diabetics. Lately, diabetes experts have also begun to look carefully at ACE inhibitors. This class of drugs seems to slow down the rate at which kidney disease develops, at least among diabetics with Type I, or juvenile, diabetes (the form that usually starts during childhood or adolescence).

WHAT TO DO: Your doctor should be aware of the fact that you're a diabetic before she prescribes any antihypertensive drugs for you—*but don't assume anything!*

When she gives you your high blood pressure prescription, be sure to ask, ''Is this okay for me to take? Remember, I'm diabetic.'' Also, you should remind her about any insulin or oral diabetes medicine you're taking.

In addition, ask specifically whether or not the blood pressure medicine is a beta-blocker. If it is, tell her you know this type of drug can be dangerous for a diabetic on insulin or oral diabetes medicine. If she insists that you stick with the beta-blocker, you may seek a second opinion. If you do take the beta-blocker—and sometimes this is the most reasonable course of action—then be sure you monitor your blood sugar levels carefully at home.

In situations like this, it's essential that you set aside any worries about offending or annoying your doctor. After all, your very life may be at stake. Don't agree to take a new prescription until you've received answers that really satisfy you.

ERROR:

Not Discussing Decreased Sexual Performance as a Side Effect of Blood Pressure Medicines

Janet became extremely depressed when, six months after her second marriage, she found herself unable to have an orgasm during sex. She didn't think of this response as a medical problem, but even if she had, she would have been too embarrassed to mention it to her doctor.

It was only by accident that she began to suspect that the cause of her sexual difficulty was her blood pressure medicine, methyldopa (Aldomet). By a stroke of luck, she developed a stomach virus and temporarily stopped taking her Aldomet. As she recovered from the virus, her libido and ability to have orgasms returned. But then, when she went back on the Aldomet, her sexual problems returned.

A few experiments of not taking her medicine a couple of days and then having sex increased her growing suspicions, and her doctor confirmed the link between the drug and her sex life when she finally asked him.

The doctor inquired, perhaps rather naively, "Why didn't you tell me about this when your sexual problems first started?"

She was too nice to respond, "Why didn't you inform me about the possible side effects?"

FACTS: I've seen more than one psyche and more than one marriage nearly destroyed when men develop an inability to start or maintain an erection after they've begun a blood pressure medicine. Who would expect that a simple diuretic, which doesn't even make your tired, could hurt your ability to have an erection? Furthermore, although men are most often the victims, women aren't immune, as the case of Janet demonstrates.

At least 95 percent of the time, blood pressure medicines will *not* harm your sex life. But most of these drugs do have sexual side effects in a small proportion of patients, say, 1 percent or less. Other drugs— notably the diuretics, Clonidine, reserpine, Minipress, and methyldopa—are more likely to cause sexual dysfunction. But even with these medications, only a minority of patients usually have problems.

WHAT TO DO: It can be misleading to put the entire blame on your doctor for failing to warn you about the possible sexual side effects from blood pressure medicines. Many blood pressure drugs list fifty or more side effects, and a good doctor is most likely to be worried about those that could potentially endanger your life. In fact, some doctors actually *avoid* mentioning sexual problems as a possible side effect. They have found that planting this idea in a patient's mind can cause worry, which may by itself become a psychological trigger for sexual performance problems!

The key issue is not whether your doctor has given you a specific warning about sexual side effects, but rather whether he is helping you monitor *all* of the problems that may arise after you go on a new drug. Good monitoring means that your doctor should ask, Have you experienced any problems or changes since taking this drug?

He may mention a few possibilities to stimulate your thinking. But he may not mention sexual dysfunction, especially if this is fairly far down on the list of possible side effects for a particular medicine.

Remember, *you* have a responsibility as well as your doctor to raise the issue of possible sexual problems after you go on an anti-hypertensive drug. Don't hesitate to say exactly how you feel: "Doc, it's a little embarrassing for me, but my sex life has been off since I went on this drug. Could the medicine be affecting me?"

Of course, your doctor may not give you a satisfactory answer. Or you may sense that he isn't interested in discussing the issue with you. In such cases, ask your pharmacist for the package insert for the drug. If you see decreased sexual performance on the list of side effects, bring that up with your doctor and tell him you'd like to try another drug. If he's still unresponsive, I think I'd change doctors.

A rule of thumb: Assume that *any* new problem might be affected by your medicines until proven otherwise. But *don't drop your medicine or change the dose on your own.* Always discuss these issues with your doctor.

Blood Thinning

Neglectful Prescribing and Overseeing the Use of an Anticoagulant, or Blood-Thinning Medication

My grandfather died thirty years ago from an overdose of warfarin (Coumadin), a blood-thinning medicine that is still used annually by more than one million patients in the United States. He had developed blood clots in the veins of his legs, and to reduce the risk from those clots, as well as to prevent any recurrence, his doctor prescribed the drug.

Unfortunately, the physician also put him on an antibiotic, a medicine that can increase the blood-thinning action of Coumadin. But the doctor didn't reduce the Coumadin dose, nor did he measure the "thinness" of his patient's blood, a procedure known as checking the prothrombin time, or the pro time.

After a week on the blood thinner plus the antibiotic, my grandfather suffered bleeding in his brain and a preventable stroke from which he never recovered.

FACTS: Blood thinners (or anticoagulants), such as Coumadin, are being used more frequently because they are effective in preventing unwanted blood clots in the legs, heart, brain, and other organs. That's the reason this drug was prescribed for my grandfather. But unlike most medicines, there is a very high chance that the blood thinner itself could be as bad as or worse than the disease. One recent study from clinics specializing in anticoagulant treatment showed that the risk of causing serious bleeding was 12 percent after one year of treatment; 20 percent after two years; and 28 percent after four years.

Doctors rarely misuse blood-thinning medications like Coumadin consciously, but the potential side effects are so dangerous that even a seemingly innocent error can be disastrous. One of the most common errors is that physicians may neglect to measure the pro time of the drug often enough, especially when they add or subtract other medicines. This test indicates the degree of blood thinning that the medication is producing in your blood. The higher the pro time, the more effective the prevention of blood clots in your body—and, also, the higher your risk of unwanted bleeding. Most authorities agree that, in most (but not all) situations, there is sufficient benefit and much less risk of bleeding if your doctor adjusts your Coumadin dose to keep the pro time on the *lower* side of the treatment range.

WHAT TO DO: If you are placed on a blood thinner or anticoagulant like Coumadin, ask your doctor to explain the prothrombin time (PT or pro time) test and to let you know the frequency with which he expects to conduct it. Learn the specific pro time level the physician is trying to achieve and whether this is near the low or high end of the treatment range.

If he plans to keep your pro time near the high end (which increases the risk of bleeding), demand an explanation from him. There are situations where relatively high doses are proper, but I would recommend that you seek a second expert medical opinion to confirm that judgment.

In addition, you should ask for your pro time value *after each test* and keep notes so that you can track the trend of the measurements. If your pro time is drifting upward, call this fact to your doctor's attention, and again, ask for an explanation. Even more important, if the pro time bounces up and down, that is, if its movements are erratic, that's a signal that you are at very high risk for bleeding. If he doesn't seem concerned or if he fails to take countermeasures immediately, you must seek the help of another doctor.

Many other factors, such as a change in your diet or illness, may change the effect of Coumadin on your body. That's the reason you should obtain a pro time test regularly if you're on this drug. Your doctor should measure your pro time approximately every three weeks and more often under these circumstances:

- When you're just starting the medication.
- When you're just discharged from the hospital.
- When you alter your other medication.

Furthermore, your doctor has an obligation to report your pro time results to you *within twenty-four hours of the test.* At this point, he should advise you about making necessary adjustments in the drug and should inform you about when you are scheduled to repeat the test.

If your doctor fails to take any of these steps or seems lax in his oversight of your health while you're on a prescribed blood thinner, make your concerns clear to him. If you're not satisfied, seek another opinion.

ERROR:

Overlooking the Interaction of a Blood-Thinning Drug with Other Medications

In my grandfather's case described under the previous error, the doctor's failure to keep track of the prothrombin time, or degree of thinness of the blood, was only one of his mistakes. While giving his patient the anticoagulant warfarin (Coumadin), this physician also erred in prescribing an antibiotic, which can increase the blood-thinning action of Coumadin.

FACTS: Coumadin is especially dangerous because of its potential to interact with other drugs, alcohol, other health conditions like congestive heart failure, and a variety of other factors. (See the accompanying boxes.)

Your physician should educate you—and you should educate yourself!—about all the factors that can alter the effect on your pro time of Coumadin or any other blood thinner or anticoagulant.

WHAT TO DO: Expect that your doctor or any qualified nurses he assigns to you will spend most of at least one visit going over drugs or situations that might alter your pro time measurements, or the degree of thinness that the anticoagulant medication is producing in your blood. The doctor should inform you what you can do to limit your exposure to these dangers. During this meeting, keep a written list to remind you about threats you may encounter and what you should do about them.

Don't take any medicines—prescription or over-the-counter drugs, including vitamins—without specifically checking with your

Selected Drugs That Interact with Warfarin (Coumadin)		
Drug	Decreases Pro-thrombin Time (Increases Risk of Blood Clots)	Increases Pro-thrombin Time (Increases Risk of Bleeding)
Adrenal steroids	X	
Alcohol	X	X
Allopurinol		X
Aspirin, ibuprofen, and other nonsteroidal antiinflammatory drugs		X
Antacids	X	
Antibiotics		X
Antihistamines	X	
Barbiturates	X	
Carbamazepine (Tegretol)	X	
Cholestyramine (Questran)	X	
Chlorpropamide (diabetes medication)		X
Cimetidine (Tagamet)		X
Digestive enzyme	X	
Disulfiram (Antabuse)		X
Diuretics	X	X
Griseofulvin (Fulvicin)	X	
Haloperidol (Haldol)	X	
Influenza virus vaccine		X
Cholesterol medications, e.g., lovastatin (Mevacor)		X
Meprobamate	X	
Methyldopa (Aldomet)		X
Methylphenidate		X
Metronidazole (Flagyl)		X
Miconazole (antifungal)		X
MAO-type antidepressants		X
Oral contraceptives	X	
Pentoxifylline (Trental)	X	
Phenytoin (Dilantin)	X	

continued on next page

continued from last page

Selected Drugs That Interact with Warfarin (Coumadin)		
Drug	Decreases Pro-thrombin Time (Increases Risk of Blood Clots)	Increases Pro-thrombin Time (Increases Risk of Bleeding)
Primidone (Mysoline)	X	
Quinidine, quinine		X
Ranitidine	X	X
Sucralfate (Carafate)	X	
Thyroid medications		X
Tolbutamide (diabetes medication)		X
Trazodone (Desyrel)	X	
Vitamin C	X	
Vitamin E (α-tocopherol)		X
Vitamin K	X	

doctor and your pharmacist about their potential effect on Coumadin. To be doubly sure, check under "drug interaction" in the package insert of each medicine you plan to use to see if it's known to effect your anticoagulant.

Some new medicines may not have been tested with regard to their possible interactions with Coumadin. So be sure that your investigation of known drug interactions is backed up by regular measurements of your blood's pro time.

ERROR:

Your Pharmacist Gives You the Incorrect-Strength Warfarin (Coumadin) Pill

A patient in California was on the blood thinner warfarin (Coumadin) for the same basic reasons as my grandfather in the previous two errors—to counter blood clots that had developed in her legs. One day when she refilled her prescription with the druggist, she received pills that were yellow in color instead of peach. She didn't think much about the color change because the same thing had happened before with other drugs. In the past she had been taking

Nondrug Factors That May Interact with Warfarin (Coumadin)		
Factor	Decreases Pro-thrombin Time (Increases Risk of Blood Clots)	Increases Pro-thrombin Time (Increases Risk of Bleeding)
Congestive heart failure		X
Diarrhea		X
Fever		X
Foods high in vitamin K (e.g., green, leafy vegetables; green tea; liver)	X	
Edema (fluid retention)	X	
Liver disease (e.g., hepatitis, jaundice)		X
Hypothyroid (low thyroid activity)	X	
Hyperthyroid (high thyroid activity)		X
Hot weather (prolonged)		X

one-and-a-half peach-colored Coumadin pills. So she continued to take that dose of the *yellow* pills every day.

At the next measurement of the level of her blood thinning (her blood's prothrombin time, or pro time), it was clear that her readings had moved too high, and she was in danger of internal bleeding.

What had happened?

FACTS: The first pills this Californian had used, the peach-colored ones, had each contained 5 milligrams of the drug. By taking one-and-a-half of these each day, she had consumed a total of 7.5 milligrams of the drug. But the new pills, the yellow-colored ones, each contained 7.5 *milligrams* of Coumadin. That meant that by taking one and a half of these daily, which was her old dose, she was getting a 50 percent higher dose, 11.25 milligrams, of the Coumadin without realizing it. This increased amount of the drug was enough to affect her pro time significantly and increase the risk of her health.

In fact, the error had occurred due to an overworked pharmacist's assistant who had put the wrong dose of Coumadin into the bottle. This mistake might not happen frequently, but it does occur often enough. I'm aware of a number of similar stories: There was a pharmacist in Texas who gave one patient a pain medicine instead of a diabetes pill because he misread the doctor's handwriting on the prescription. And my aunt in Florida had her digoxin pill switched and wound up in the hospital with a severe overdose.

WHAT TO DO: This sort of mistake should never happen, but pharmacists filling prescriptions or physicians handing out pills from their samples cabinet do become tired or distracted. They can easily lapse into the error of failing to double-check the precise medicine that's being given to ascertain that it is precisely in the dosage and on the schedule that you're supposed to be using.

To prevent this problem, you should take these simple steps. Every time you get a new bottle of your medication, check these points:

- *The dose strength on the tablet,* which will be indicated by a number. This number should remain constant, from prescription to prescription, unless your physician has changed your dose. If he has changed it, be sure that you know why and are aware of any new instructions that should be followed with the adjustment.

- *The color of the tablet.* If it's different from the pills you've been taking in the past, find out why from your pharmacist or doctor before you begin the medication.

- *The brand name on the tablet.* Different manufacturers may have different ways of indicating dosages.

If you discover any discrepancies or changes in one or more of these items, don't take the blood-thinning pill until your physician and pharmacist have satisfied you completely.

ERROR:

You Are on a Blood Thinner, and Your Doctor Fails to Train You to Detect and Report Signs of Bleeding

Al, an executive in his fifties, was placed on the blood thinner warfarin (Coumadin) because of excessive narrowing that had been detected in his arteries as a result of a buildup of plaque. He experienced no apparent negative reactions to the drug, but within a couple of weeks, he did notice that some of his bowel movements seemed to be black in color. Also, he periodically felt dizzy, but the sensation usually went away fairly quickly, and in most cases, he thought he could link it to his having stood up too quickly from a sitting position.

These changes didn't bother him particularly, though he did mention to a friend, "We've been eating more vegetables lately because my wife thinks I need a lower-fat diet. It must be those vegetables that are causing these differences in me."

A month later, Al suffered a hemorrhagic (bleeding) stroke.

FACTS: Doctors and nurses easily fall into the trap of assuming that what is common knowledge to them is also known to you. Or they may think that someone else has taught you the basics of monitoring your own bodily functions before you come under their care.

In the case of blood-thinning agents, the mistake is assuming that a patient like Al has been taught how to recognize when he might be bleeding internally. Of course, red blood in your stool would sound an alarm for almost anyone. But red blood isn't normally the main symptom when blood begins leaking from the upper parts of the intestines or from the stomach. In most cases, the genuine sign of bleeding is black, tarry-colored stool after a bowel movement. So it's always important to check your stool when you're on a blood thinner.

Caution: Iron pills, beets, spinach, and Pepto-Bismol can all cause the same black effect, and so it's usually necessary for your doctor to do a lab test on your stool to be sure that what you're observing is really blood.

Early symptoms of internal bleeding may include feeling weak, light-headed, dizzy, or sweaty. A rapid heartbeat or low blood pressure may also indicate this problem. Later symptoms may be abnormal bleeding from the gums, nosebleeds, blood in the urine, excessive bleeding from cuts, spontaneous or severe bruising, or excessive vaginal bleeding.

WHAT TO DO: Expect that your doctor or nurse will discuss all the possible signs of internal bleeding with you when you start Coumadin or another blood thinner. Also, the doctor or nurse should always check to be sure that you understand how to detect bleeding and that you are following through on your self-monitoring. Report any of the above-listed signs of possible internal bleeding immediately.

If your doctor fails to instruct you about how bleeding may occur with a blood thinner, you're not getting the supervision that you need. Detecting early signs of bleeding might have saved Al from having that stroke—and may save your life.

Stroke

Failing to Recognize the Most Important Early Warning Sign of a Stroke

One day, Margot, a 64-year-old public relations executive, began to experience some dizziness, and she had a tendency to slur her words when she spoke. Also, even though she seemed to be unaware of it, she shuffled slightly when she walked.

When Don, her husband, pointed out some of the physical changes, she indicated she had not really been aware of most of them, but she was concerned about the dizziness. So at his suggestion, she agreed to see a physician. They made an appointment for the following week to discuss her dizziness.

By the day of the appointment, all of the symptoms had disappeared. The doctor checked her over and then said, "It might have been an inner ear virus that threw off your balance. Or it might have just been stress. Try to relax more, and I'm sure you'll be all right."

Two months later, Margot suffered a stroke, which left her partially paralyzed on the right side of her body and also impaired her ability to speak. What happened?

FACTS: Strokes can occur at any age, but their frequency doubles each decade after age 60. Factors that increase stroke risk in young adults include all forms of heart disease, cocaine and related drugs, oral contraceptives, acquired immunodeficiency syndrome (AIDS), high blood pressure, and conditions in which there is an increase in the clotting tendency of the blood. In people older than 60, stroke risk increases with the presence of such factors as high blood pressure, elevated cholesterol levels, diabetes, cigarette smoking, alcohol abuse, and heart disease.

Many, though not all, strokes give an early warning signal known as a *transient ischemic attack,* or TIA, which involves a short-term reduction of the blood flow to the brain. These attacks produce only temporary debilitation, usually for a period of less than a half hour. In almost every case, all the symptoms disappear within 24 hours. (For a list of typical signs or symptoms of a TIA, see the accompanying box.)

A source of major medical errors is that TIA symptoms may be ignored or misdiagnosed by doctors as the patient's supposed response to anxiety, migraine, hypoglycemia (low blood sugar), or some other condition.

In Margot's case, her doctor focused too narrowly and quickly on her dizziness complaints, which often are the result of stress or an inner ear virus. I'm sure that the possibility of a TIA didn't even enter his mind. If it had, he would certainly have asked Margot about her slurred speech or weakness—both classic warning signs of TIA. As for Margot, she may have made a mistake herself in not bringing Don with her to the visit. Don had a sense that her slurred

---

Symptoms of a Transient Ischemic Attack (TIA), the Most Important Signal of an Impending Stroke

Common symptoms of a TIA include

- Weakness of a particular arm, leg, or area of the face.
- Numbness or tingling of a particular arm, leg, or area of the face.
- Loss of vision in one eye or in part of a visual field.
- Dizziness or loss of balance.
- Inability to speak or think clearly.

Obviously, many people experience one or more of these symptoms for reasons other than a TIA. But if any of the symptoms persists for fifteen minutes or longer, you should see your physician immediately. By definition, TIA symptoms, though similar to those of a full-blown stroke, are temporary. Typically they disappear completely within twenty-four hours.

speech and foot dragging might be important. But unfortunately, Margot didn't push the issue.

WHAT TO DO: When I was a resident, I was taught that there wasn't much that could be done for patients with strokes except to keep them alive and wait to see how much neurological (brain and nerve) function they could recover. Now, this passive attitude is beginning to change as doctors recognize the stroke-blocking effects of aggressive, early treatment, and as both doctors and their patients are learning to become more alert to the physical responses that may signal a TIA or stroke.

If you notice any of the TIA symptoms listed in the box opposite, you should report them right away to your doctor. It's particularly urgent for you to act if the symptoms seem markedly intense or if they have occurred in the past. If your doctor seems unconcerned, if her explanation seems inadequate to you, or *especially* if you have other risk factors for stroke (such as high blood pressure), ask for a consultation with a neurologist, who is a specialist in diseases of the nervous system.

ERROR:

Automatically Treating a Stroke Patient with a Blood Thinner

Paul noticed a loss of vision in his right eye and also a weakness in his left arm and hand. The doctor correctly diagnosed Paul's problem as a stroke. He prescribed the blood thinner warfarin (Coumadin). But he did not order a computed tomography (CT) scan of Paul's brain. The CT scan provides a detailed picture of the brain that can show hemorrhaging as well as tumors and other abnormalities.

After taking the blood thinner for a couple of days, Paul's symptoms worsened, and a belated CT scan revealed that he had a massive area of bleeding in his brain as a result of a hemorrhagic (bleeding) stroke. He was immediately scheduled for surgery, but the hemorrhaging had progressed too far. He was permanently paralyzed and died within four months.

FACTS: Like many heart attacks, the large majority of strokes result from narrowed arteries or clots that block the flow of blood to the brain. If the source of a stroke is indeed clogged arteries or a clot, blood-thinning medications can stop the stroke by increasing the flow of blood to the brain. Furthermore, if the drug is administered early enough, blood thinners can even prevent the stroke.

But about 10 percent of all strokes are caused *not* by a clot, but rather by bleeding (hemorrhaging) in the brain. A smaller proportion results from a brain tumor or from an aneurysm (swelling) of an artery in the brain. In these cases, taking an anticoagulant medication (blood thinner) like Coumadin or even aspirin can make the stroke worse and can easily be fatal.

How can you know the type of stroke that's involved? All stroke victims should have an emergency CT scan to determine whether the problem arises from bleeding or clotting. If a CT scan isn't available, a spinal tap, though less accurate than a CT, may also be helpful to determine the type of stroke. On the other hand, a diagnostic tool like magnetic resonance imaging (MRI) is not as sensitive as a CT for detecting early bleeding into the brain, though this procedure is excellent in diagnosing other conditions.

WHAT TO DO: You or your affected family member *must* have a CT scan of the brain—or a good explanation to the contrary—before aspirin or stronger blood-thinning agents are used after a possible stroke. If the scan indicates that the stroke has occurred as a result of a hemorrhage or bleeding in the brain, blood thinners should be avoided during treatment.

On the other hand, if a CT scan establishes that the cause of the stroke involves some form of clotting, then it's appropriate to employ a blood thinner. For example, if the problem is thrombosis (a blood clot in the arteries of the head or neck), most neurologists give aspirin to thin the blood and prevent a recurrence. Ticlopidine, a new blood-thinning agent, is an option for people who can't take aspirin.

For aspirin, usually a moderate dose is used, such as one 325-milligram one to four times daily. More vigorous anticoagulation therapy, such the drug heparin, is routine after a stroke due to an embolism (a traveling clot, which may originate elsewhere in the body, especially the heart).

Another popular anticoagulant, dipyridamole (Persantine), has been widely used, but recent studies suggest it's not very effective in preventing the recurrence of a stroke. Be sure to question your physician about his rationale if he prescribes this drug. If his explanation seems unconvincing or leaves your questions unanswered, seek a second opinion.

ERROR:

Your Doctor Not Testing for a Traveling Blood Clot (Embolism) as the Cause of a TIA or Stroke

Tina experienced a classic transient ischemic attack (TIA) that resulted in strokelike symptoms, including weakness on the right side and slurred speech. These problems disappeared after one day. When she went in for a medical checkup immediately after this incident, her doctor correctly recognized the problem as a TIA. He also ordered a CT (computed tomography) scan to be sure that the symptoms didn't arise from bleeding in the brain, and that test came back negative. In addition, there appeared to be no clogging of the carotid arteries on the sides of her neck, which fed blood to her brain. So the physician placed her on aspirin therapy and sent her home.

Shortly afterward, against all Tina's and the physician's expectations, she suffered a massive stroke.

What went wrong?

FACTS: Tina's TIA resulted from an embolism, a traveling blood clot that had originated in her heart. Everyone who experiences an unexplained TIA or a stroke should have not only a CT scan, but also an echocardiogram, which tests for abnormalities of the valves or chambers of the heart. Blood clots, which may form in enlarged chambers or abnormal valves within the heart, can be "sprayed" (embolized) through the arteries. Pieces of the clot may end up in the head and cause blockage and localized bleeding in the brain. Infections on the heart valve, known as *vegetations*, can also break off and travel to the brain. Another useful test, a 24-hour heart rhythm monitor, can detect irregular heart rhythms. These can also cause blood clots in the heart that can embolize to the brain.

Patients who suffer these embolic strokes have to receive special treatment, which may involve intravenous anticoagulation (blood thinning) or intensive treatment with antibiotics. The outlook for such patients can be excellent *if* further embolisms can be prevented.

WHAT TO DO: A traveling embolism as cause for a stroke shouldn't be overlooked by the doctor during her diagnosis. If a friend or loved one has a stroke, you should always ask the question, Have you checked for a traveling clot or embolism?

If the answer is no, then ask that a test be performed. Putting this question to the attending physician might be especially important in an HMO setting, where the incentive is to provide fewer diagnostic tests and procedures rather than more.

If the answer to your first question is yes, then ask, Does that mean you've ordered an echocardiogram? If the doctor says no, then you should insist that one be done.

Just reminding your family doctor or neurologist should be enough to have the test performed. If you meet resistance or are dissatisfied with the response you're getting, ask for a consultation with a cardiologist (a heart specialist).

ERROR:

Sloppy Medical and Nursing Care Sets Back Recovery from a Stroke

Karen was bedridden for several weeks after her stroke. During this period, she developed pneumonia and blood clots in her legs. Could these complications have been prevented?

FACTS: Those who are bedridden after a stroke are vulnerable to a host of complications, many of which can be prevented by more attentive care. Here are some of the most common problems and solutions:

Problem 1: Aspiration (or breathing into the lungs) of food, which can cause pneumonia.
Solution: Medical personnel should check to see if the patient can swallow three ounces of water without coughing or developing a wet-hoarse-sounding voice. A speech therapist can evaluate the quality of the voice. If the patient is unable to pass this test, additional attention must be paid to preparation of food and eating habits to guard against aspiration of food. (This was Karen's problem, which resulted in her pneumonia.)
Problem 2: Blood clots in the legs and ultimately the lungs.
Solution: Because inactivity promotes this problem, a physical therapist, nurse, or even a trained family member should help the patient keep the limbs moving. Also, the doctor may prescribe a blood thinner.

Problem 3: Malnutrition or dehydration.

Solution: A record should be kept showing how much the patient actually eats and drinks. The patient should be weighed, preferably every day. Family members can help oversee this record and also assist in feeding the patient. In addition, it's important to be sure that the patient is urinating several times a day and is also having regular bowel movements. If both of these functions are being performed well, malnutrition and dehydration are unlikely.

Problem 4: Bed sores.

Solution: Nurses should change the patient's position frequently and observe, massage, and lubricate the skin over points exposed to the bed. Egg crate mattresses or more expensive pressure-limiting beds and devices can help. Four-inch-thick egg crates work, but the two-inch-thick type is worthless. Also, the so-called doughnut devices shouldn't be used.

Problem 5: Physical deconditioning, weakness, or muscle shortening (contracture).

Solution: To counter these difficulties, even sitting in a chair is much better than lying in the bed. Ask the nurse to show you how to move the patient's limbs gently through a passive "range of motion." (Of course, the nurse should be doing this routinely without your asking.) Once the acute danger period is past, insist that a physical therapist attend the patient's physical therapy needs. Better still, ask for a consultation with a physiatrist—a physician who specializes in rehabilitation medicine—to supervise the physical therapist's work.

Problem 6: Losing independence.

Solution: You should consult a physician who specializes in rehabilitation (usually a physiatrist) to help you plan for the patient's rehabilitation needs. A physical therapist can help the individual regain basic skills, such as moving to a chair and sitting down. A speech therapist can assist with swallowing and speech. Rehabilitating these and other simple skills will help greatly in providing the patient with a greater sense of independence.

Problem 7: Depression.

Solution: Many stroke victims become depressed for both neurological (physical nerve) and psychological reasons. This problem can be alleviated through antidepressants, the presence of a supportive family, occupational therapy, and advice from chaplains and psychological counselors.

WHAT TO DO: The chances are that you'll be in a position to deal best with this error as a concerned family member rather than as a patient. Stroke victims benefit more than most patients from having a strong, well-informed advocate to oversee the care given by the medical staff. All else being equal, you're best off at a hospital with a distinct set of beds designated as a "stroke unit," or one with a well-organized stroke rehabilitation program. That way you can be confident that the hospital staff is well trained in the special needs of patients with stroke.

The risk of your parent's or other family member's being harmed by any of the above problems will be considerably lower if you stay on the case while he or she is in the hospital. Most of the errors at the rehabilitative stage of a stroke occur because proper care is time-consuming and not at all glamorous. It's easy for a nurse or aide to become slack, and it's up to you to be sure that they all stay alert.

I'd suggest that you use the above problems and solutions as a checklist. If you see any of the listed problems developing, start asking questions until the deficiency is corrected.

Finally, don't forget to ask about hospital discharge planning. Many patients just begin to make some progress when their insurance coverage runs out and they are told they have to leave. Damage that can be inflicted by an abrupt, unexpected departure can be limited if you ensure that the discharge planning begins by the second or third day of the hospital stay. You should ask about the number of days left in the hospital and also about the availability of a rehabilitation facility, nursing home, and outpatient physical therapy.

Cholesterol

ERROR:

Your Doctor Relies Only or Mainly on Total Cholesterol Measurements to Prescribe Cholesterol-Lowering Medications

A wife and husband, Jane and Carl, both in their midforties, had almost the same total cholesterol levels: approximately 260 milligrams per deciliter. Noting that the risk of heart disease increases greatly as total cholesterol levels move above 200, their physician prescribed the same cholesterol-lowering medication for each spouse.

In fact, he should have given the medication to Jane but not to Carl. What was his mistake?

FACTS: Much has been made of the total cholesterol number and the importance of keeping it at 200 milligrams per deciliter or below. But evaluating the risk posed by cholesterol is a much more complicated and subtle matter than just focusing on the total cholesterol reading.

For one thing, this doctor failed to take into account the importance of the "good" cholesterol levels—the subcomponent of the total cholesterol known as high-density lipoprotein (HDL) cholesterol. Higher HDL cholesterol levels have been associated with a lower incidence of atherosclerosis, or clogging of the arteries. Conversely, low HDL levels have been linked to a higher risk of atherosclerosis. Jane had a low HDL level of 33 milligrams per deciliter, while Carl had a high level at 84 milligrams per deciliter. (See the accompanying box, General Cholesterol and Triglyceride Guidelines.)

General Cholesterol and Triglyceride Guidelines

Cholesterol

Total cholesterol. This number is important only as a very rough screening guide. It consists of several subcomponents, including "bad" LDL cholesterol, "good" HDL cholesterol, and VLDL (very low-density lipoprotein) cholesterol. VLDL also carries most of the blood's content of triglycerides (see below).

In general, your total cholesterol should be below 200 milligrams per deciliter, and studies have shown that for every percentage point increase in cholesterol above 200, the risk of heart disease in the American population increases by 2 percent. But total cholesterol is only the first thing you should consider.

LDL cholesterol. LDL cholesterol, also known as "bad" cholesterol, is the subcomponent most closely associated with the buildup of fatty deposits (plaque) in the arteries. If your LDL is less than 130 milligrams per deciliter, then your LDL-related risk of heart disease is low. If the figure is between 130 and 159, your risk is higher, and you should work to reduce the fat and cholesterol in your diet.

If your LDL is 160 or higher, you are at high risk for heart disease. At this level, try a rigorous low-fat, low-cholesterol diet for six months. Also, if you have excess body fat—a factor that can raise cholesterol levels—lose the extra weight. Your diet should be designed and supervised by a qualified physician or dietitian. If your LDL fails to drop below 130 within six months, and if you also have other risk factors for heart disease, your doctor may prescribe cholesterol-lowering drugs in addition to the diet and weight-loss program.

If your LDL is 190 or higher, you are at very high risk for heart disease. For six months, you should try a vigorous low-fat, low-cholesterol diet designed and supervised by a qualified physician or dietitian. Also, you should lose excess body fat. If this diet doesn't bring your LDL down into the 130 to 159 range within the six-month period, you should consider starting cholesterol-lowering medications even if you have no other heart disease risk factors.

HDL cholesterol. High levels of HDL cholesterol, also known as "good" cholesterol, have been associated with a low risk of atherosclerosis and heart disease. People with HDL levels below 35 (about 20 percent of all men and 5 percent of all women) are, on average, at high risk for developing heart disease *even if their total cholesterol is under 200.* Those with HDL levels of 75 or higher are usually at fairly low risk for heart disease even if their total cholesterol is in the 300 range.

Those with HDL levels of 50 milligrams per deciliter or above have a relatively low cholesterol-related risk of developing heart disease if they can keep their total cholesterol levels around 200 or below. Many physicians base their evaluations of a patient's blood fat profile on the ratio of total cholesterol to HDL cholesterol. So if your total cholesterol is 200 and your HDL cholesterol is 50, your ratio is 4.0. In general, those with a ratio of 4.0 or below have very good protection.

One exception to these rules of thumb: Those on an extremely low-fat or vegetarian diet may have low HDL levels without an increased risk of heart disease.

Triglycerides

Triglycerides are another type of blood fat that, like cholesterol, has been associated with an increased risk of heart disease.

In general, triglycerides below 250 milligrams per deciliter don't pose an undue risk. Those in the 250 to 500 range may represent an increased risk of atherosclerosis and heart disease, especially where the person has a personal or family history of heart of circulatory disease or very low HDL cholesterol. Triglycerides above 500 have been associated with a higher risk of heart disease as well as short-term risk of damage to the pancreas and other organs.

Also, Jane's "bad" LDL (low-density lipoprotein) cholesterol was over 200 milligrams per deciliter, a result that is well into the high-risk range for heart disease. Carl, in contrast, had LDLs of less than 150—moderately too high but nothing to panic about.

Finally, the physician neglected to give adequate weight to other heart disease risk factors before prescribing medication. Specifically, he overlooked the fact that Jane had a family history of heart problems (her mother had experienced angina pains beginning at age 53). Carl had no such family history.

Heart disease experts recommend very detailed cholesterol and triglyceride guidelines, adjusted according to age, sex, and other factors. That approach can be helpful for those with particular blood fat problems. But in the accompanying box, General Cholesterol and Triglyceride Guidelines, I've used a simpler approach to provide a more general "snapshot" that will enable you to keep the major danger areas in mind when you have a blood test. This information is based on findings by the National Institutes of Health and other authorities. You'll note that, first, there are guidelines for cholesterol and its subcomponents. Then, I've included guidelines for triglycerides, another important but often overlooked blood fat that can be a risk factor for heart disease.

WHAT TO DO: The husband and wife in our example, Jane and Carl, should have received quite different kinds of treatment from their physician. Jane, whose mother developed angina (chest) pains by age 53, should have had her cholesterol tested once more within a month. Then if the results were similar, she should probably have been placed on a cholesterol-lowering medication. Carl, who has no family history of heart disease, should not have been put on drugs but, instead, should have been instructed to embark on a low-fat, low-cholesterol diet. Their physician made a mistake by lumping the two patients together for the same treatment after looking only at their respective total cholesterol levels.

Jane and Carl might have protected themselves from the oversight by their physician if they had been prepared to ask him a few basic questions about the meaning of their cholesterol report.

1. What are the measurements for every component of my blood fats: total cholesterol, LDL cholesterol, HDL cholesterol, triglycerides, and the ratio of total cholesterol to HDL cholesterol? (See the accompanying box.) What do these measurements mean?

2. What bearing do my *other* heart disease risk factors have on my blood fat profile? In particular, you should ask your physician about the impact of these important risk factors:

- Any family history of heart disease, especially if a parent or sibling has had a heart attack, angina, stroke, or artery disease of the leg before age 55.

- Male sex or early menopause.

- Tobacco use.

- High blood pressure.

- Diabetes, or high blood sugar.

- Excessive body fat.

- Sedentary lifestyle.

- Hurried, high-stress lifestyle or feelings of chronic anger or hostility.

3. When can I have another blood test performed just to be sure that there is no error in this test?

I still occasionally see patients who have begun cholesterol-lowering medicines after having only one measurement with a high cholesterol reading. Like any lab test, cholesterol exams are subject to mistakes. By current standards, readings of 195 and 210 on the same tube of blood are considered to be within acceptable variation. That's not so reassuring when the official dividing line between an okay and a high cholesterol result sits on the razor-thin edge of 200 milligrams per deciliter.

There are also cases where labs mix up tubes of blood or make other gross errors. So accept no final treatment decisions until you have been tested twice and the two tests are fairly close in results.

Note: Be sure that you take nothing into your body but water for at least ten to twelve hours before your test, or the results—especially the triglycerides and the LDL cholesterol—may be affected.

ERROR:

Undertreatment of Patients with Low Levels of "Good" HDL Cholesterol

Three separate blood tests revealed that Will's total cholesterol averaged 190 milligrams per deciliter, but his "good" HDL cholesterol was quite low at 25 milligrams per deciliter. Also, Will had borderline high blood pressure, and his father had died of a heart attack at age 49. But Will's doctor, after glancing at the results, pronounced his cholesterol "fine" and suggested no further steps for treatment.

What was wrong with the doctor's response?

FACTS: Although Will's total cholesterol was below the 200 milligrams per deciliter upper threshold recommended by many experts, his HDL cholesterol was far below the minimum of 35, which moves a patient into the high-risk category. (See box, pp. 88–89.) In fact, a person with an HDL of 25 who has a total cholesterol in Will's range faces a 7 to 10 percent probability of developing heart disease within the next four years! Furthermore, the risk increases if that person has other heart disease risk factors, such as Will's high blood pressure and his family history of heart disease.

WHAT TO DO: If, like Will, you have unusually low HDL levels and also one or more of the heart disease risk factors (listed under What to Do in the previous error), you and your doctor must not become complacent just because your total cholesterol level seems low. There are two steps you can take to improve the balance of HDL and total cholesterol. Bring these up with your doctor, and if he seems unresponsive or lacks knowledge, find another physician.

Step 1: Try various lifestyle options to improve the level of your HDL cholesterol. These include the following:

- If you're overweight, lose weight and keep it off. HDLs will rise after weight loss, but usually only many months after the extra pounds have been eliminated.

- Develop a regular program of vigorous endurance or aerobic exercise. In many people, this type of activity will raise HDL levels.

- Avoid smoking, which lowers HDLs.

- Avoid male hormone drugs, such as body-building steroids, which lower HDLs.

- Consider taking estrogen supplements if you're menopausal or past menopause. These tend to raise HDL levels.

- Be aware that small amounts of alcohol—in the range of one to two drinks a day—can raise HDL levels. But if you do drink, don't drink in larger quantities because imbibing extra amounts won't help your HDLs and may very well create other health problems.

Step 2: If you find you can't raise your HDL cholesterol by the above measures, consult a physician with special expertise in heart disease prevention (a cardiologist) to see if you should take cholesterol-lowering drugs. Many of these medications can also raise HDL cholesterol.

There are two schools of thought on such treatment. Some respected authorities advocate using medicines to increase very low HDL levels even if the total cholesterol is normal at 200 milligrams per deciliter or below that level. They recommend this step only if the patient has other heart disease risk factors, such as the family history of heart attacks and high blood pressure that characterized Will's condition.

Most authorities would not recommend drug treatments in this situation, but I'm quite sympathetic to the arguments posed by the minority of physicians who take the more aggressive stance. They feel that increasing a person's HDL through drugs could actually help prevent heart attacks. And they note that the medicines used—mainly the same ones used to treat high cholesterol—are reasonably safe.

Caution: One concern, expressed by a number of experts, is that the drugs used to lower cholesterol or raise HDL cholesterol may also lower total cholesterol to unreasonably low levels. Several studies have shown that lowering cholesterol through medications can result in lower rates of heart disease, but several of these studies have also found more deaths from other causes such as suicide, homicide, and accidents in the group taking cholesterol-lowering drugs. It's not clear whether there is a cause–effect relationship between these factors or just coincidence. But until more is known about this issue, I would recommend not lowering total cholesterol below 160 milligrams per deciliter through drugs.

In any event, there is relatively little to lose and perhaps much to gain by getting those HDL levels up as high as possible. Certainly, if very low HDL levels are left untreated, we do know that patients in this category face a high risk of developing heart disease within a relatively short time.

ERROR:

Your Doctor Ignores Your Triglyceride Levels

Anne had a blood test, and she noticed that values were provided for total cholesterol, LDL cholesterol, HDL cholesterol, and triglycerides. Her doctor said that her cholesterol profile "looks great," but he ignored the triglyceride result, which was 340 milligrams per deciliter. When Anne asked about this measurement and pointed out that it had been tagged as high on the lab report, the doctor said, "Don't worry about that. The cholesterol is the important thing."

What was his mistake?

FACTS: As you've seen in the box on p. 89, many experts feel that triglyceride levels below 250, measured after a water-only fast of ten to twelve hours, are not usually a problem.

On the other hand, most (but not all) experts believe that triglycerides above that level—and especially those above 500 milligrams per deciliter—can increase the risk of atherosclerosis and heart disease. Among other things, they may drive down the levels of "good" HDL cholesterol and may also contribute to the buildup of fatty deposits and plaque in the arteries. The threat posed by high triglycerides is magnified in those people who have other heart disease risk factors, such as those described under What to Do in the error Your Doctor Relies Only or Mainly on Total Cholesterol Measurements to Prescribe Cholesterol-Lowering Medications (p. 87). Also, very high triglycerides are associated with a short-term risk of damage to the pancreas and other organs.

WHAT TO DO: If your triglycerides are in the higher ranges, be sure to undergo a second blood test performed after at least a ten- to twelve-hour water-only fast. Also, if you are a drinker, avoid all alcoholic beverages for at least three days. Many people dramatically raise their triglycerides after only a few drinks.

Because very high triglycerides can pose a significant threat to health, you should begin a rigorous low-calorie, low-alcohol (or no-alcohol) regimen designed and supervised by a qualified physician or dietitian. Also, being overweight can elevate triglyceride levels. So can unrecognized diabetes.

If changing your diet and losing weight don't work, you may be a candidate for triglyceride-lowering medications. Drugs become especially important if you have other heart disease risk factors, such as a family history of cardiovascular problems.

$$\boxed{\text{E R R O R :}}$$

Mistakes Involving Cholesterol-Lowering Medications

Bob's total cholesterol level was 320, and his "good" HDL level was only 35—a situation that made him a candidate for a cholesterol-lowering medication. The doctor prescribed a low-fat, low-cholesterol diet; a weight loss program; and 4 grams (4,000 milligrams) per day of timed-release niacin capsules. He said that niacin, a B vitamin, could be purchased over-the-counter at a much lower price than prescription drugs, and also, the timed-release variety would help prevent flushing, a common niacin side effect.

The doctor then said, "You might want to check back with me in about three months to see how your cholesterol level is doing."

Bob did have his cholesterol checked at a walk-in clinic three months later and found that the program was lowering his cholesterol nicely. His total cholesterol level was now 230, and his HDL level was up to 45. He sent the results over to his doctor but didn't have any direct response from the physician.

What did the doctor do wrong?

FACTS: Niacin is often quite effective in lowering cholesterol and triglyceride levels and raising the HDL level, and it's by far the least expensive cholesterol drug. But this B vitamin also poses the highest toxicity risk of all the current cholesterol medicines. Here are some of the problems:

- At least 30 percent of those who take niacin in effective doses stop taking it because of symptoms like flushing, itching, nausea, hyperacidity, diarrhea, or dry eyes.

- Also, there may be more serious side effects, such as liver inflammation, increased blood sugar, and increased uric acid. These problems are more likely to be aggravated by the timed-release type of niacin than by the shorter-acting regular niacin. (However, the regular niacin causes more vigorous flushing.)

- Niacin can be dangerous for people with a high risk for such problems as a past or current history of ulcers, gastritis, hepatitis, diabetes, and gout.

- The risk of side effects of niacin increases dramatically in doses above 3 grams (3,000 milligrams).

WHAT TO DO: The main mistake that Bob's doctor made is that he failed to insist on a firm schedule to test Bob's liver function, sugar levels, and uric acid after prescribing a relatively large dose of 4 grams of niacin per day. If your doctor prescribes niacin, be sure to follow these guidelines:

- Notify your doctor if while taking niacin you develop loss of appetite, nausea, acid indigestion, general malaise or flulike aches. These can be signs of niacin toxicity.

- Always start with a low dose of niacin, e.g., 100 mg, then, under medical supervision, work up to doses in the 1,500 to 3,000 mg range over many weeks or months.

- *Always* ask that your blood exams include tests for liver function, sugar levels, and uric acid. These tests should be performed about monthly as your dose increases, then at least once every six months once your dose is stable.

- Avoid niacin if you have a past history of ulcers, gastritis, hepatitis, diabetes, or gout.

- Take niacin only with meals. This will reduce the chances that you'll have a stomach or intestinal upset.

- Take at least part, if not most, of your daily dosage in the evening, preferably with your evening meal. Because your body makes most of its cholesterol at night, cholesterol-lowering medications tend to be most effective at that time of day.

- Taking an aspirin thirty minutes before you take a dose of niacin can reduce flushing.

- Although regular, rapid-release niacin may cause more flushing, this problem tends to diminish after your body gets used to the dose. Also, the regular release type is considered safer than the timed-release niacin, which is more likely to cause liver problems.

- Look for generic niacin tablets rather than brand-name pills, which can cost ten times as much.

Pros and Cons of the Main Types of Cholesterol-Lowering Medications

There are four main types of cholesterol-lowering medicines now in use: (1) niacin; (2) HMG-CoA reductase inhibitors; (3) fibric acid derivatives; and (4) bile acid resins. You've already been introduced to the main pros and cons of niacin in the error Mistakes Involving Cholesterol-Lowering Medications. Now, here is some practical information on the other three types.

HMG-CoA Reductase Inhibitors

Names of medications: Lovastatin (Mevacor), pravastatin (Pravachol), and simvastatin (Zocor).

Advantages: This group of cholesterol-lowering medications is very well tolerated by more than 95 percent of patients. They are extremely effective in lowering LDL levels and moderately good at lowering triglyceride levels. HDL levels are often increased. HMG-CoA reductase inhibitors can be taken once or twice daily.

Disadvantages: They are expensive. One to two percent of people develop liver inflammation. Perhaps 1 in 200 develop muscle inflammation, which, if not recognized, can cause kidney failure. HMG-CoA reductase inhibitors definitely slow progression of atherosclerosis and may cause a reversal. But definite proof that they actually prevent heart attacks is, so far, less solid than with other types of cholesterol-lowering drugs.

Most frequent errors

- Failing to give most of the dose in the evening. A dose at dinner is much more effective than the same dose at breakfast, because the body makes most of its cholesterol at night.
- Not educating patients that generalized muscle aches could be a symptom of dangerous toxicity.
- Not checking liver and muscle enzyme blood tests regularly.
- Combining these drugs with gemfibrozil (Lopid). This combination *may* be done in very special situations, but taking the

drugs together can markedly increase the risk of muscle inflammation.

Fibric Acid Derivatives

Names of medications: Gemfibrozil (Lopid), clofibrate (Atromid).

Advantages: Fibric acid derivatives are usually well tolerated by patients. They lower triglyceride levels and raise HDL levels.

Disadvantages: They are expensive. Fibric acid derivatives have a mediocre effect on reducing LDL cholesterol and might cause gallstones. Clofibrate (Atromid) reduces the risk of having a heart attack but increases the proportion of heart attacks that have a fatal outcome. Atromid also increases cancer risk. Neither of these problems applies to gemfibrozil (Lopid).

Most frequent errors

- Prescribing Atromid at all. It remains on the market, but disadvantages far outweigh advantages.

- Using gemfibrozil as the main treatment for high LDL cholesterol.

- Not recognizing that some patients who experience lower triglyceride levels while on Lopid may suffer a rise in LDL cholesterol as a side effect. (This action can be prevented by combining Lopid with a bile acid resin, as indicated below.)

- Failing to check on gallbladder symptoms, such as nausea, right upper abdomen distress, and pain radiating to the right back or shoulder.

Bile Acid Resins

Names of medications: Cholestyramine (Questran, Questran Light); colestipol (Colestid).

Advantages: Bile acid resins are not absorbed into the body and so there is little potential for systemic side effects, such as damage to liver functions or alteration of blood sugar levels.

They lower LDL cholesterol and sometimes raise HDL cholesterol.

Disadvantages: They are expensive. They come as a messy
powder that takes some effort to prepare. There is a moderate
frequency of gas and constipation or diarrhea, especially when
you're just starting the medication. Bile acid resins reduce absorption of medicines given within a few hours and also reduce
absorption of vitamins and minerals. They may increase the
blood triglyceride level.

Most frequent errors

- Not giving careful preparation instructions and schedule for
  taking this medication. For example, stomach or intestinal
  upset can be reduced by taking wheat bran or Metamucil
  with the drug. Also, it should be taken one hour before meals,
  with the most effective time being just before the largest meal
  of the day.

- Not realizing that rising triglyceride levels may be a side effect
  of these drugs. This can be prevented or treated by combining
  the bile acid resin with gemfibrozil (Lopid).

- Not spacing other medicines at least one hour before or four
  hours after taking a bile acid resin.

- Not assessing vitamin and mineral status. (I routinely recommend a multivitamin mineral supplement to be taken three
  or four hours apart from the bile acid resin doses.)

ERROR:

Your Doctor Fails to Monitor Fish-Oil Capsules, Vitamins, and Other Alternative Over-the-Counter Cholesterol Medications

Don, who had a distressingly low "good" HDL cholesterol (about
34 milligrams per deciliter) and relatively high total cholesterol
(above 250 milligrams per deciliter), was put on a cholesterol-
lowering medication by his doctor.

Don was sufficiently worried about his cholesterol that he also started taking one aspirin a day, high doses of fish-oil capsules, and also a regular regimen of antioxidant vitamins—including vitamins E and C and β-carotene (a precursor of vitamin A). He called his doctor to let him know the additional alternative measures he was taking, but his doctor gave no response.

At his next blood test about six months later, Don's cholesterol level had improved. However, he also started noticing that his stool was looking black after a bowel movement—a sign of possible internal bleeding. What had gone wrong?

FACTS: Some over-the-counter alternative medications may be helpful, and others may be decidedly dangerous. The problem is that scientific research is in an early stage regarding fish oil, antioxidant vitamins, small aspirin doses, and the like. As a result, practicing physicians must do their best to keep abreast of the breaking medical news and make the soundest recommendations they can, knowing at the same time that they can't be 100 percent certain right now about the impact of some of the vitamins and other supplements.

Here's what we do know right now about some of these alternative approaches to preventing heart disease:

Fish oil. Most doctors don't know a thing about omega-3 fatty acids, which are the active treatment component of fish oil. These acids decrease triglycerides and also thin the blood—a process that may account in part for the low heart disease rates among Greenland Eskimos, who eat a diet that is very high in omega-3 oils.

Although omega-3 fish-oil capsules—the type that Don was taking—are readily available without prescription in most health food stores, you should be aware of the potential dangers before you put your money down. Though they rarely present a problem in practice, fish-oil capsules could, theoretically, make your blood *too* thin if you take too much, if you already have a potential bleeding disorder, or if you take fish oil in combination with other blood-thinning medicines such as aspirin or Coumadin. Also, high doses of omega-3 oils sometimes increase "bad" LDL cholesterol and elevate blood sugar.

Fish oil also poses a problem in quality control. Like other unsaturated fats, fish oil, when stored, is easily oxidized to a state of rancidity unless substantial amounts of vitamin E or other antioxidants are added.

My recommendation: Eat plenty of salmon or other fatty deep-sea fish, which contain abundant amounts of the omega-3 oils. But stay away from fish-oil capsules unless you have the specific approval and supervision of a physician who really knows what she's doing.

Aspirin. "Sticky" or clotting blood often precedes a heart attack. A nationwide study involving 22,000 middle-aged male doctors has shown that taking one adult aspirin (325 milligrams) every other day can reduce heart attack risk by about 40 percent. Another study of 87,000 female nurses found that women who take one to six aspirins a week had 32 percent fewer heart attacks than did women who took no aspirin. Although other studies failed to show this benefit from aspirin, most experts believe that aspirin can decrease heart attack risk, perhaps even at doses as low as one baby aspirin (about 80 milligrams) every other day.

On the other hand, taking regular aspirin, even in low doses, on a daily basis can increase the risk of bleeding from the stomach. This over-the-counter medication can also raise the risk of bleeding into the brain (also known as a *hemorrhagic stroke*), especially among people with severe high blood pressure.

My recommendation: I think that most middle-aged men and women who are at high risk for heart disease should take low-dose (80-milligram) aspirin daily or every other day. However, people who are at low risk for heart disease should not take aspirin routinely, nor should those who are at high risk for aspirin's bleeding complications (e.g., people with very high blood pressure, a history of ulcer or bleeding tendency, or a high alcohol intake). But because each situation is individual, it's essential for you to get the go-ahead from your physician before you start a regular aspirin routine.

Antioxidants. Vitamin C, vitamin E, β-carotene, selenium, and a number of other vitamins and minerals are known as *antioxidants* because they have the power to block the damaging effects of certain caustic chemicals known as *oxidants*, or oxidizing agents. Oxidants are produced by the body's metabolic reactions or are introduced by certain foods, such as improperly stored or overcooked fats and oils.

Oxidation causes damage to many body tissues, in effect turning them rancid. Oxidant injury is currently being studied as a probable contributor to heart disease, cancer, stroke, and many other conditions, including the aging process itself.

Cholesterol, for example, is relatively nontoxic to arteries in its natural state. When oxidized, however, cholesterol is very damaging according to a number of research reports in recent years. Specifically, the oxidation of "bad" LDL cholesterol is increasingly regarded as a major factor in atherosclerosis, or the clogging of the arteries with fatty deposits. When antioxidants are introduced into the body through the diet or as supplements, they can help keep our cholesterol in its nonoxidized, less toxic state.

My recommendation: Taking antioxidant vitamin supplements is probably a good idea for most of us. Even though we don't yet know for sure, there's a reasonably good chance that they will help lower your risk of heart attack. At the same time, there is very little risk of doing harm by taking them. But as with aspirin, be sure to get clearance from your physician before you begin a vitamin regimen because there are a few possible dangers: Vitamin A, a close relative of β-carotene, can be toxic at fairly low doses, especially in pregnancy. Vitamin C often causes gastrointestinal upsets, and in a few people with specific metabolic abnormalities, it can cause kidney stones. Also, vitamin E should not be taken with blood thinners or by people with bleeding problems, unless your doctor specifically approves it.

WHAT TO DO: Don's doctor should have been alert to the potential of fish-oil capsules, together with even low doses of aspirin, to increase the tendency toward bleeding. Of course the bleeding in his stool might well have been due to aspirin alone or to a coincidental stomach or intestinal problem. But its intensity could easily have been made worse by the fish oil's blood-thinning effects.

As I mentioned earlier under Facts, I personally would avoid fish oil at this time, but still I advise eating plenty of fish. Also, you might consider taking antioxidant vitamins C and E and β-carotene under the doctor's direction. It's also wise to discuss the possibility of taking a baby aspirin once a day or every other day, especially if you've experienced a prior heart attack and don't have a history of internal bleeding or very high blood pressure.

Heart Attack

Your Doctor Fails to Rehearse You for a Heart Attack

These three incidents, all ultimately the result of a combination of patient and physician error, recently came to my attention. In each case, the individuals were under the regular care of a doctor, and each had undergone a general physical examination within the year before their mishap.

- Frieda, a healthy 72-year-old, had three episodes of pressure in the pit of her stomach about one week apart. Each ended with a burp, and so she assumed it was indigestion. The fourth episode was a massive heart attack that might have been prevented.

- Jerry, a 56-year-old department store manager, suspected that the tightness that began in his chest one Saturday night might signal a heart problem. But when he learned that another physician was covering for his own, who was away on a holiday, Jerry decided to wait it out until Sunday morning.

  A crushing chest pain hit at 4:00 A.M. and made it necessary for his son to rush him to the local emergency room. But the damage to his heart was too great, and he died of heart failure later that morning.

- Jim, a 46-year-old long-distance runner, experienced numbness in his left arm and brief heart palpitations for three to four minutes at the end of a workout. The thought of heart disease occurred to him, but he was sure that his physical condition was too good for that sort of problem.

Jim was lucky. He lapsed into unconsciousness during a mid-morning run but was resuscitated by a passerby trained in cardiopulmonary resuscitation (CPR). The diagnosis at the hospital was an electrical rhythm disturbance of the heart, which had been caused by insufficient blood flow through a partially blocked artery. After a bypass operation, Jim recovered completely and is now running again.

What common threads of error run through each of these incidents?

FACTS: Can you imagine giving an important speech without rehearsing it first? "Rehearsing" your first heart attack is infinitely more important than rehearsing a speech. Yet most doctors neglect to prepare their patients to recognize the early warning signs and symptoms of a heart attack so that they can respond effectively when the real emergency occurs.

Rehearsing your ability to recognize symptoms and respond to them is primarily important because this exercise can increase your speed in getting proper medical treatment. Fast treatment is essential for a number of reasons, such as these:

• Most heart attack victims die within the first hour of an attack because of an excessively fast, slow, or irregular heart rhythm. But if you can make it to a hospital, emergency room, or even a well-equipped ambulance and if you can be brought under medical monitoring before the heart rhythm problem progresses too far, the danger can be minimized.

• Damage to heart muscles during a heart attack—and the accompanying risk of dying—can be dramatically reduced by treatment with intravenous clot-busting agents, such as streptokinase and tissue plasminogen activator (TPA). But these drugs are most effective only if they are given during the first six hours of a heart attack—and the sooner the better.

So time is of the essence. A heart attack rehearsal supervised by your physician can be a life-saving form of preparation.

WHAT TO DO: If you are over age 50 (or age 40 if you have high heart disease risk factors such as high cholesterol, high blood pressure, diabetes, or smoking), don't wait for your doctor to raise the subject of rehearsing for a heart attack. Instead, schedule a visit with him to discuss how you can recognize early warnings signs. Here's a typical rehearsal I conducted with a patient in my office a few days ago. It's presented in a question-and-answer format, which I find to be the most helpful way of getting this action-oriented information across. The patient is asking the questions, and the doctor is answering them.

Question: When should I be concerned that I might be heading toward a heart attack?

Answer: The problem could be your heart if you feel a pressing physical discomfort of many types. This feeling may involve pain, or pressure or tightness in the chest. Typically it occurs in the center of your chest or in the left arm, left shoulder, neck, jaw, teeth, or upper abdomen.

Take no chances and call an ambulance immediately if

- The discomfort is intense.

- You feel sweaty or faint or short of breath.

- Your pulse is weak, rapid, fast, or irregular.

- Symptoms persist for more than ten minutes, whether they occur at rest, during sleep, or during or after physical exertion, mental stress, or a large meal.

Question: Is every twinge I feel in the vicinity of my heart an emergency?

Answer: No. Often these discomforts are not heart-related at all. But it's better to be safe. When people have angina (heart-related chest pains) or other heart disease symptoms, they can go on with a stable heart condition for years or even decades. The key thing is to become familiar with your personal pattern. You should hear alarm bells only if the pattern is changing; for instance, is it becoming more intense, occurring more frequently, lasting longer, or happening at lower levels of exertion or during periods of rest? Call the ambulance if the pattern changes, especially if the change occurs in a marked, crescendo fashion.

Question: Isn't a pain in the chest usually the result of gas or indigestion?

Answer: Yes, it is, but every year I hear a story of a person who thought he or she had indigestion but turned out to have angina or a heart problem. Angina pain can even trigger belching or gas.

You should first ask yourself, Is it *possible* this could be my heart? Be particularly suspicious if the "indigestion" seems new or different in its pattern or intensity. If you feel justified in answering that it's possible your heart is involved, then raise the question with your doctor.

Always call me with any suspicious symptoms if you're a middle-aged adult or older and particularly if you have other heart disease risk factors. (See the list on pp. 113–114.)

Finally, if the cause isn't obvious assume that the problem is your heart until proven otherwise. There's little to lose by going over to the emergency room in the first hour of such symptoms, and there's a great deal to gain if you do have a cardiac problem.

Question: If I suspect a heart emergency, should I call you first or go to the emergency room?

Answer: Call me first if the problem seems mild and your suspicions of a heart attack are low. But if your symptoms grow worse or if you can't reach me or my covering doctor, don't wait. Go to the emergency room.

If there's a rescue squad or ambulance serving your town, call this service rather than trying to drive directly to the emergency room. Of course, in many parts of the country, calling 911 connects you immediately to a police emergency service with the ability to dispatch an ambulance instantly. You'll receive heart monitoring and treatment more quickly by waiting for the rescue team, and by resting at home instead of trying to drive for help, you'll also cause less stress to your heart.

Now let me ask you a question: Do you know the number of your local ambulance or rescue squad? If not, find out by checking the phone book or asking at the police station or your local hospital. Put that number by your telephone, and also jot down a copy to carry with you at all times in your wallet. If you have a choice of more than one ambulance service, talk to all the candidates. Choose the one that carries a heart defibrillator machine in the ambulance and also maintains routine radio contact with doctors at the hospital.

Question: If I have a choice of several hospitals during a heart emergency, which one should I choose?

Answer: As a practical matter, a rescue squad will probably be required to take you to a specific hospital, usually the closest one with a qualified emergency room. Since time is of the essence, that's usually the right direction.

If for some reason a family member decides to drive you to a hospital, it's wise to find out in advance which emergency facility is nearest to your home or office. There's no advantage to trying to reach a world-famous heart center an hour away when you have a capable emergency room ten minutes down the road. Also, don't drive yourself. That can be dangerous.

It's also advisable to do a dry run one day by driving over to the emergency room and checking to see where the entrance is and exactly how you enter. If you or your driver has to ask directions during a heart attack, you lose valuable time and may be jeopardizing your health.

By going through these questions and answers with your physician—and by encouraging him to raise and answer others with you—you'll be well rehearsed in case a real emergency strikes.

ERROR:

Failing to Follow an Effective Emergency Room Drill

When Mark felt the heavy pain hit him in the center of his chest, he was fairly certain he was having a heart attack. But being the sort of person who didn't want to "put anybody else out," he went to his supervisor at work, mentioned he was feeling ill, and asked for permission to go to the hospital. The supervisor was concerned and offered to have someone accompany him to the emergency room, but he waved her off and indicated he could handle things by himself.

Mark did make it to the emergency room, but as he was checking in, he couldn't seem to impress on any of the staff that he might have a serious problem. He said, "I'm really feeling bad, and I think this could be serious," but they were concentrating more on people who were lying on stretchers, some of whom seemed to have been injured in car accidents or gunplay.

Finally, growing frustrated and angry, he shouted, "Look, I think I'm having a heart attack. I have a terrible pain in the center of my chest, and my left arm is growing numb. You've got to help."

That got action, but not soon enough. Mark died of a massive heart attack within the hour.

FACTS: Anyone who has been in an emergency room knows the ease with which a serious problem can be overlooked. It's essential that you assume a high profile *immediately* with those in charge so that your case will become a priority. If they learn you might be having a heart attack, they'll put you at the front of the line, but the message has to be gotten across to them.

After they are alerted, emergency room staffers become very good at sorting through patients with possible heart attacks. They recognize about 98 percent of true impending heart attacks and incorrectly send home only one heart attack victim in fifty. One reason for such mistakes is that inexperienced residents, especially new residents working during the midsummer vacation months, may be giving care without adequate supervision. They might send a patient home because his symptoms seem vague or atypical or because his electrocardiogram seems almost normal. In fact, electrocardiogram abnormalities can be very subtle or absent in the early stages of a heart attack and escape the eye of even an experienced physician.

WHAT TO DO: Your own doctor should brief you on distinctive emergency room procedures in your area. Well before you ever find yourself in an emergency room, it's important to ask her what the customs and level of competence are at the emergency room where you're likely to go during a crisis. Also, you might actually want to visit the emergency room and ask a few questions, such as who a patient should talk to first to get immediate attention when there's a true emergency. With this sort of information, you'll be in a much better position to make a smart decision if you yourself end up as an emergency room heart attack patient.

Your physician should then help you plan how you'll deal with an emergency room situation if and when the need arises. Here are some of the considerations that you should keep in mind as you discuss this matter with your physician:

- If you arrive by ambulance, you'll be in a much stronger position to get good treatment because the rescue squad will already have started working on you. In effect, they become your advocates and give you a status superior to those who arrive on their own or with a family member.

- If you arrive on your own and not by ambulance, it will be up to you to impress the staff immediately with the message that you believe you're having a heart attack. When this idea sinks in, they will put you at the front of the line.

- If you're alone when you arrive, you'll have to get this message across by yourself, as Mark tried to do in the above example. But it's much better to ask someone to accompany you even if you think you may be "putting them out," as Mark did. The last thing a heart attack victim needs is to get into an argument with a clerk or hospital aide. Emotional upsets can trigger heartbeat abnormalities, which may in turn be fatal. Your job as the patient is to keep calm. Your companion's job is to make sure that you are seen within minutes of your arrival.

- If the emergency room doctor doesn't seem to be taking your case seriously, you or your companion should demand to see a cardiologist. Most residents or nurses are happy to share the responsibility of making important decisions with a specialist.

A good question to ask in the emergency room is, Am I going to receive clot-dissolving medication? After you are hooked up to a heart rhythm monitor, the most urgent decision the emergency room physician must take is whether to give you an intravenous clot-dissolving agent. This medication could save your life if you're having a heart attack, but it may also cause internal bleeding and even a stroke. (See pp. 70–78.)

The best approach is for a cardiologist to see you immediately and give the go-ahead before starting clot-dissolving drugs. But this procedure can cause delays if a cardiologist isn't readily available. The current trend, which involves a very well trained emergency room staff, is to allow the emergency room physicians to make the decision and initiate treatment.

In any event, if you find yourself in an emergency room as a heart attack victim, you should inform the physician about personal factors that might increase your risk of bleeding, such as abnormal bleeding tendencies, ulcers, gastritis, severe high blood pressure, regular intake of alcohol, or regular use of aspirin or other antiinflammatory medications. You might also request that the emergency room physician at least *talk* to a cardiologist before making a decision about blood-thinning medications.

ERROR:

Assuming a Lax Approach to Patient Care After a Heart Attack

Dr. G., a 70-year-old internist who was still practicing full-time, had always believed that when one of his patients had a heart attack, only three things were absolutely essential. He would tell them:

- "Take it easy; don't exert yourself too much."

- "Keep taking the medicines they gave you when you left the hospital."

- "After a couple of weeks, when you feel stronger, make an appointment with me and we'll see about giving you another electrocardiogram."

This loose system of monitoring seemed to work rather well—until an elderly patient who had suffered one heart attack neglected to contact Dr. G. for several months. One day Dr. G. learned from a family member that she had suffered a second heart attack, this time a fatal one.

FACTS: When I was a resident twenty years ago, most heart attack patients went home from the hospital with few medicines or instructions beyond those offered by Dr. G. A number of older physicians still practice this way despite tremendous advances in medication and diagnosis that can help predict and, in some cases, prevent second heart attacks. Some critics of our modern, high-tech approach may wax nostalgic about the good old days. But the current standard of care requires a far more active approach than that used by Dr. G.

WHAT TO DO: Before you are discharged from the hospital and also during your first follow-up visit with your doctor (which should occur within a few days after your release), be sure that your doctor reviews with you the following post–heart attack topics:

Postattack Topic 1: Treatment with medicines that might directly prevent a future heart attack. These include beta-blockers, aspirin or other blood thinning agents, and angiotensin-converting enzyme (ACE) inhibitors. You should receive a written list of all medicines you'll be taking with an indication of what each one is for, the dosage, and the schedule for taking them. Also, your doctor should indicate the major side effects that accompany these drugs and what can be done if they occur.

Postattack Topic 2: The stress test issue. Your doctor must decide if you should have a mini exercise stress test before you leave the hospital (one that may involve a relatively short, low-intensity session of exercise). Or he may choose a full exercise stress test (usually a fast walk of longer duration on a moving treadmill) six weeks after your discharge. Or he may want you to undergo both procedures. The purpose of these tests is to identify the patients who remain at high risk and who thus might benefit from more aggressive treatments.

Postattack Topic 3: Symptoms you should watch for that might indicate the onset of a second heart attack. You should contact the doctor immediately or enter an emergency room if you have recurring or increasing chest pain; very rapid, slow, or irregular heart rate; fainting; or severe shortness of breath. You should contact your doctor within a day if you experience weakness, fatigue, anxiety, or depression.

Postattack Topic 4: The pace at which you may increase physical activities. When can you go outside, drive a car, have sexual relations, or return to work? Also, your doctor should tell you whether or not he recommends a formal, medically supervised exercise rehabilitation program.

Postattack Topic 5: Any specific treatment you may need for heart disease risk factors, such as high cholesterol, high blood pressure, excessive body fat, diabetes, or cigarette smoking. Your doctor should identify the subjects that are of the greatest concern and tell you when they will be discussed with you in detail.

ERROR:

Unnecessary Invasive Tests for Heart Disease

Jeanne, age 55, consulted her family doctor because she couldn't keep up with the pace of her weekly tennis game. She had also noticed a vague tightness in her chest that occurred sometimes during exercise, sometimes after eating. She had no other symptoms.

An electrocardiogram her doctor ordered was normal, but she wanted to be sure she wasn't missing something, and so she suggested a consultation with a cardiologist. The cardiologist, who was very well respected, had Jeanne undergo a stress test, which was borderline abnormal. A similar borderline reading resulted from a more sophisticated and expensive version of the stress test, which involved the injection of thallium into her blood.

The cardiologist then decided to take another more aggressive step. He ordered an arteriogram, which required the injection of an X-ray dye through a catheter tube, which was inserted by ''catheterization" directly into the arteries of Jeanne's heart. This test revealed that Jeanne's coronary arteries were in good shape, with no significant heart disease. It was obvious that her shortness of breath and chest pressure were due to some reason other than a cardiovascular problem.

Unfortunately, however, as the test was being completed, a blood clot formed around the catheter, broke off, and passed up to Jeanne's brain, causing a mild stroke. Today, her left arm is partially paralyzed.

Did the doctor make a mistake ordering this test?

FACTS: For better or worse, borderline stress test results are a common fact of life. Given the equivocal findings of Jeanne's stress tests, her cardiologist estimated that the odds that she actually had heart disease were less than fifty-fifty. But he reasoned that if she did have a problem, it would be better to find it early and deal with it rather than allow it to progress to the point that she might have a heart attack. He knew that there was about a 1 in 500 chance that there would be any serious complications from the arteriogram, and 1 in 1,200 that death would occur. These risks seemed to him small enough to justify the test.

Some cynical critics of American medicine would argue that Jeanne's doctor's decision to do a cardiac catheterization was likely influenced by his knowing that he would earn $1,000 for doing this procedure. Or they might suggest that he was motivated, at least in part, by the fear of being sued if he did *not* do the procedure and Jeanne later had a heart attack.

Knowing the doctor in this case, I'm almost certain that neither reason entered his conscious decision-making process. Physicians, with only a few exceptions, have a strong personal and professional commitment to the ethical principle that their job is to serve the patient's best interest, not their own.

Still, subconscious incentives might be at work. Expensive "high-tech" procedures are certainly done more often under fee-for-service payment systems than under managed care, where incentives are reversed to favor cost control.

Some health care experts believe that the prevailing tendency of American cardiologists, as a group, is too aggressive in favoring cardiac catheterization and then cardiac surgery. For example, one research group from the Harvard School of Public Health estimated that about half of the one million heart catheterizations each year aren't really necessary. They pointed out that catheterization and surgery are done much more frequently in the U.S. than in any other country.

Other equally respected experts cite flaws in the Harvard study and point to other research which shows benefits from invasive heart procedures for many types of patients. They give examples of individual patients from their own experience who they say would have gone on to a heart attack or sudden death had they not intervened aggressively.

The bottom line, of course, is not national statistics but what's the best choice for *your* individual case. Was Jeanne's trip to the "cath lab" a good medical judgment? Should she have resisted?

While I can appreciate the desire to find out for certain whether Jeanne actually had heart disease, given the risks of the procedure and the equivocal evidence that was creating her doctor's worry, I think that watchful waiting would have been a better choice. Then, if later stress tests became more abnormal or progressive symptoms developed, an arteriogram of her heart would have been in order.

Fortunately, most patients fit reasonably well into relatively clear-cut guidelines that indicate when a heart catheterization should or should not be done. Unfortunately, there are always in-between cases where we have to rely on our judgment—and the informed patient's preferences for dealing with risk and uncertainty.

WHAT TO DO: My experience tells me that when it comes to major health decisions, nearly all physicians take their ethical responsibilities very seriously. You can assume that they don't recommend potentially dangerous procedures just to make money. At the same time, you as a patient must be cautious. Insist on a full explanation of the pros and cons of each option, and don't hesitate to seek a second opinion when you're facing something as serious and invasive as an arteriogram.

Here are some guidelines that you and your physician should keep in mind as you decide whether or not to have the catheter test. Lean *toward* doing a cardiac catheterization if

- You have angina (classic heart-disease-related chest pains) or other known symptoms of cardiac disease, and they have been worsening despite medical therapy.

- You have other recurring chest pains or pressure, and the cause can't be determined despite your having been checked for other potential causes such as heartburn, anxiety, and hyperventilation.

- You've recently had a heart attack and have not experienced a prompt, complete recovery from it.

- You've had a recent exercise stress test that was severely abnormal.

On the other hand, you should lean *away* from a catheterization if

- You have not had a definitely abnormal stress test using newer and more sophisticated techniques, such as thallium.

- Your angina or heart symptoms are long-standing and stable.

- You have other symptoms that are somewhat vague or hard to pin down to a cardiovascular problem.

ERROR:

Your Doctor Oversells Heart Surgery or Angioplasty

Edward, a business executive, underwent a cardiac stress test as part of his annual physical. It indicated that there was an abnormality in blood flow in the coronary arteries leading to his heart. An arteriogram, which was appropriate in this situation, confirmed that there was a narrowing in two of the vessels, one of them being 70 percent blocked and the other, about 80 percent blocked. But Edward had experienced no symptoms of heart disease, such as angina pains.

Still, his doctor said, "You really can't delay taking care of this. You're in a dangerous situation."

So with Edward's agreement, the physician scheduled an angioplasty procedure, which involved enlarging the narrowed vessels with a balloon-tip catheter that was inserted into the coronary arteries. Although the procedure seemed to be successful at first—widening the narrow arteries—within six months after the procedure the blockage in the vessels became worse than it had been initially. As a result, the doctor referred Edward for a coronary bypass operation, which involved grafting veins onto the heart so that blood could be shunted around the blocked vessels. This surgery has also provided only temporary benefits, and now Edward is considering whether to accept a second bypass operation.

Did the doctor make a mistake in ordering the first angioplasty procedure?

FACTS: Doctors sometimes oversell angioplasty and bypass procedures with what I call the "ticking time bomb" argument. They emphasize that your narrowed arteries are in effect ready to "explode" in your body within weeks, months, or, at the most, a year or two.

Those who are most likely to benefit from these operations usually have severe angina symptoms, poor heart muscle contraction, or an alarming, abnormal exercise stress test result. An arteriogram will often show that these people have severe narrowing of their coronary arteries at locations that threaten to block off the flow of blood to large areas of the muscle of the heart. Most experts agree that such patients with such severe disease are likely to live longer and enjoy a better quality of life if they receive early bypass surgery or angioplasty.

But this approach doesn't apply to other patterns of blockage, which may include blood vessels that are less clogged or those that have remained stable for five or ten years or longer. A narrowing of the artery doesn't have to be corrected just because it's there—especially if the patient has only mild heart-related symptoms.

In many cases, surgery and angioplasty do a better job than medication in reducing angina symptoms and can give a new lease on life to patients who find their symptoms causing disability. But for many common patterns of blockage, patients live as long and, on average, incur no higher rate of heart attacks if they choose to be treated with medication rather than surgery or angioplasty.

Also, as Edward learned, angioplasty and surgery may not provide a permanent cure—and may even make a stable situation worse. After angioplasty, early relapses often occur, with about 30 percent of blockages recurring within six months to a year. After coronary bypass surgery, vein grafts may close off in as many as 40 percent of patients within five to ten years. Furthermore, because of the increase in scar tissue and the damage initially done to organs and vessels, reoperating is almost always more difficult than performing the first operation.

WHAT TO DO: If you are presented with a choice between an invasive coronary procedure or surgery and sticking with medication, keep this basic principle in mind: You should be surgically aggressive if medical treatment is failing. But you should play for time—be more inclined to delay surgery or angioplasty—if your situation is stable.

Another essential strategy in making this serious decision is to seek a second opinion. Edward might very well have been told by a second independent physician that he would have been wise to wait rather than have angioplasty. He might even have sought a third opinion to help him with this weighty issue; I know I certainly would have!

Here's another interesting source of advice and information that you should consider: Cardiologists and heart surgeons in hospitals typically meet weekly to discuss difficult cases of educational value, and yours may very well fall into this category. So ask that your cardiologist present your case and your heart catheterization films before his department's educational conference. (Most cardiologists do so routinely, without having to be asked.) Also, ask him to provide you with the details of what the other doctors said. This approach will give you plenty of professional feedback on which to base your final decision.

ERROR:

Your Doctor Refers You for Heart Surgery, Angioplasty, or Another Invasive Procedure to a Specialist with Less Than Optimal Experience or Skill

Geri's family doctor determined that she needed a coronary arteriogram, and so he sent her to the local hospital, where a physician friend of his worked. He didn't mention to Geri that she had a choice among several hospitals and that this particular institution did relatively few arteriograms—only about one hundred per year.

In any event, Geri went to the hospital her doctor suggested. During the procedure, she suffered a ruptured blood vessel, which caused some internal bleeding but, fortunately, didn't cause permanent damage.

How could she have protected herself better?

FACTS: There's an old saying that only the operating room nurses and anesthesiologists know who are the best and worst surgeons and specialists in various procedures. Hospitals do keep statistics on deaths and complication rates from their operations and procedures. Unfortunately, except in New York State and Pennsylvania, where some data are made public, this information isn't available to patients. Even your cardiologist can't get these numbers except perhaps by making quiet inquiries with a personal contact.

But there are some ways that you can make independent checks when you're facing an elective procedure, such as an arteriogram, angioplasty, or bypass surgery. Here are two checkpoints you should keep in mind as you make your decision:

Checkpoint 1: Ask your family doctor, cardiologist, or another doctor or nurse who might have information about the reputation of the doctor recommended for your procedure. Is that doctor considered the best or only so-so? Would *you* (the doctor you're talking to) use this person if you were or your mother were undergoing the procedure?

Checkpoint 2: When you meet with the specialist who is doing the operation or procedure, ask her about her training, the number of cases she does annually, and her death or complication rates. If she won't discuss these matters with you, get another physician.

The number of procedures the doctor does each year is very important for two reasons. First, it takes experience to gain and maintain the technical skill needed for surgery, angioplasty, and other complicated cardiac procedures. Second, a high volume of activity means that the doctor is respected by her colleagues who are referring many cases to her.

Also, it's reassuring to me when the doctor's *hospital* also handles a high volume of similar cases. This means that your doctor isn't the only one she knows doing this particular procedure, but instead, she's in an environment where she can consult with other experts.

How many cases should an expert doctor and her hospital be handling annually? Here are some guidelines:

For a coronary arteriogram: Most guidelines recommend that a cardiologist should do a minimum of 50 procedures per year to keep up his or her skill level. However, all else being equal, you will better your odds if you prefer a cardiologist who does at least three cases each week, or 150 per year. The hospital should do at least 300 per year to keep the "cath lab" staff in top form. Major cardiac centers may do 1,000 arteriograms annually. I recommend the 150-procedures-per-year standard for two reasons—typically, doctors become more skilled at procedures the more often they do them. Also, those cardiologists who receive the most referrals have been given a high vote of confidence in their skills by the referring physicians.

For angioplasty: The doctor should have done at least 200 procedures in her career and regularly perform at least 75 annually. Many
physicians have done more than 1,000 angioplasties. Her hospital
should perform 200 per year.

For coronary bypass surgery: The doctor should do at least 150
operations each year—though many heart surgeons don't meet this
standard. The hospital should handle at least 350 operations annually, with many top centers doing more than 1,000 per year.

Although some experts would disagree, I believe that cardiac surgery and angioplasty treatment is often as good and in some cases
better in many excellent community hospitals than at more famous
medical school centers. But if you choose a local doctor or institution, be sure that they are well recommended and also meet the
minimum requirements for the procedures and operations mentioned above.

Special note: If you are considering a heart procedure in New York
State, write to Cardiac, Box 2000, New York State Health Department, Albany, NY 12220 for the number of patients operated on in
your hospital and the outcomes of the operations. Statistics about
individual surgeons are not disclosed.

> ## ERROR:

Your Doctor Concludes That Worsening Heart Symptoms Always Mean That Your Heart Disease Is Getting Worse

Betty, who was 58, had never had a heart attack, but after many
years of indifferently treated very high blood pressure, she developed marked symptoms. These included both chest pains with exertion (angina pectoris) and shortness of breath due to fluid
accumulating in the lung (congestive heart failure).

With a combination of medication and a low-fat dietary program,
Betty did very well for two years. She was able to hold on to her job
and, in general, lead a normal life. But then her condition began to
slide, with increasing chest pains and more shortness of breath.

Betty's doctor doubled her medications, and then doubled them
again. She was scheduled to be admitted to a hospital for a cardiac

catheterization as a final prelude to possible cardiac surgery when her preadmission blood tests disclosed a surprise.

What went wrong with this diagnosis?

FACTS: Betty's doctor neglected to review her health history closely enough to see that something other than a heart problem was affecting her health. Her blood work six months before had shown that she had mild anemia. If the anemia had progressed, that might account for her worsening symptoms. Sure enough, the hospital's preadmission lab tests showed that Betty was severely anemic. She had been slowly leaking blood from her stomach, probably as a result of antiinflammatory medicines she had been taking for her arthritis. This noncardiac condition, increasing the strain on her heart—not worsening heart disease—had been responsible for the shortness of breath and chest pains.

WHAT TO DO: If you have a heart condition that seems to be deteriorating, the cause may indeed be your cardiovascular condition. Both you and your doctor need to review your *entire* case, including factors that may be at work outside your heart and blood vessels, to find the correct answer to your problem. Such a review should include the following:

- A detailed history of all symptoms you have, including those that have changed.

- An evaluation of all prescription and over-the-counter medications you're taking, with special attention to recent additions or subtractions of drugs.

- A review of all the potential side effects of your medications.

- Any changes you've made in your diet.

- A thorough medical examination, including chest X ray and electrocardiogram.

- Lab work and blood exams, including these tests: SMA screening panel (a set of chemical tests that measure liver and kidney function as well as sugar and various mineral levels in the blood), thyroid test, blood levels for all measurable relevant drugs (e.g., digoxin and antidepressants), urinalysis, and sedimentation rate.

In addition, you should check the accompanying boxes, which include noncardiac conditions and medications that can worsen heart disease or its symptoms. If you notice that you have any of these conditions or take any of the medications, call this to the attention of your doctor immediately. You may very well find that by eliminating these factors, you'll also reverse the worsening of your symptoms.

ERROR:

Outdated Treatment for Congestive Heart Failure, Heart Enlargement, or Ventricular Hypertrophy

Frank had been diagnosed as having congestive heart failure (indicated by fluid accumulating in the lungs which is visible on a chest X ray) and was placed on a combination of digitalis and diuretics by his doctor. But Frank noticed in a health column in his local newspaper that other drugs were being used for his condition, and he brought this to his doctor's attention.

Noncardiac Conditions That Worsen Heart Disease Symptoms

Anemia.
Over- and underactive thyroid.
Overweight or recent weight gain.
Lung disease, such as bronchitis, emphysema, pneumonia, and asthma.
Influenza and other viral illness.
Inflammatory disease, such as arthritis and muscle inflammation, temporal arteritis, or polymyalgia rheumatica.
Kidney failure, whether mild, moderate, or severe.
Vitamin deficiencies.
Psychological distress.
Inadequate sleep.
Subtle infections of the urinary tract, lung, sinuses, or prostate.
Blood clots in veins (phlebitis) or in lungs (pulmonary embolism).
Low blood potassium.
Low blood magnesium.
Caffeine.

Common Medications That Worsen Heart Disease		
Type of Medication	Worsens Angina	Worsens Congestive Heart Failure or Promotes Fluid Accumulation
Appetite suppressants	Yes	No
Aspirin and nonsteroidal antiinflammatory agents	No	Yes
Asthma, bronchodilator, or theophylline medication	Yes	No
Beta-blockers	No, except with abrupt withdrawal	Yes
Calcium channel blockers	No	Yes
Cortisone-type medication	No	Yes
Digitalis overdose	Yes	Yes
Estrogen hormones	Yes (if abnormal blood clotting)	Yes
Hydralazine (Apresoline), a blood pressure medication	Yes	No
Migraine (ergot-type) medications	Yes	No
Thyroid hormone	Yes	Yes

His doctor's response: "These new treatments come and go, and it's important not to jump too soon at every new thing you read about. The medications you're on are used all over the country, and they've been working well with thousands of patients for many years."

What was wrong with this answer?

FACTS: For two generations, up until just a few years ago, treatment for congestive heart failure didn't change. The standard regimen was, as Frank's doctor said, digitalis and diuretics.

These two drugs still work, but recent research now makes it clear that another category of drug, known as vasodilators, can be very beneficial in reducing the need for hospitalization *and* in prolonging life. Vasodilators relax or dilate the arteries and veins, thus reducing the resistance against which the heart must pump.

ACE inhibitor drugs, which are now among the most popular treatments for high blood pressure, are one of the most effective vasodilator treatments. Other medications for vasodilator effects include prazosin and hydralazine as well as nitroglycerin, the traditional treatment for angina chest pain. Ironically, beta-blockers are also being explored as treatments for congestive heart failure in certain cases despite the fact that weakened heart muscle contraction and fluid congestion in the lungs can also occur as a beta-blocker side effect.

In addition to helping with congestive heart failure, the vasodilators can be used effectively to treat those who have an enlarged heart (as shown on a chest X ray) or left ventricular hypertrophy (thickness of the heart muscle wall as indicated on an electrocardiogram or echocardiogram).

WHAT TO DO: If you have a heart problem of any kind, ask your doctor if the problem involves heart enlargement, heart muscle wall thickening (hypertrophy), weak heart muscle contraction, or congestive heart failure. If you have any of these conditions, inquire if your treatments include a vasodilator-type medicine. If they don't, there may be a good reason. (See the accompanying box on possible errors that may be made with different heart disease medications.) But given the proven benefits of vasodilators, you should be sure that you understand your doctor's reasoning.

You can obtain a summary of federal governmental guidelines for patients with congestive heart failure by calling the Agency for Health Care Policy and Research (AHCPR) at 1-800-358-9293, or by writing to AHCPR Publications Clearinghouse, P.O. Box 8547, Silver Springs, MD 20907.

Common Errors and Smart Patient Responses Related to Popular Heart Disease Medications

Digitalis (digoxin)

Common Errors or Oversights: Digitalis overload can cause heart failure or heartbeat irregularities, which are potentially fatal. Conditions that may change the blood level of digitalis or otherwise increase risk of digitalis toxicity include alcohol use, beta-blockers, asthma bronchodilator medicines, calcium channel blockers, cortisone drugs, diuretics, epilepsy medicines, kidney disease, low blood magnesium, nasal decongestants, low blood potassium, quinidine and various antibiotics.

Patient Response: Ask your doctor to recheck your digitalis blood level periodically, especially after any change in another medication.

Diuretics

Common Errors or Oversights: These drugs decrease blood potassium, though the so-called potassium-sparing types do not. Low potassium increases the risk of heart rhythm abnormalities. Digitalis may also drive the blood pressure too low.

Patient Response: Ask your doctor to check your blood potassium periodically. Many, but not all, experts believe that the blood potassium level should be kept in the high normal range, because potassium depletion can become fairly advanced before blood potassium falls below normal readings. Check your blood pressure shortly after starting this drug to be sure it's not dropping abnormally.

Beta-blockers

Common Errors or Oversights: Though a main treatment for certain heart rhythm abnormalities, beta-blockers can cause a slow heartbeat (heart block) in vulnerable patients. Beta-blockers can also bring out asthma and congestive heart failure and mask the presence of low blood sugar in diabetics taking insulin. Also, this drug may drive blood pressure too low.

Patient Response: Have an electrocardiogram done before starting a beta-blocker. Use the drug cautiously, if at all, with asthma, congestive heart failure, or a diabetic condition being treated with insulin. Report to your doctor if your heart rate drops below 50 beats per minute or if you feel weak, light-headed, or short of breath. Check your blood pressure and pulse shortly before starting the drug.

Calcium Channel Blockers

Common Errors or Oversights: Calcium channel blockers can trigger a slow heartbeat or congestive heart failure and low blood pressure.

Patient Response: Obtain an electrocardiogram before starting the drug. Report any slow heart rate or feelings of weakness, light-headedness, or shortness of breath. Check your blood pressure and pulse shortly after starting the medication to see if there has been any change.

ACE Inhibitors

Common Errors or Oversights: ACE inhibitors cause kidney failure if kidney function is already impaired. They tend to increase the blood potassium level and may reduce blood pressure excessively. They also promote hives. In rare cases, ACE inhibitors may damage white blood cells. They often create a throat-clearing cough, which is not dangerous but can be annoying and may confuse the doctor.

Patient Response: Use them cautiously if at all with kidney disease or if you have a history of hives or allergic swelling (anaphylaxis). Check your blood pressure, blood count, potassium, and kidney function periodically. One possible exception: Despite their potential for harming kidneys, ACE inhibitors may actually help protect the kidneys of juvenile-onset diabetics, many of whom eventually develop kidney failure.

Nitroglycerin

Common Errors or Oversights: Nitroglycerin may lower blood pressure excessively. Stopping the drug suddenly may trigger angina pains. Headache is a common side effect. Long-acting oral nitroglycerin and nitroglycerin patches lose their effective-

ness when taken around the clock. (One sign that the drug is
no longer working may be that you stop getting headaches.)
Taking too much may reduce or eliminate the drug's effectiveness in reducing angina pains.

Patient Response: Discuss with your doctor proper scheduling
of times to take the drug. A nitroglycerin-free period of ten to
twelve hours is usually enough to restore its effectiveness.
Check your blood pressure shortly after starting to be sure it's
not dropping too low.

PART TWO

The Question of Cancer

Special Alerts: Cancer

- The darker area surrounding your nipple (the areola) becomes more dimpled, and you call this to your doctor's attention. But your doctor indicates you shouldn't be concerned: "After all, you are a 38-year-old woman, and changes in the body do take place as we get older." (See error, p. 146.)

- Although vaginal cancer is rare, your doctor fails to check your vagina carefully for signs of possible cancer even though your records show that you were born between 1945 and 1971. (See error, p. 155.)

- You notice that your clothes are becoming tighter around the abdomen, and you are puzzled because you exercise regularly and have been watching your diet closely. During your regular medical checkup, you jokingly mention to your doctor that you may have to start some spot reducing. He shrugs and goes on with the exam, failing to recognize the change in your body as a possible sign of ovarian cancer. (See error, p. 160.)

- Your stool sample has been chemically tested for occult blood on several occasions in the last few years, and in every case, the results have been negative. Your doctor has told you that if you want, you can also have a flexible sigmoidoscope exam, which involves inserting a tube with a viewing mechanism into your rectum and up into the lower part of your large intestine (colon). But from your discussions with her, it's been obvious that she doesn't think it's really necessary. She has also failed to ask about your daily vitamin intake, which involves large doses of vitamin C. A few months later, blood appears in your stool, and a subsequent exam reveals that you have cancer of the colon. (See error, p. 163.)

- Your annual routine checkup by your internist doesn't include a systematic viewing of all your skin surfaces—an absolute prerequisite for detecting the deadly skin cancer, malignant melanoma. (See error, p. 173.)

- You complain to your doctor about frequent difficulty in swallowing and also report an increasing tendency to have a hoarse throat. Your physician fails to refer you to a specialist. (See error, p. 138.)

- You are diagnosed as having breast cancer, but you are not informed about the importance of measuring estrogen and progesterone receptors of the breast cancer tissue. (See error, p. 184.)

Prevention and Early Detection of Cancer

Your Doctor Tries to Cover Too Many Health Concerns in One Checkup and Fails to Focus on Cancer Risks

One of my patients, a 60-year-old whom I'll call Susan, was being treated for asthma, migraine headache, high blood pressure, high cholesterol, and anxiety. When she came in for an exam, I often felt like asking, "Okay, what fire do we put out now?"

Her treatment requirements were so demanding that I failed to pay close attention to one area of preventive care—the condition of her skin. I didn't give her a thorough visual exam of every surface of her body. So I was quite disturbed when she reported to me that she had been to see a dermatologist about a mole she'd found on her ankle and had learned that it was a malignant melanoma, a potentially deadly form of skin cancer.

Susan's thoroughness and alertness in watching her own health had saved the day—and filled in a medical gap created by my oversight. Happily, her melanoma was at an early stage, and the current outlook is that she will be completely cured.

FACTS: Although I pride myself on advocating preventive medicine, when push comes to shove with a patient like Susan, I'm vulnerable to the same trap that catches most doctors. The squeaky health wheel gets the grease, and preventive exams are too often deferred or forgotten.

The basic rule of thumb is that you should receive thorough cancer-screening exams regularly and with increasing frequency as you grow older. See the accompanying boxes, which contain guidelines based on American Cancer Society recommendations for early detection of cancer in symptomless, average-risk men and women.

Other medical groups recommend cancer screening guidelines which are less aggressive than the American Cancer Society's. There is a legitimate debate on this topic. But for now, I think that the odds of your benefiting still remain best with an aggressive program for finding cancer early, such as that recommended by the American Cancer Society.

WHAT TO DO: Schedule a visit with your doctor to discuss setting up a sensible schedule of exams and tests that will cover all the major cancer risks. Then, be responsible to make sure that you follow through, year after year, to be sure that these tests are performed. If there's time to include part of your cancer exams during a checkup for some other health problem, by all means take advantage of this opportunity. There's no rigid rule that says you have to have all cancer tests at the same time.

But don't allow this piecemeal approach to cause you to forget

---

Guidelines for Early Detection of Cancer in Symptomless, Average-Risk Men

Age 20 to 39:

Have a cancer-related checkup every three years, which should include general cancer counseling and examination of the mouth, thyroid, skin, lymph nodes, and testes.

Age 40 to 49:

Have a cancer-related checkup yearly, which should cover all of the above areas, plus a yearly rectal examination, with palpation of the prostate.

Age 50 and Older:

Have the yearly exams, which include the above tests for younger age groups, plus a yearly prostate-specific antigen (PSA) blood test. In addition, you should have both an annual chemical stool blood test and flexible sigmoidoscopy of the lower colon every three to five years.

Guidelines for Early Detection of Cancer in Symptomless,
Average-Risk Women

Age 20 to 39:

Have a cancer-related checkup every three years, which should
include general cancer counseling and examination of the
mouth, thyroid, skin, lymph nodes, and pelvic organs. In addition, you should do a personal breast self-examination each
month; have a physical breast exam by your doctor every three
years; and have a baseline mammogram at about age 40. You
also need a Pap test and pelvic exam every year, but after three
or more annual consecutive satisfactory exams, the Pap test
may be done less frequently, at the discretion of your physician.

Age 40 to 49:

Have a cancer-related checkup that includes all the procedures
recommended above for younger women. Also, you should
undergo these exams:

- A rectal examination yearly.
- A breast physical exam yearly.
- A baseline mammogram at age 40, to be repeated every one
  to two years.
- At menopause, an endometrial tissue sample should be analyzed for women at high risk for uterine cancer. (See the
  box, How to Tell If You're at High Risk for Different Cancers,
  pp. 135–138.)

Age 50 or Older:

Have all the tests and procedures listed above plus the following:

- A chemical stool blood test every year.
- A flexible sigmoidoscopy every three to five years.
- A mammogram yearly.

any important tests or checkups. If necessary, do as Susan did: See a specialist, such as a dermatologist, to deal with areas of cancer risk that your doctor seems to lack time or expertise to handle.

ERROR:

Failing to Consider Family History Factors That Put You at High Risk for Certain Forms of Cancer

Kay's mother and older sister had died from breast cancer. But Kay did not inform her doctor of this history because the questionnaire that she had been given at her first examination years earlier hadn't caused her to think that this information was important. When she was 48 years old, Kay discovered a lump in her breast, which turned out to be malignant. She had to have the breast surgically removed.

FACTS: Most doctors tend to be too busy to cover all the bases with every one of their patients. In this case, as in my own situation described in the previous error, Kay's doctor had focused so much on Kay's other problems, including allergies and migraine headaches, that he just never got around to evaluating her cancer risk factors.

Of course, the doctor should have taken the time to analyze her family history. If he had done so, he would most likely have noted the high risk for breast cancer and would have recommended a more aggressive cancer-screening program. For example, it would have been appropriate to schedule a physical breast exam every six months and mammography annually from age 40 onward. He should also have put the cancer-screening procedures at the top of his agenda every time Kay came in to see him.

The overwork and excessive time pressure that beset most physicians these days make it imperative that *you*, the patient, fill in the gaps in order to protect yourself from serious health problems.

WHAT TO DO: You should first learn what the main risk factors are for the most common types of cancer. Then, if you find that you are at higher than average risk for any form of cancer, inform your doctor immediately. Remind him to take this information into account to help you plan your preventive medicine schedule, including various cancer-screening tests and procedures. (See the accompanying box.)

How to Tell If You're at High Risk for Different Cancers

Breast Cancer:

All women should consider themselves at relatively high risk for this disease because about one in nine eventually develops the condition. But your risk is even higher if

- Your mother or sister has had breast cancer, especially if the disease occurred before menopause (in this situation, the risk doubles to quadruples).
- Any of your aunts or cousins have had breast cancer.
- You began your menstrual periods before age 12.
- Your menopause was delayed until about age 55.
- You have had no children, or the first birth occurred after you were 30.
- You're 20 percent or more above your ideal body weight.
- You have had a previous cancer of the breast.

Cervical Cancer:

Cancer of the cervix develops in about nine women per thousand. Your risk is higher than average if

- You began sexual activity when you were quite young (16 or younger).
- You've had multiple sexual partners.
- You're a cigarette smoker.
- You've been infected with the human papilloma virus or had genital warts.

Uterine Cancer:

Your risk is higher than average if

- You have abnormal vaginal bleeding, especially at or after menopause.
- You have a family history of uterine cancer.

- You have a personal history of breast cancer.

- You are taking tamoxifen for breast cancer.

- You are obese (more than 30 percent above your ideal body weight). This factor triples your risk.

- You have diabetes.

- You are older than age 40 and have never had a full-term pregnancy.

- You have had problems with your ovaries, causing chronically irregular or frequently missed periods (such as polycystic ovary syndrome).

- You've had estrogen treatment without progesterone.

- You've undergone X-ray treatments on your pelvis.

Vaginal Cancer:

This cancer is rare except in women born from 1945 to 1971. Many pregnant women during that period were exposed to diethylstilbestrol (DES), an estrogen-type hormone, during their mother's pregnancy. DES treatments in pregnant women have been linked to a high incidence of vaginal cancer in their offspring.

Ovarian Cancer:

This cancer, which affects 1.3 percent of all women, can pose a higher than average threat if

- Your mother or sister had ovarian cancer. (But more than 97 percent of victims of this disease don't have any such family history.)

- You're a white person (African-Americans and Hispanics have a lower risk).

- You have no children.

- You are on a high-fat diet (i.e., more than 30 percent of the calories you consume each day come from fats).

- You've previously had breast cancer.

Colon and Rectal Cancer:

These diseases affect about 6 percent of all men and women. You have a higher than average risk if

- Several members of your family have had colon cancer or multiple tumors or polyps of the colon. (Members of these very high-risk families have a 50 percent probability of developing bowel cancer.)
- A parent or sibling has had colon or rectal cancer, a fact that increases your risk by two to three times.
- You have a personal history of adenomatous polyps of the colon (where a glandlike growth occurs within the colon).
- You have a personal history of ulcerative colitis, a condition that increases your risk by twenty times.
- Your diet consists of a high intake of red meat and fat, with a low intake of fiber or vegetables.

Lung Cancer:

You are at above-average risk if

- You are a smoker.
- You are exposed regularly to secondhand smoke from others.
- You have been exposed to asbestos.
- You have a low dietary intake of β-carotene (a precursor of vitamin A) and vitamins C and E.

Melanoma Skin Cancer:

You're at above-average risk if

- You have fair skin.
- You've had heavy sun exposure, especially with repeated sunburns.
- You have a family history of melanoma.

- You have many moles or freckles.
- Your skin has unusual looking or atypical moles.
- You have a personal history of melanoma.

Prostate Cancer:

About 10 percent of all men will be diagnosed with prostate cancer at some point in their lives, and 2 to 3 percent will die from it. A much higher proportion have microscopic cancer in their prostates by age 80—perhaps as high as 40 percent of all in that age group. (But it's not known if these microscopic cancers will eventually cause problems.) Your risk of prostate cancer is above average if

- You've had a vasectomy. (This risk factor is not 100 percent proved but recent evidence points to it.)
- Your racial background is African-American.
- You are 70 years old or older.
- You have a family history of prostate cancer.
- You are on a high-fat diet (more than 30 percent of calories each day from fats).

Thyroid Cancer:

Your risk is above average if you were exposed as a child to X rays of the neck.

ERROR:

Your Doctor Fails to Ask You About Common but Frequently Overlooked Cancer Symptoms

Lillian was having some difficulty swallowing her food, and she also had experienced frequent bouts of hoarseness even when she knew she didn't have a cold or other respiratory infection. She mentioned these concerns in passing to her physician. He examined her throat and told her that he didn't see any signs of disease or other abnormality.

"Keep me posted if the swallowing or hoarseness gets any worse," he said. He also recommended that she cut her food up into tiny pieces and chew it even more thoroughly before she tried to swallow it.

Six months later, Lillian was diagnosed as having cancer of the esophagus (the part of the digestive tract leading from the throat to the stomach), a disease with little hope for cure. She died a few months later.

FACTS: Difficulty in swallowing may be caused by relatively unthreatening conditions, such as a natural, though abnormal narrowing of one portion of the esophagus or by spasms occurring at the point where the esophagus is connected to the stomach. But swallowing problems, especially when combined with ongoing hoarseness, can also be a sign of esophageal cancer and *must* be dealt with on that basis until the possibility of cancer has been eliminated.

Doctors may delay in taking the complaints of patients seriously when reasons other than cancer are most likely to be the source of the complaints. So it's imperative for the patient as well as the doctor to know some of the danger signals that may indicate *either* mild or nonemergency health concerns *or* life-endangering cancer.

WHAT TO DO: Certainly, you don't want to become a hypochondriac, overly worried every time you develop a little cough or hoarseness. On the other hand, if certain symptoms continue to nag or get worse, they should be brought to your doctor's attention. One of the reasons that I like the idea of a routine annual physical for those over 40 is to give them time to review issues that are usually omitted during regular, problem-focused medical visits. Cancer detection and prevention are much easier to accomplish if you're in the habit of seeing your doctor every year and if you plan to go to her office regardless of whether or not you have symptoms.

It's helpful for every patient to do a self-analysis before these annual exams. To this end, it's extremely helpful to keep in mind the seven early warning signs of cancer, which have been publicized by the American Cancer Society. They can be remembered with the acronym THIS WEB:

T—Thickening or lump in the breast or elsewhere.

H—Hoarseness or coughing, which may nag or recur.

I—Indigestion or difficulty in swallowing.

S—Sore that doesn't heal.

W—Wart or mole that undergoes obvious changes.

E—Emission of blood or other discharge.

B—Bowel habits change.

Before each visit with your doctor, repeat THIS WEB, and use the acronym as a checklist. This way, you can be more effective in evaluating yourself to see if you are experiencing any of these signs or symptoms.

In addition, before each visit to your doctor, look over the accompanying box, Common Symptoms That Could Arise from Cancer or Other Causes.

If you notice that you have any of these symptoms—and especially if they seem to be chronic or growing worse—be sure to tell your doctor. Even if you have other symptoms or a definite sense that "something is not right" with your body or health, tell her exactly how you feel. She may be able to help you sort through the seriousness of your concerns.

You can obtain additional excellent information about early cancer detection and prevention from your local American Cancer Society chapter or from the society's national office in Atlanta (1-800-ACS-2345).

ERROR:

During a Routine Medical Exam, Your Doctor Fails to Ask You to Show How You Examine Your Own Breasts

When Paula came in for her routine physical, the physician noted that she had a noticeable lump in her breast. He immediately scheduled a mammogram, and subsequent tests revealed that she had a malignant tumor that required surgery. Nearly two years had passed since her previous examination, but the doctor was puzzled about how such an obvious mass could have developed without her being aware of it. He had shown her how to examine her own breast, and

Common Symptoms That Could Arise from Cancer or Other Causes		
Symptom	*Type of Cancer*	*Other Causes*
Loss of appetite	Stomach, pancreas, colon	Low thyroid, depression, ulcer
Darkening spot on skin	Melanoma	Age spot
Blood spotting in stool	Rectal, colon	Hemorrhoids, polyps, diverticulosis
Constipation bloating, or feeling full without eating much	Colon, ovary, stomach, esophagus, pancreas	Too little fiber, too little exercise, low thyroid, depression
Shortness of breath	Lung	Asthma, heart disease, anxiety
Decreased urine stream, blood in urine	Prostate, bladder, kidney	Benign prostate enlargement, side-effects of medicine, urine infection
Fatigue	Any cancer	Almost any disease, physical or psychological
Swollen glands	Lymphoma	Mononucleosis, low-grade infection, sinusitis, acquired immunodeficiency syndrome
Nagging cough, hoarseness	Esophagus, larynx, lung	Upper respiratory infection, colds, allergy symptoms

she had assured him several times that she was following the exact procedure that he had suggested.

What went wrong?

FACTS: Paula didn't conduct her self-examination properly. Instead of going systematically over her entire breast slowly, section by section, she consistently did an incomplete job, skipping about and poking here and there. Too often, she allowed months to go by between these self-checkups. As a result, the tumor went undetected for more than a year.

Because many women submit to gynecological and related examinations only reluctantly—and because most doctors are aware of this fact—many male doctors are reluctant to say to a female patient, "Okay, now please *show* me how you examine your breast."

Although this approach may seem overly aggressive on the part of the physician and may even be resented by some patients, it's an absolutely necessary part of effective screening for breast cancer. Most women do find their own breast cancer, but many don't examine their own breasts because they lack confidence that they can do so correctly. Also, many women do the self-exam incorrectly by skipping areas as they move from section to section of each breast. Or they may feel with the tips of their fingers or with the palms of their hands rather than the pads of their fingers, which are more sensitive.

Ironically, another key reason why many women avoid breast self-exams is because they fear they might find a lump that might be cancer. Fortunately, the vast majority of breast lumps are not cancer. Even those that are referred for biopsy usually turn out to be benign.

WHAT TO DO: Every physician should show female patients how to do a proper breast exam or should have a qualified nurse teach the technique. The patient should also be provided with instructional pamphlets, which are available through the American Cancer Society.

But the final and most important element in monitoring the patient's technique is to have her show the physician or nurse exactly how she does it. If Paula had been given this opportunity by her doctor, she would probably have discovered the tumor when it was in an early stage, and she might have saved her breast.

ERROR:

Your Doctor Says You Shouldn't Worry About a Small Hard Spot in Your Breast Because It Hasn't Shown Up on Any Mammogram

Both Alice, a 36-year-old who had relatively large, dense breasts, and her doctor were able to feel a very small, hard knot in her left breast, but two mammograms failed to produce a picture of the spot. Her doctor said, "Don't worry at this point. We'll just keep watching it."

Within a year, the lump had grown significantly larger, did show up on a mammogram, and was established as malignant by a biopsy. As a result, Alice had to undergo a mastectomy.

Did the doctor make a mistake?

FACTS: Yes, the doctor did make a mistake. About 15 percent of breast cancers can be felt on a physical exam but don't show up on a mammogram. One study of more than 1,000 proven breast cancer patients revealed that mammograms had been misinterpreted as benign for one case in twelve. Furthermore, the proportion of missed tumors is higher among women before menopause, when relatively dense breast tissue can make mammography less sensitive. Alice, who had large breasts, was in this category.

Unfortunately, despite these clear benefits of a physical exam, a study from the National Cancer Institute has shown that even though more women are getting mammograms, the proportion who have also had a physical exam of their breasts has decreased. This trend should raise a red danger flag for both patients and physicians.

WHAT TO DO: Insist on an annual *physical* breast examination by your doctor even if you've had a mammogram with a negative result. If your physician finds a lump of any type on the physical exam, you and your doctor must take this discovery seriously, even if the lump is undetectable or appears benign on the mammogram.

If your breasts tend to be dense or heavy, you should also ask your doctor about a *xeromammogram*, a picture done with a special mammography machine from Xerox. This procedure provides more sensitive pictures for women who have dense breast tissue or who have silicone implants. But the radiation dose is higher for this test than for standard mammography. So I would recommend it only for evaluating a mass that has been detected by physical palpation (feeling) or a regular mammogram. Eventually, magnetic resonance imaging (MRI) technology may supplant regular mammography, especially for women with dense breasts. But MRI mammography is currently in the experimental stage and is much more expensive than the standard test.

In many cases, further examination of the lump will require a biopsy (removing and analyzing a portion of the lump or mass for malignancy). But there are some other tests that a qualified doctor can perform short of a biopsy. One of these is a sonar or ultrasound study of the breast, which will show whether the mass is solid or hollow (cystic). If the mass is hollow, the doctor might withdraw (aspirate) fluid through a needle placed into the mass.

If clear fluid comes out, then the mass is probably a harmless cyst. In the event that the cells from this fluid look benign under a microscope, and the cyst collapses and does not refill, the probability of cancer is very low. But if *no* fluid comes out, the breast mass is probably solid, and a biopsy will probably be necessary. If the mass reappears or is otherwise suspicious, then a biopsy is essential, even if the fluid looks clear under the microscope.

If your doctor recommends against a biopsy, you should ask him about the probability of your having cancer, regardless of how low that probability may be. Then insist on making the final biopsy decision yourself. Usually, a series of tests and examinations will present you and your doctor with a situation where you have to estimate the odds and decide whether you can live with some degree of uncertainty or whether you should go ahead with the biopsy to be sure.

ERROR:

Your Doctor Tells You That Because You've Had One Baseline Mammogram Before Menopause, There Is No Reason for You to Have Another Mammogram Until You Are Past Menopause

Trisha, a 44-year-old with no breast lumps that could be detected by physical exam, had undergone one mammography procedure when she was 40. This test was performed as a *baseline* mammogram, which would establish that her breasts were healthy and would provide her doctor with a standard picture to show the normal condition of her breasts.

Trisha had read in a women's magazine that women should have regular mammograms after they are 40, and she asked her doctor about this. He replied, "There's no need for you to have another mammogram before you reach 50 or go through menopause." And he cited a Canadian study of 50,000 women, age 40 to 49, who experienced no decrease in their death rate from breast cancer as a result of having had mammography.

Two years later, Trisha discovered a lump on her breast during a self-examination, and subsequent mammography and a biopsy proved it to be malignant.

Where did the doctor slip up?

FACTS: The National Cancer Institute and many American radiologists have found fault with the Canadian study in question, in part because modern mammography machines are more accurate now than when the Canadian study was conducted.

In light of the weaknesses in the Canadian study, the American Cancer Society is sticking with its previous recommendation that a baseline mammogram be done at age 40, and that mammography be performed every one to two years from age 40 to 49.

One argument against early mammography concerns the fear that, over time, repeated X-ray exposure will actually increase the risk of developing breast cancer. This risk is real but very small. Current mammography involves extremely low-dose exposure to X rays—much lower than with the less sophisticated machines available in the 1960s and 1970s.

It's been estimated that the very low doses of radiation from mammography may cause 1 case of cancer for every 34,000 women under age 40; 1 case in every 130,000 for women age 40–49; and 1 in 210,000 for women age 50 and older. These long odds, when compared to the benefits of having a mammography, have prompted most experts to come down on the side of more frequent mammograms.

WHAT TO DO: I tell my patients—and I would have told Trisha— that if they are at high risk for breast cancer, they should follow the current American Cancer Society guidelines. I believe these are more appropriate than the more restrictive recommendations advocated by some cancer experts and insurance companies who are influenced by the Canadian study. This means having a baseline mammogram at about age 40 and then regular exams every one to two years from age 40 to 49. (For a summary of the factors that may put you into the high risk category for breast cancer, see the box How to Tell If You're at High Risk for Different Cancers, pp. 135–138.)

For my female patients who are only at average risk, I tell them that it's all right to delay the first baseline mammogram until their early forties. Then, after they have the baseline, they should proceed with the standard guidelines, which require mammography every one to two years up until age 49. After that, the procedure should be performed without fail each year. Women at very high risk for breast cancer, of course, should talk with their doctor about a more aggressive screening program.

When you're dealing with your doctor, it's her prerogative to advise you about the likely benefits, costs, and risks of medical testing. But if you initiate a serious discussion of the issues we've been exploring under this error—and you conclude that you would be most comfortable with more frequent mammography—she should be willing to accommodate your wishes.

ERROR:

You've Noticed Some Changes in the Appearance or Shape of Your Breast, but Your Doctor Tells You Not to Worry

Diane noticed that her right breast had become somewhat more dimpled around the nipple and areola, the darker area surrounding the nipple. She pointed out this change to her doctor, but he said, "Don't be concerned about that. After all, you are a 38-year-old woman, and changes in the body do take place as we get older."

Diane underwent mammography about a year later, and the test revealed a tumor, which turned out to be malignant.

FACTS: The majority of breast lumps and other changes in the shape, size, or appearance of the breast are benign, that is, they don't involve cancer. But some telltale signs should trigger further study, including a recommendation of mammography or other test. These include

- A lump or thickening in or near the breast or in the underarm area.

- A change in the size or shape of a breast.

- A discharge from the nipple.

- A change in the color or feel of the skin of the breast in the area surrounding the nipple (areola) or in the nipple itself. For example, the nipple may become puckered, dimpled, or scaly.

Doctors and nurses tend to make two types of mistake in dealing with a woman whose breasts have these signs or symptoms. First, as Diane's doctor did, they may discount what seems to be a slight or minor change on the grounds that the change is probably a normal result of aging, which for the time being should just be "monitored" or "watched." Second, doctors and nurses may be sensitive to the seriousness of a particular change, but they may erroneously assume that any normal patient will call these changes to the doctor's attention, when in fact many patients won't be so assertive. Ironically, many women notice important changes and sense they may have a problem, but they don't seek medical attention because they fear finding out that the abnormality they have noticed might be cancer!

One reassuring fact: The large majority of breast lumps that are biopsied actually turn out to be benign.

WHAT TO DO: Any changes in your breast should be brought to your doctor's attention immediately, as Diane did. But unlike Diane, don't be satisfied with doing nothing or "watching" the condition unless your physician has satisfied you completely that the change you've noticed isn't a possible malignancy. If you remain unconvinced by his explanations, seek a second opinion.

ERROR:

Your Doctor Sends You to an Unqualified Mammography Center

Frieda, who lived in a small town, was referred to a local clinic that had just installed a mammography center. During the course of the examination, the female technician told her that she was one of her first patients. When Frieda expressed some concern about her expertise, the technician said, "You can check with the radiologist. He knows about my background." But the radiologist, a qualified medical doctor, wasn't scheduled to be at the clinic until the following day.

Frieda again expressed her concern about the mammography when she spoke to her doctor on the phone the next day. But he said, "Believe me, those people know what they're doing. The radiologist is fresh out of his residency, but he's bright and he knows his business. Besides, I'm a part owner in that clinic, and you can be sure I keep close track of what they're doing."

FACTS: Government studies indicate that there has been substantial variation in the quality of exams given by the thousands of mammography centers around the country. Although this situation should improve as a result of new federal certification procedures instituted in the fall of 1994, both doctors and their patients should always be careful about the way the tests are conducted.

Top-level mammography requires a combination of important factors in addition to good equipment. Most important are the professional training of the radiologist and staff as well as the volume of their experience. (See the following "What to Do" section for a checklist of these factors.)

WHAT TO DO: You should ask these questions as you prepare to choose your center:

- Is the center accredited by the American College of Radiology (ACR)? Many centers are not. About 30 percent of centers that apply for this credential are turned down the first time. You can locate an ACR-accredited facility through your local chapter of the American Cancer Society or the National Cancer Institute's information service (call 1-800-4-CANCER).

- How qualified is the radiologist who actually reads the mammograms? The ACR requires that the radiologist be board certified and read at least 480 mammograms a year. Obviously, Frieda's center didn't meet this requirement. Unfortunately, the ACR doesn't actually test a radiologist's skills. This weakness in the system can be important since many radiologists complete their residency without much supervised training in mammography. *My recommendation:* Rely heavily on the volume of mammograms done by the radiologist.

- What is the volume of the mammography center? For most medical procedures, quality tends to improve with increased volume and experience. A busy mammography center will do at least 2,500 examinations a year (about 50 a week). Many do considerably more. Again, Frieda's center falls short.

- Will the radiologist be physically present when the mammography is done? There's an advantage to this practice, which wasn't followed by Frieda's radiologist: When the radiologist is on the spot, marginal studies can be repeated immediately instead of your having to be called back for a second test. Even better, some centers have the radiologist read the film and give you the result right away instead of having to wait.

- Is the mammography device "dedicated" for use only for mammography and employed for no other purpose? Machines designed for multipurpose use expose you to more radiation than machines designed solely for mammography.

- Are the technical personnel registered and state licensed?
- Does your physician schedule you for visits to the same center each time you get a mammogram? This way, past films can be compared. If you have to go to different centers, you have an absolute right to obtain a copy of your films to bring to another physician or mammography center if you wish.

A word on mobile mammography machines: These devices, often found in shopping centers, have the advantage of convenience, but the disadvantages far outweigh the advantages. First of all, movement of the van may affect the delicate equipment. Also, there's usually no radiologist on the premises. And there's the danger that a particular unit with the record of your films and medical history may not be available next year.

ERROR:

The Technician Fails to Ask You If You Have a Silicone Breast Implant Before Giving You a Mammogram

Kristine visited a walk-in clinic for a mammogram, but the technician on duty forgot to ask if she had any silicone breast implants. On adjusting the paddle to flatten Kristine's breast for the exam, the technician applied too much pressure. The implant was ruptured, and Kristine had to be rushed to the local hospital for immediate surgery.

FACTS: Silicone breast implants block the ability of the mammogram to visualize the full breast. Some cancers will be missed, though most will still be seen. A technician must be aware of the presence of implants in order to exercise the special care that's necessary to manipulate the breast properly as the mammogram is being done. Otherwise, a section of the breast may be hidden from view.

Also, if the technician isn't aware of the implant in advance, she may put a setting on the mammography machine that will flood the breast with an overdose of X rays. And there's also the danger of what happened to Kristine: excessive compression of the paddle leading to rupture of the implant.

WHAT TO DO: Tell the radiologist *and* the technician about your implants in advance.

ERROR:

Neglecting to Schedule a Pap Smear for Very Young or Very Old Patients

Heather, a 14-year-old, was still seeing her pediatrician, and he regularly gave her checkups when she came in for viral infections, athletic injuries, and other youthful complaints. What he failed to ask her about—and what she didn't tell him—was that she had already become sexually active.

Heather's grandmother, a 74-year-old widow, had moved to a retirement community in Florida after her husband's death ten years before. She also went for regular medical checkups, and her physician concentrated almost exclusively on controlling her mild hypertension and her elevated cholesterol. What her doctor also failed to ask about—and what Grandma didn't tell him—was that she, too, was continuing to be sexually active.

The granddaughter had never had a Pap smear, and the grandmother had not undergone one since she was in her late fifties.

FACTS: Deaths from cervical cancer have fallen dramatically in the decades since Pap smears became the centerpiece of women's preventive medical exams. Still, some 5,000 deaths, most of them completely unnecessary, occur each year because Pap smears are not done or because they are done and read incorrectly.

Why is it so important to know a person's sexual habits when you consider recommending a Pap test? Cervical cancer is a sexually transmitted disease. All women who are or were sexually active are at risk. Furthermore, the earlier the age of first intercourse and the larger number of male partners, the higher the risk. With sexual activity these days often beginning in the teenage years or early twenties, women are increasingly being struck down by cervical cancer before they reach age 30.

Young, single, sexually active women—especially teenagers—often don't seek Pap smears, and frequently doctors are too embarrassed to ask about sexual habits. So the women at highest risk for cervical cancer are the least likely to get a Pap.

On the other hand, cervical cancer can appear after decades of slow incubation. About one-quarter of new cases and about 40 percent of all deaths are in women over 65. Doctors and patients may become lax in scheduling Pap smears for this age group because they think of cervical cancer as a young woman's disease. They may also underestimate the amount of sexual activity among older people. Until just recently, Medicare actually refused to cover a Pap smear—a misguided policy that has now been corrected!

WHAT TO DO: If you're old enough ever to have had sex, you should be sure you're scheduled for a regular Pap smear. Current American Cancer Society guidelines call for a Pap test and pelvic exam for sexually active women every year. After three or more consecutive annual exams that are normal, the Pap test may be done less frequently at the discretion of your physician.

I personally recommend that my patients under age 65 have a Pap smear every year regardless of previous normal tests. As a practical matter, however, I accept the fact that this policy often translates into every year and a half to two years. Women 65 or older should continue to have Pap smears at least every three years. Most gynecologists argue for annual exams for older women whether or not they are or have been sexually active, in part because a yearly visit allows an opportunity for a review of any symptoms. Also, more frequent checkups help the doctor detect signs of ovarian, uterine, or vaginal cancer, and other female concerns.

ERROR:

Your Doctor Fails to Order a Second Pap Test After a Normal First Test, Even Though You Are Experiencing Spotting or Other Symptoms Between Periods

Zelda was experiencing occasional spotting between her periods, and her doctor ordered a Pap test. Because the test came back negative and the spotting involved only small amounts of blood a few times during the month, the doctor said he thought it would be all right for her to "sit tight and we'll check you again when you come in for your next checkup."

When Zelda came in for her next checkup nearly a year later, the Pap smear was positive, and she was diagnosed as having cervical cancer.

FACTS: I've heard all kinds of horror stories from medical insiders about women who have developed cervical cancer that went undetected on a Pap smear. Some of these results were due to physician error, such as not getting a good enough sample of cells from the opening of the cervix. Other times, the mistakes were attributed to slips at the laboratory reading the smears. Still other errors occurred because of simple, everyday oversights, such as a failure by the physician or nurse to see or respond appropriately to an abnormal Pap report.

Problems can occur in the doctor's office if she isn't able to visualize the cervix clearly through the speculum she uses for the procedure. There is evidence that suggests that the yield of good cell specimens is higher when the doctor uses a device called an *endocervical brush*. This tool enables her to sample cells from inside the cervix as well as outside.

Since 1992, laboratories doing Pap smears have had to meet rather strict federal standards, including actual testing of the labs' ability to process known Pap smears submitted by government regulators. The error rate at individual clinics, which before the 1992 rules varied from about 2 percent to 30 percent of all Pap smears submitted to a given clinic, is believed to have been reduced. But all practicing physicians know that the potential for Pap smear error is still present and that the results of all tests have to be monitored closely. If there are any suspicious symptoms, such as the spotting that Zelda was having or bleeding after intercourse, a complete reexamination should be done promptly, including a second Pap smear.

WHAT TO DO: As with all other lab tests, you should insist on being notified of the result of your Pap smear by phone or mail or by calling your doctor's office. If you have any abnormal symptoms, such as spotting between periods or bleeding after intercourse, keep pursuing the cause even if your last Pap was normal. If you've had one mildly abnormal Pap smear and the next one is okay, you'll need to *confirm* that good news with *another* Pap smear at your next scheduled exam. Of course, if the Pap smear is very abnormal or if your cervix looks suspicious to your doctor, then she will probably move directly toward more vigorous diagnosis by examining your cervix with a small portable microscope, a procedure known as a *colposcopy*.

Finally, ask your doctor if she uses an endocervical brush as one of the instruments for obtaining a Pap smear. If she doesn't, and fails to give a good explanation, you might say that you have heard that many doctors now favor the brush as more accurate than the traditional "wooden scraper" instrument. Obviously, your doctor can't stop to order a new instrument during the middle of your Pap smear, but you should consider the nature of your doctor's response. Is she curious about your remarks rather than uninterested? Is she open to discussion rather than defensive? Does she place a priority on keeping up to date?

Another quick tip: If you're not too distracted during your exam, watch to see if your doctor or nurse sprays the Pap slides with a fixative within a few seconds after the procedure. This keeps the specimen well preserved. Waiting several minutes or longer for this treatment can make the slide difficult to read.

ERROR:

Endangering a Woman's Ability to Have a Successful Pregnancy by Not Referring Her for a Colposcopy Procedure After an Abnormal Pap Smear

Kay's Pap smear came back with a class III rating, which indicated an intermediate-grade abnormality. Her doctor, "to be on the safe side," referred her for a cone biopsy, a relatively extensive and invasive procedure that involves removing part of the cervical tissue, which is then tested for malignancy. This procedure involves the removal of larger sections of the cervix than a regular biopsy.

Kay, who was in her early thirties, had planned on becoming pregnant before she reached 35, but she found after the cone biopsy that she couldn't become pregnant. She and her husband are now being counseled by a fertility expert.

FACTS: Kay may be having problems getting pregnant because of the cone biopsy, which is known to cause complications with future pregnancies. In many situations, such as the one that Kay faced, a less dangerous alternative to the cone biopsy begins with a diagnostic procedure called *colposcopy*.

A colposcope is a device that's essentially a portable microscope, which enables a doctor to examine the cervical area very closely for possible malignancies. With this tool, he can decide more easily whether a biopsy is necessary, and if it is, he can identify more precisely the section of the cervix from which the tissue should be extracted. With the aid of colposcopy, the abnormal section of the cervix can often be removed with a more limited procedure than the traditional cone biopsy. (This procedure is known as a LEEP, or loop electrosurgical excision procedure.)

Although the use of colposcopy is rapidly becoming standard for gynecologists and even family physicians, there do remain many internists and family physicians who are unwilling or unable to alter old habits. So it may be necessary for you to be referred by your doctor to a specialist who has one of these devices.

When should your doctor send you for a colposcopy? To answer this question, you first have to understand the scoring system that is used for Pap smear results. You'll note that Kay's test involved a class III result. Until recently normal smears were rated class I, and outright cancers class V. Most abnormalities range from almost normal (class II) to almost cancer (class IV). As you can see, Kay's result was right in the middle. Recently, most laboratories have switched to a new scoring format called the Bethesda system. This system describes the slide's appearance in more detail than do the traditional Pap classes. The translation from Pap to Bethesda reports is described in the box below.

Unless there is an obvious ulcer or other change on the cervix, which can be biopsied directly, women with intermediate-grade abnormalities on the Pap smear need to be evaluated further, such as by colposcopy. In general, you shouldn't be sent in for a cone biopsy without first undergoing the less serious colposcopy procedure. And you definitely shouldn't be sent in directly for a hysterectomy without these preliminary procedures unless the doctor considers your situation a true medical emergency.

WHAT TO DO: If your Pap smear is abnormal, ask for the grade or class of the result. If it's class III or higher, you should definitely expect further action. If you hope to have children, a colposcopy exam, plus a regular biopsy if necessary, is the best option. Usually, a more extensive cone biopsy or hysterectomy should be performed only after the colposcopy has been done. Under the Bethesda reporting system, Pap's class III is replaced by four separate categories. (See the box below.)

With the aid of colposcopy, it's often possible to take out the suspicious area with the LEEP. This is less invasive than a cone biopsy and less prone to complications. Laser surgery also seems to work well, but it's much more expensive than the LEEP and no more effective.

ERROR:

You Were Born During the Period 1945 to 1971, and Your Doctor Fails to Check Your Vagina Carefully for Cancer

For years, Pat's results were negative for Pap smears of her cervix and other visual exams performed by her doctor. But on one recent visit to the doctor's office, she was found to have advanced cancer of the vagina—a condition that should have been picked up years before. What went wrong?

Translating Old Pap Names into the New Bethesda System for Pap Smears	
Pap System	Bethesda System
Class I	Within normal limits
Class II	Reactive or reparative damage
Class III	Squamous epithelial lesion
	Atypical squamous cells of undetermined significance
	Atypical glandular cells of undetermined significance
	Squamous intraepithelial lesion
	Low-grade
	High-grade
Class IV	High-grade
Class V	Squamous cell carcinoma
	Glandular cell abnormalities
	Adenocarcinoma
	Nonepithelial malignant neoplasm

FACTS: Because vaginal cancer is rare, there is a tendency among many doctors to focus on higher-risk areas, such as the cervix, when doing Pap smears or other tests. The problem is that women who were born during the period 1945 to 1971 may have been exposed in the womb to DES. This is a crystalline compound similar to estrogen that was given orally or by injection to pregnant women during those years as a treatment to prevent miscarriage.

Unfortunately, what was thought to be good for the pregnancy was *not* good for the daughter. Female infants born during this period have suffered an unusually high incidence of vaginal cancer, which is triggered by the early prenatal exposure to DES.

WHAT TO DO: If you are a woman born during the period 1945 to 1971, your physician should take a thorough prenatal history on you and try to determine whether or not you were exposed to DES. She should also check your vagina carefully as she does the other parts of your body for signs of malignancy. If you are a man who was born in the same period, you should also inform your doctor. Although potential complications from DES are less likely for men, certain genital abnormalities have been reported in male DES babies.

Women who are known to have been exposed to DES—or even if there is a possibility of such exposure—should be checked regularly (at least annually) by a gynecologist who is skilled in colposcopy. They should also have a careful Pap smear performed specifically on their vagina and a careful visual examination of their vagina on a twice-a-year basis.

ERROR:

Your Doctor Fails to Ask If You Are Experiencing Any Itching or Other Discomfort in the Vulva Area

Sue, who was 51 years old, had always gone in to her doctor for an annual physical examination, including regular Pap smears. But she had been reluctant to bring up a sensitive subject: that for nearly a year she had been experiencing periodic itching around her vulva, the entrance to her vagina.

Finally, the condition was becoming so aggravating that she decided to mention it to him after a visit when she was about to leave his office. But he passed her complaint off as "probably just dry skin, or it may be that you're going through menopause."

He said, "You're already dressed now, so why don't you just see how it goes for a while. If it gets worse or fails to go away in a couple of weeks, call me and I'll send you to a dermatologist."

The condition did grow worse, and a meeting was scheduled with a dermatologist. He discovered small tumors around the vulva and diagnosed her problem as cancer of the vulva.

FACTS: Cancer of the vulva isn't very common, but it's enough of a threat to warrant a regular examination of the vulva by your doctor. Although most vulval cancer victims are over age 60, about 15 percent of the malignancies occur in women under 40. Also, your doctor should ask you to report any symptoms you're experiencing in any part of your body. The most attentive doctors will give you examples of these symptoms and signs, such as itching, bleeding, or any sort of new growth or knot.

With cancer of the vulva, itching is the most common early symptom. In the later stages, there may also be bleeding, ulcers, or growths, such as small tumors.

WHAT TO DO: You must *not* allow embarrassment or hypersensitivity to prevent you from bringing up problems or symptoms you've noticed in your genital or reproductive area. If you're a woman and you feel shy about talking to a male doctor about these matters, find a female doctor. By the same token, if you're a man and find it's hard to discuss your private parts with a female doctor, then by all means go to a man!

The important thing is that you disclose any persisting irritation, discomfort, pain, or change in your body to your physician. He or she has been trained to link those observations to specific health conditions and diseases. If you fail to share your knowledge with your doctor, the consequences for your health could be serious, if not fatal.

ERROR:

Relying Only on a Pap Smear and Pelvic Exam to Check for Cancer of the Uterus

Meg, an obese single woman who was 49 and had just been through menopause, noticed some vaginal bleeding on several occasions.

She reported this symptom to her doctor, who scheduled her for an exam that week. He did a thorough Pap smear, which came back negative, and he also performed a pelvic exam but noticed nothing unusual.

"Probably, the problem is just related to menopause, or maybe the bleeding is just the result of an abrasion or some other temporary problem," he said.

He recommended that they wait a few months until her next regular checkup before doing further tests. In the meantime, Meg experienced more bleeding. At her next checkup, she was examined more thoroughly and found to have cancer of the uterus.

Could the doctor have caught this problem sooner?

FACTS: About 35,000 new cases of cancer of the uterus occur each year, and 90 percent of them are in women who are approaching or are past menopause. This disease can be diagnosed early and can usually be cured surgically *if* the doctor is alert in his exam or if the patient knows what signs and symptoms to bring to his attention.

Bleeding is a particularly important symptom and risk factor. Any woman with an episode of bleeding at least one year after menopause must be considered to have possible uterine cancer. In fact, uterine cancer will be the cause of bleeding in about 25 percent of such cases.

But there are exceptions: If you take estrogen hormones, you may bleed as a result of these hormones. In fact, women who take estrogen plus progesterone on a cyclical basis should *expect* to bleed in a regular pattern—usually at or just after the end of the progesterone cycle. On the other hand, bleeding early or through the progesterone phase is abnormal and should prompt an evaluation for uterine cancer. A pus-type discharge from the vagina or pain in the pelvis can also be a warning sign for cancer of the uterus.

Whether or not there are bleeding abnormalities, the first thing a doctor should know is the risk factors that are present in his patient. You'll recall from the box on pp. 135–138 that these include:

- Abnormal vaginal bleeding, especially at or after menopause.

- A family history of uterine cancer.

- A personal history of breast cancer.

- Taking the drug tamoxifen for breast cancer.

- Obesity, a condition that triples the risk.

- Diabetes.

- Being over age 40 and never having had a full-term pregnancy.

- Chronic lack of ovulation, which may result from a condition like polycystic ovary syndrome.

- Undergoing estrogen treatment without progesterone.

- Having had X-ray treatments of the pelvis.

As you can see, Meg had several of these risk factors: postmenopausal bleeding, obesity, and never having been pregnant. Also, her doctor either overlooked the fact or did not know that her mother had suffered from cancer of the uterus.

A Pap smear can detect some cases of uterine cancer, but this test is not nearly as sensitive for this problem as for cancer of the cervix. More advanced screening for uterine cancer should be done with high-risk patients. This may require a procedure called an *endometrial biopsy.*

In performing this test, which is usually done in the doctor's office, the physician does a standard Pap smear and then inserts a small device through the cervix into the uterus and removes a sample of uterine tissue. In some cases, the doctor can't obtain tissue from the uterus using this relatively simple procedure, and he has to do a *D and C*—a dilatation and curettage, which involves dilating and scraping the uterus while the patient is under general anesthesia. This test is normally done in the outpatient department of a hospital.

WHAT TO DO: If you find yourself in a situation like the one that confronted Meg, that is, you are experiencing symptoms like bleeding or have one or more of the risk factors for uterine cancer, you should undergo an endometrial biopsy. Or as an alternative, you could have a D and C. Normally, a gynecologist will perform these tests. In any event, don't accept the response "We'll wait and see if it happens again."

If you have not had abnormal bleeding but do have high-risk factors for uterine cancer, be sure to discuss your situation with your physician to see if an endometrial biopsy should be added to your Pap smear routine. Many cancer experts feel that an endometrial biopsy is too expensive to be offered to all women routinely, perhaps even including those with some risk factors. But this should be *your* decision with your physician, depending on your personal risk profile and how strongly you feel about protecting your health.

"I don't do a biopsy" is not a good reason for not doing one, though you might hear this from many internists and some family doctors who have not been trained in this procedure. Furthermore, it's not up to your health insurance plan to decide on a cost–benefit basis whether the traditional Pap smear and pelvic exam is sufficient. Rather, the decision must be made in consultation with you in light of what is best for your health.

ERROR:

Overlooking Subtle Health Signals That May Indicate the Presence of Ovarian Cancer

Doris had been pursuing a rigorous aerobic and calisthenics program for several years and also had been quite conscientious about sticking to a low-fat, near-vegetarian diet. A childless 49-year-old career woman, she had apparently completely recovered from a small malignant breast tumor that had been removed at an early stage. She had also been using talcum powder around her genital area since the early 1960s.

Despite her active lifestyle and healthy diet, Doris had found that her stomach frequently seemed bloated and her clothes fit much more tightly around the waist than they had a few years before. This development puzzled her because she had noticed no increase in her body fat; on the contrary, she could pinch much less fatty tissue around her stomach than when she had been much younger.

"Well, our bodies do shift in shape as we grow older," her doctor said when Doris called these changes to his attention.

But Doris wasn't willing to accept advancing age as the final explanation for these alterations in her looks. Her response was to work out even harder; she actually doubled and then tripled the number of sit-ups she did each day. But her stomach remained the same size and shape.

Eight months later, she was diagnosed as having advanced ovarian cancer. The malignancy was too far along to make surgery worthwhile. A complete case history that was compiled on her revealed that her sister was also a victim of this disease.

FACTS: The late comedian Gilda Radner brought ovarian cancer to the public's attention when she was struck down by the disease in her thirties. News reports revealed that she had been caught unawares by the disease, in part because she had not known that ovarian cancer ran in her family. Such a background greatly increases the risk of developing this cancer at a young age.

Family history, when positive for ovarian cancer, is the most important risk predictor. In fact, many cancers can be family linked, including cancer of the breast, uterus, ovary, large intestine, and skin (malignant melanoma). So it's important for you to know your specific family history of diseases and to communicate that information to your doctor. Unfortunately, even people with no family history of a specific cancer may develop it, though at a lower rate statistically. For example, even though ovarian cancers occur in many members of certain cancer-prone families, the majority of ovarian cancers can occur among women with no family history of this disease.

Records of ovarian cancer-prone families maintained by Dr. M. Steven Piver of Roswell Park Cancer Institute, Buffalo, New York, reveal that there is about a 50 percent risk of your developing ovarian cancer if you have two first-degree relatives with the disease (i.e., mother, sister, or daughter). If you have one close relative with ovarian cancer, as Doris did, that more than quadruples your risk from about 1.4 percent for the average women to about 6 percent. If you have a cousin or aunt with ovarian cancer, your risk triples to about 4 percent.

Other important factors that may double your risk include not having had children, being on a high-fat diet, and having a previous history of breast cancer. Doris, of course, had two out of these three in her personal medical history. In addition, taking fertility-inducing drugs may increase the risk of ovarian cancer as might a long history of using talcum powder around the vaginal area. Before 1970, there was no restriction on the amount of asbestos, a cancer-causing mineral, in most talcum powders.

Some women with ovarian cancer also have odd symptoms, such as abdominal bloating, clothes becoming tighter, or pelvic discomfort. These symptoms can complicate the diagnosis because they may arise from many other causes, including intestinal gas, diverticulitis, emotional stress, or, in some cases, the natural process of aging. In addition to overlooking danger signs in her medical records, Doris's doctor also missed the significance of her abdominal bloating.

To avoid her mistakes, the best strategy for patient and doctor is to assemble a complete "package" of symptoms and family history. Then, at as early a stage as possible, the physician should investigate more thoroughly if the patient seems in a high-risk category for ovarian cancer.

Ninety percent of patients with early ovarian cancer can be cured. But unlike uterine cancer, where early bleeding is common, or cervical cancer, which can be found with a Pap smear, early ovarian cancer triggers only vague, equivocal symptoms and leaves no telltale signs. That's why most cases aren't found until they have spread beyond the ovary. At that advanced stage—which is where Doris found herself—less than 10 percent can be cured.

The problem is not so much that patients fail to seek care or that doctors fail to give it. Rather, the methods available to detect ovarian cancer aren't very precise. Screening more aggressively would certainly save lives but would cost the health system more than $10 billion a year.

WHAT TO DO: Before your next medical exam, interview your relatives to determine whether your mother, a sister, an aunt, or a cousin may have developed ovarian cancer and at what age. Inform your doctor about your findings, and ask how this information might affect her cancer screening recommendations.

Notify your doctor about any symptoms that may be linked to ovarian cancer, including abdominal bloating, a tighter fit of clothes without obvious increase in body fat, or any pelvic discomfort. Be sure to stay up-to-date with your pelvic exams.

If you are at high risk for ovarian cancer and especially if you have a definite family history of the disease, your doctor can give you a blood test called *CA-125*. The results of this test will often, but not always, indicate the presence of the disease.

Also, transvaginal ultrasonography, a kind of radar scan of the pelvis, may have some value in screening women who are already known to be at high risk. In one study among 1,100 high-risk women, four early ovarian cancers were detected.

Combining CA-125 and transvaginal ultrasonography also has possible merit. In another study of 20,000 women, 258 had an elevated CA-125 blood level. Of these, 22 were also abnormal when tested with ultrasound. Of these 22, one-half had ovarian cancer.

Finally, a new ultrasound technique called *transvaginal color-flow Doppler ultrasonography* may be able to improve the rate of detection while reducing false-positive diagnoses. But at its current cost of about $450 per exam, it would take roughly $1 million to detect only one early-stage cancer of the ovary.

For more information on ovarian cancer, call the Gilda Radner Familial Ovarian Cancer Registry, Roswell Park Cancer Institute, Buffalo, New York, at 1-800-682-7246.

ERROR:

Relying Only on a Negative Stool Sample Test in Screening for Colon and Rectal Cancer

Warner, who was 54 years old, usually had a chemical stool sample test done whenever he went in for his regular annual physical. In every case, including the most recent, the test had come back negative, indicating that no blood was found in the sample. (The presence of blood may indicate colon or rectal cancer.)

His doctor had mentioned that if he wanted, Warner could also have a flexible sigmoidoscope exam. This involves inserting a tube with a viewing mechanism into the rectum and up into the lower part of the colon, or large intestine. But the doctor had obviously not been too enthusiastic about the test and said he didn't perform the procedure. Instead, Warner would have to go to a gastroenterologist, a specialist in disease of the stomach and intestines.

Warner decided that the sigmoidoscopy sounded rather uncomfortable, and so he chose to skip the extra hassle and expense of going to the specialist. The doctor moved on to the next area of the checkup without asking Warner anything about his eating habits. As a result, he failed to pick up the fact that Warner was on a high-antioxidant supplement regimen, including large daily doses of vitamin C (about 2,000 milligrams per day).

A few months later, blood appeared in Warner's stool, and an exam his doctor scheduled immediately afterward revealed that he had cancer of the colon.

FACTS: Colon and rectal cancers are a major killer of both men and women—striking down many more women than do ovarian cancer, uterine cancer, and cervical cancer combined. The tragedy is that some simple early-detection screening tests can help an alert physician identify and treat colon and rectal cancers at an early stage.

The chemical testing of the stool for hidden blood is the first line of defense. It's a simple, cheap screening procedure, which the American Cancer Society has long recommended be done annually on everyone 50 years of age or older. Several studies have questioned the value of the test, but recently, a large thirteen-year study from Minnesota found that those who received stool testing every few years had a one-third reduction in colon and rectal cancer death rates.

But there are a few factors that may cause the test to produce a wrong result:

- Taking high doses of vitamin C in the few days before testing can turn a stool test that should be positive for blood into one that tests negative. That's what happened with Warner, whose colon cancer was masked too long by his vitamin C intake.

- Shipping stool tests through the mail allows them to dry out, a process that can cause samples with blood in them to test false negative—unless a drop of water is added to the sample before actual testing.

- Eating red meat in the few days before testing can leave blood in the stool that is from the meat, not from your colon or rectum.

- Aspirin, related painkillers, and alcohol often cause internal bleeding in the absence of cancer.

- Bleeding hemorrhoids and menstrual flow may contaminate a stool sample.

Most important of all, among the many middle-aged or older people who have blood in their stool, only about 2 percent have cancer, though 30 percent of those with blood do have polyps in their intestines that sometimes develop into cancer.

If blood is found in your stool, you should take the next step, which is to undergo the above-described flexible sigmoidoscope test. Those at very high risk, perhaps because of a family history of intestinal cancer, may have a colonoscopy, which requires having a tube passed all the way around the large intestine (the flexible sigmoidoscope can cover only about one-third of the colon). (See p. 137 for the factors that may place you at high risk for colon cancer.) Aggressive physicians recommend that every person over age 50 who has unexplained blood in the stool should be looked at with a colonoscope.

If you are at high risk for this type of cancer, your checkups should be more stringent than those for the average person. For one thing, you shouldn't wait for blood to show up in your stool to undergo more extensive testing. Stool tests should be followed by a flexible sigmoidoscope exam and perhaps a colonoscopy or a barium enema. Even if your risk profile is okay, you should still have a yearly stool test beginning by age 50 plus a yearly rectal examination. You should also undergo a sigmoidoscopy at age 50 and have it every three to five years thereafter.

WHAT TO DO: Report any major change in your bowel habits to your physician, such as constipation, diarrhea, abdominal pain, or narrowing of the stool. Black, tarry-colored stools may mean bleeding from the stomach or intestine, though this coloring may also result from spinach, beets, iron pills, or Pepto-Bismol.

When you go in for your annual checkup, have the chemical stool sample test done if you have the opportunity. In any event, it should be performed every year from age 50 on. Be sure to tell your doctor about any vitamin C before you take the stool test. (Also avoid red meat for several days, since this can give a falsely positive test for blood in the stool.)

If your doctor regularly offers the flexible sigmoidoscope exam to her patients, by all means take it. You'll have to fast the night before to clear out your bowels on the morning of the exam with an enema. But the discomfort is worth the additional assurance that you are likely to be free of cancer of the lower colon or rectum. Or if you are found to have one of these cancers, you'll be in a better position to have it treated successfully at an early stage. What may seem like a hassle at the moment might actually save your life.

ERROR:

You Are Injured During a Sigmoidoscopy or Colonoscopy by an Unskilled Physician

Ted was asked by his doctor if he wanted to be checked with a new sigmoidoscope that had just been delivered to the doctor's office. Although Ted agreed to the procedure, he did ask his doctor about the safety of the procedure—and whether or not the physician really felt comfortable using the new instrument.

"Oh, sure, I used to do a lot of these," the doctor said. "This new device is almost exactly like the older ones."

In fact, properly used, the new instrument is better and more comfortable than the older sigmoidoscopes, which had wider, less flexible tubes that had to be inserted into the colon. The problem in this particular situation was that the doctor had not yet mastered the new technique—despite his experience with the older "straight" instrument. Ted's test was agony, both during and afterward. Intestinal cramping and gas triggered by the exam continued to plague him for the rest of the day. The doctor didn't even thread the sigmoidoscope as far as he needed because Ted's ashen face persuaded him to quit before he had completed the exam.

FACTS: When I was trained to be a physician, sigmoidoscopy was done with a short, straight metal tube, which was passed about one foot into the colon. A sharp twist of the bowel about halfway up the rectum could be difficult to negotiate with this instrument and often resulted in a physician's getting stuck and sometimes perforating the wall of the colon.

Today, the standard sigmoidoscope has essentially become obsolete and has been replaced by the more sophisticated flexible sigmoidoscope. The flexible sigmoidoscope is a two-and-a-half-foot-long soft, flexible tube, whose direction can be guided by controls at the handle. It's less painful than the old sigmoidoscope and, with training, can be easier to use. Many internists and family physicians have become skilled at flexible sigmoidoscopy, but on average, you'll tend to get the test performed more quickly and easily with a gastroenterologist.

Despite the improvements in the new flexible sigmoidoscope, there is still a very small danger of a perforated colon, especially when patients have diverticulitis or diverticulosis (small outpouchings along the surface of the bowel). A much more likely problem is a painful or incomplete exam when the instrument is in the hands of an unskilled physician, such as the one who treated Ted. Generally speaking, you can assume that a physician is skilled if he has done at least fifty flexible sigmoidoscope procedures and if he is using the instrument on an ongoing basis. Of course, as with most medical skills, the more a doctor does, the better he gets.

Colonoscopy is done almost exclusively by gastroenterology specialists or by colon and rectal surgeons. It involves the use of a much longer version of the sigmoidoscope and causes enough pain to require it to be done with moderate sedation, usually in the outpatient department of a hospital. The procedure requires considerable skill and is not risk-free, but it can be quite successful in detecting early colon cancer, as happened a number of years ago with President Ronald Reagan.

If a doctor is unskilled either with the sigmoidoscope or colonoscope, a perforation of the colon becomes a potentially life-threatening complication. This disastrous error occurs on average in about 1 case in a 1,000. A few physicians perforate more than others—sometimes because of lack of training and sometimes because of a "cowboy" attitude that makes the doctor keep pushing forward even though the bowel is resisting. I am aware of one physician who was alleged to have perforated the large bowel of three colonoscopy patients within just a few years. Yet some physicians in the community, either because they didn't know of the incidents or didn't want to judge a fellow physician, continued to refer patients to him.

Another potential problem that may arise with inexperienced or inattentive physicians is infection with diseases like hepatitis. These conditions may be transferred from one patient to another through improperly cleaned sigmoidoscopes. But so long as you choose an expert to do the test, your risks of such problems are minimal.

WHAT TO DO: Don't hesitate to undergo a flexible sigmoidoscope exam if blood is found in your stool, you're at high risk for colon or rectal cancer (see p. 137), or you're 50 or older.

But before you have the test, be assertive in checking the experience of your physician. If your family doctor or internist has done the minimum fifty procedures with the instrument being used, then I would recommend that you stick with her. If your doctor has less experience than this or if you've had previous problems with polyps or other gastrointestinal disease, then you should have the test performed by a gastroenterologist.

There's no need to have a colonoscopy or barium enema unless your risk of having colon or rectal cancer is high or you have clear symptoms of possible disease of the large intestine. For the best results, any colonoscopy should be done by a gastroenterologist who has performed at least 150 procedures and who is approved by your primary care physician.

ERROR:

Your Doctor Omits the Rectal Exam as a Screening Procedure for Prostate Cancer

Andy, who was in his late fifties, was in the habit of going in every year or so for a regular medical checkup with his family doctor, an old friend with whom he socialized. The doctor always conducted a blood test, checked Andy's blood pressure, listened to his heart with a stethoscope, and thumped here and there on his chest and back.

But the physician never conducted or even suggested a rectal examination, which would have involved the insertion of a gloved finger, and Andy was relieved that the subject never came up. He knew that other doctors performed this procedure, but he suspected it wasn't very important and he thought it certainly would be uncomfortable, if not painful.

Two years later, the force of Andy's stream of urine decreased noticeably, and when he mentioned this problem to his doctor, a visit was scheduled with a urologist, a specialist in matters of the urinary and genital area. He was found to have cancer of the prostate, the nutlike male gland that lies just behind the outlet for the urinary bladder.

FACTS: Prostate cancer is a nightmare for health care administrators who are trying to limit medical costs since the number of potential prostate cases may turn out to be staggering. At least 40 percent of all men, and possibly more, develop cancer cells in their prostate if they live long enough. Furthermore, advanced cases of this cancer can kill, though often the disease tends to be slow moving and may not become lethal before a man dies of some other cause. We are not sure whether early detection and treatment of prostate cancer actually saves many lives. However, most (but not all) experts believe that the more effective we can be in screening for early prostate cancer, the more likely it is that an epidemic of this disease can be contained as our population grows older.

The old-fashioned way to detect prostate cancer is for the doctor to put on a glove, ask the patient to bend over, and then insert a gloved finger into the rectum. The doctor then feels for hardness or lumps in the prostate, which can be detected through this procedure. This approach is still the mainstay of early discovery of prostate problems.

This test isn't comfortable for the patients and isn't particularly appealing for the doctor either. Typically, neither looks forward to it. But if you're a man over 40, the rectal exam *must* be done, and the older you get, the more important the test becomes.

It's best to schedule your prostate exam as an integral part of an overall checkup or even as part of a special visit for planning your long-term prostate cancer screening strategy. On the other hand, I recommend against trying to slip this exam in quickly, say, at the end of an exam for another problem. A cursory evaluation could cause the doctor to miss an important diagnosis.

Many patients assume that you really don't have to worry too much about the prostate until certain symptoms begin to appear. And it is true that in the later stages of a prostate problem, there may be rectal or low-back pain or symptoms of prostate enlargement, such as slow urination, frequency of urinating in small amounts, or dribbling of urine. But there are usually no early symptoms for prostate cancer—and it's early detection that you want if you hope for the best odds of receiving treatment.

WHAT TO DO: When you, as a man, reach age 40, schedule a visit with your primary care physician to check your prostate and to establish a plan for prevention of the disease. You should expect to have the rectal finger exam every year. Also, go over the possible signs and symptoms of possible prostate cancer with your doctor and be sure you understand them. In addition, you and your doctor should discuss your being checked with the sensitive prostate specific antigen (PSA) blood test. (See the following error.)

ERROR:

You Aren't Given a PSA Blood Test to Check for Prostate Cancer

Pierre, a 55-year-old carpenter, was given a rectal examination by his doctor as part of the screening procedures for prostate cancer. But he was not offered a PSA blood test because, the doctor said, "Those blood tests are wrong too often. I can pick up anything serious with the rectal."

Was Pierre's doctor right?

FACTS: No, Pierre should have had the PSA. This blood test can often detect prostate cancer *before* it can be felt on a physical exam. But it is true that the test can sometimes be misleading or mistaken.

A very high PSA result—more than 10 on the scale—means the risk of cancer is high and usually requires referral to a urologist for ultrasound imaging and a biopsy. But when the reading is in the lower abnormal range, say, 4 to 9 on the blood test scale, the result may indicate either prostate cancer or an entirely different condition known as *benign prostatic hypertrophy*, or BPH. This is the noncancerous enlargement of the prostate that affects most men over 50 to one extent or another.

With readings in this range, a doctor may tell you to wait three or four months and then repeat the PSA. Or she may refer you to a urologist for further tests. An abnormal PSA should always be repeated just to be certain that a gross lab error hasn't occurred.

WHAT TO DO: Do undergo a PSA test. A normal test (0–4) is reassuring, but you should be aware that men with localized prostate cancer can often have a normal PSA; so your doctor should still pay attention to any lump felt on your prostate when she examines with a gloved finger.

An abnormal test might mean prostate cancer, but don't panic. Most of the PSA elevations in the 4–9 range are due to benign prostatic enlargement (hypertrophy—BPH) or prostate infection (prostatitis), both noncancerous conditions.

What to do about a moderately elevated PSA depends in part on your and your doctor's tolerance for living with uncertainty. If the PSA abnormality is slight and its level does not rise on repeated measurements, "watchful waiting" may be an option. Even so, I strongly recommend that a urologist participate in the process, since a urologist will have more experience with this problem than will your family physician or internist. This advantage, I believe, outweighs the specialist's inherent bias toward action and higher costs, especially in a fee-for-service payment system.

If the PSA level is above 10 or is lower but increasing, then further testing by a urologist is mandatory, including an ultrasound examination of the prostate and biopsies of the prostate (a relatively simple procedure done in the office).

ERROR:

You Are a Smoker, and Your Doctor Fails to Recommend a Chest X Ray During Your Regular Checkup

Larry, who had been smoking a pack of cigarettes a day for years, read an article about some controversy over whether or not a smoker should have a regular chest X ray. He called his doctor to ask for advice but was told, "X rays are not routine these days. Several scientific studies say they aren't necessary."

Was the doctor right or wrong?

FACTS: When I first started practicing medicine, most patients and all smokers were given a chest X ray routinely along with their annual physical. As Larry's doctor correctly indicated, the practice is no longer routine—even for smokers—because several large studies have shown that finding lung cancer earlier by X ray or by cytology (a kind of Pap smear of phlegm coughed up from the lung) doesn't improve the average patient's chances for survival.

On the other hand, other experts—and I'm personally sympathetic to this group—argue that you are an individual, not a statistic. Most doctors can point to at least one or two patients (usually smokers—John Wayne was one) who appear to have been cured of lung cancer after the problem was picked up on a routine X ray.

A side benefit of undergoing this procedure: An X ray can often be a powerful motivation to get smokers to quit their habit.

WHAT TO DO: If you are at high risk for lung cancer due to a smoking habit, asbestos exposure, or some other factor, you might possibly improve your odds of surviving lung cancer by detecting it earlier with an annual chest X ray or cytology exam.

Are these simple exams worth the cost? Or in the lingo of the economist, are they cost-effective? That depends on your point of view. From society's viewpoint, the answer is no because statistically speaking, the cost will be high, and the benefits, low. But if you're a potential lung cancer victim who is at high risk, you might possibly be saved by detecting a cancer early. In such circumstances, it may be well worth your time and money to obtain extraordinary medical screening.

ERROR:

You Are a Smoker, but Your Doctor Never Hassles You About Your Habit

Eric, a regular cigarette smoker, had received a mild reprimand from his doctor several years ago for his habit. But the doctor never brought the subject up again, and Eric was grateful. He had already decided that if the doctor nagged him, he would switch to another physician.

FACTS: Eric's doctor was lax in his professional responsibilities. Physicians often assume, erroneously, that patients who smoke won't stop smoking if the physician recommends they quit. Also, they worry that the patient will be offended if they keep bringing it up. So they let the subject slide by.

In fact, most cigarette smokers have mixed feelings about their habit. Many studies show that about 5 percent of smokers are so close to the edge of giving it up that just a request from their physician is enough to trigger a serious effort to stop.

WHAT TO DO: If you're a smoker, bring up the subject with your doctor. She's there to protect your health, and sometimes that means making you uncomfortable. After all, you're not paying her to tell you only what you want to hear! Your doctor may be reluctant to initiate this potentially sensitive subject, but she should be helpful if you ask for advice.

Another reason for asking her advice is that she has access to information that can make it less painful for you to quit. One thing she should tell you about is how nicotine patches and gum can ease any withdrawal symptoms. Other medicines and techniques, including hypnosis, may also be helpful.

But the average doctor is often limited in being able to deal effectively with habitual behaviors that trigger an urge for a cigarette. Also, she sometimes lacks the background to help you develop alternative stress management skills and weight control strategies once you try to give up the habit. For this sort of help, I frequently recommend that my patients get involved in support programs like these:

- Freedom from Smoking, a twenty-day, do-it-yourself program sponsored by the American Lung Association, 1740 Broadway, New York, NY 10019.

- Quit Smoking Clinics, sponsored by local chapters of the American Cancer Society. Check your local phone book, or call or write to the American Cancer Society, 1599 Clifton Road, Atlanta, GA 30329, phone 1-800-ACS-2345 or 1-404-329-7629.

- SmokEnders, a commercial eight-week course that's available in different parts of the country. Call their Philadelphia headquarters at 1-215-332-8813.

ERROR:

Your Regular Medical Exam Doesn't Include a Systematic Viewing of All Your Skin Surfaces

Arlene, a fair-skinned woman who was in her early thirties, disliked going in for a checkup by her doctor, who was male, because she felt uncomfortable being partially undressed in his presence. Although he was completely businesslike and always had a nurse present when he was examining a woman, he sensed her discomfort. As a result, he did all he could to keep most of her body covered and still perform an adequate checkup.

One day midway between checkups, Arlene noticed an irregular, reddish mole on her hip. Although she had many moles on her body, this one looked so different that she thought it might not be a mole at all. She suspected it might be a scratch or a bruise. But after a few weeks, when it didn't go away, she contacted her physician. The mole turned out to be a deadly skin cancer, a malignant melanoma.

FACTS: With all the things to do when you're at your doctor's office, one exam that's often forgotten or given short shrift is the close, systematic viewing of the skin. A good dermatologist will always follow this procedure—and not a few have been suspected of being "dirty old men" because of the practice.

Family physicians and internists often neglect this part of the exam because of the very situation faced by Arlene and her doctor: The patient feels uncomfortable, and the doctor doesn't want to be misunderstood or criticized. Consequently, this all-important part of the physical may be omitted—and a malignant melanoma may be overlooked.

I remember back in the 1970s when a physician colleague informed me that a mutual acquaintance had been diagnosed with malignant melanoma. We shook our heads sadly, because in those days, the diagnosis was roughly equivalent to a death sentence. Today, enormous progress has been made in melanoma treatment, in part because both doctors and patients have educated themselves to recognize melanoma at its earliest stages, when there's still time for a cure. The bad news is that melanoma frequency has increased dramatically—actually tripling over the last forty years. It's the number one cancer among white Americans in their late twenties.

Most early melanomas are first noticed by people who bring their concern to the attention of their physician. Unfortunately, however, too many patients wait too long, in part because their physicians don't check them thoroughly enough or don't instruct them in what to look for in their own self-exams.

One study found that melanoma patients waited an average of sixteen and a half months before notifying their doctors after noticing a change in the size or color of a mole. They even waited an average of six months after noticing that a mole was growing in height, and they waited four months if the mole became ulcerated or tender or started to itch! When bleeding occurred, patients tended to react more quickly, but bleeding melanomas are already likely to have reached an advanced stage of malignancy.

How can you recognize a malignant melanoma at an early stage? Physicians have a useful mnemonic device to help them remember what to look for—the acronym ABCD:

A—Asymmetry. Melanoma moles are usually not perfectly round.
B—Irregular borders. The outline of a melanoma is usually notched, scalloped, or blurred, not smooth.
C—Color. Melanomas are often moles with two or more colors. Black or blue moles are especially alarming, but shades of brown, red (as Arlene had), tan, or white are also significant.
D—Diameter, which is often greater than 6 millimeters (about one-fourth of an inch). Early melanomas can be smaller than this, however.

WHAT TO DO: Schedule a visit for cancer detection that includes completely disrobing for an inspection of your entire skin surface. If you feel uncomfortable with a physician of the opposite sex, choose your physician accordingly.

If you are at high risk for melanoma, this exam should be done by a skin specialist, a dermatologist. Characteristics that put you at high risk include being very fair skinned, having a family or personal history of melanoma, having been sunburned frequently, or having many freckles or moles on your body. If you don't have any of these risk factors, the exam may be conducted by your family physician.

You should also conduct your own self-examination for melanoma at least once a month. If you have trouble seeing certain parts of your body, ask somebody else to check you in those places. Any skin mole or freckle that changes in size, regularity, shape, or color or becomes itchy or tender should be examined by your doctor.

If you or your doctor have any questions about a mole or spot, it's best to go directly to a dermatologist. I see many skin lesions that don't look typical of melanoma but do appear to be odd in various ways. Because some melanoma spots don't look typically abnormal, I refer most of these cases to the dermatologist for a second look.

So far, none of these has been cancer, and perhaps I'm being too cautious. Still, despite reading many articles and looking at numerous pictures of early melanoma, I don't feel confident in evaluating some unusual freckles or moles. Even dermatologists, who are experts in this subject, can have difficulty making a decision.

If there's any doubt at all, it's usually best to obtain a skin biopsy, a simple procedure that any dermatologist, surgeon, or even some family physicians can perform in the office. When melanoma is a likely possibility, the doctor will probably do a complete excision of the blemish, with a narrow margin of normal-appearing skin being removed as well. In other cases, she'll do a simple punch biopsy by extracting a small portion of tissue from the middle of the mole.

Treatment of Cancer

You Are Being Treated for Cancer, and Your Doctor Fails to Refer You to an Oncologist

Charlie was diagnosed as having prostate cancer and underwent surgery by a urologist, a specialist in diseases of the urinary and genital area. After the operation, he continued to go to the urologist.

Charlie was never referred to an oncologist (a cancer specialist) either before or after the operation. After the operation, he discovered that he was impotent.

FACTS: Although your urologist may be highly skilled at treating your prostate cancer surgically, he may or may not give equal consideration to nonsurgical alternatives, such as radiation. In Charlie's case, radiation might have been a better alternative in that the cancer might have been controlled and his sexual potency might have been maintained.

About 30 percent of cancer patients never see an oncologist, and with a very few exceptions, this is almost always a mistake. With a serious health condition that can be treated in more than one way, you need a complete picture of the full range of possibilities. If you only see a surgeon, you'll usually get a prosurgery recommendation. If you see a radiotherapist, you'll most likely receive a proradiation recommendation. With cancer, an oncologist can help you sort through the options and make the best decision.

Charlie's operation for prostate cancer took place a few years ago. Today, many urologists have been trained in a new operative technique for removing the prostate called potency-sparing surgery. Although impotence remains a complication for a minority of patients, its rate is much reduced from that of traditional prostate surgery. Unfortunately, all urologists are not well trained in the new surgical method, especially many older urologists, who are years past their residency training. So, if prostate surgery is being considered, critically important facts to find out are whether your urologist uses the newer potency-sparing method, how many cases he has done, and what proportion of his cases have had complications such as impotence.

WHAT TO DO: If you are found to have cancer, always consult an oncologist early on, preferably before any aspect of treatment is decided. This advice holds whether the actual treatment is done by your personal physician, a radiotherapist, a surgeon, or some other specialist.

Does it matter where your oncologist practices or what his hospital affiliation is? For simple cancer cases, which have an excellent prognosis of cure, such as very localized breast cancer, an oncologist associated with a local community hospital will usually be just fine. On the other hand, with very serious or complicated cases, you should at least seek a second opinion from an expert at a larger regional cancer facility. (For a reference to one of the regional centers in your area, call the National Cancer Institute hot line, 1-800-4-CANCER.)

This second opinion should not be done behind the back of your local oncologist, but, rather, should be shared with your local specialist. If the local facility lacks the technology or expertise to treat you adequately, then you'll have to make regular trips to a better-equipped regional center for your treatment. But it's not at all unusual for a regional cancer center's recommendations to be implemented or monitored by a local community oncologist.

In the case of prostate cancer, how can you tell if your urologist has mastered the techniques of potency-sparing surgery? One option: ask him. Where did he train in the technique and for how long? How many supervised cases did he do in training, how many has he done since? What is his success rate? A respected local oncologist who works with prostate cancer patients should be in a position to know which urologists in your community have an excellent track record.

Key Questions to Ask
When You Are First Diagnosed with Cancer

1. Is there any doubt at all about the diagnosis of cancer or the type of cancer I have? Is this a type of cancer which is at all likely to be confused with any other? No diagnosis is certain without examining a piece of cancerous tissue under the microscope. Even then, the diagnosis might not be clear-cut.

2. What kind of cancer do I have? What specific subtype, aggressiveness, and stage? Thus, cancer of the lung is not enough. There are specific types (e.g., adenocarcinoma and squamous cell), degree of malignancy, and stages of spread. If there's any doubt about the biopsy report, tissue specimens should be submitted for review to a leading national center such as the armed forces Institute of Pathology.

3. Were any special tests done on the tumor? For example, breast cancers should be tested for the presence or absence of receptor sites for the hormones estrogen and progesterone.

4. Do I need further diagnostic testing before obtaining a recommendation for treatment? Further tests may be needed to determine whether your tumor is localized or has spread or whether you are likely to respond to a particular treatment.

5. What are *all* my treatment options including surgery, radiotherapy, and/or chemotherapy? Which do you recommend for me and why? Is the choice clear-cut or do different alternatives have some advantages? Is thinking among cancer specialists fairly uniform or is there controversy as to which approach is best?

6. What is my likely prognosis (survival and quality of life) without treatment? And with the recommended treatment? What are the risks of the treatment? How serious and frequent are they?

7. Should I obtain another opinion before making a decision? Should my second opinion or treatment be at a regional cancer center? A second opinion is almost always advisable. An opinion from a regional center is especially important if your tumor is rare or has a poor prognosis; when the regional cancer center is likely to recommend a different approach than is done locally; or if the treatment is new, difficult, experimental, or requiring especially sophisticated equipment.

ERROR:

You Are Scheduled for Breast Surgery and Your Doctor Offers You a Mastectomy Rather Than a Lumpectomy

Lois, a Texas resident, was diagnosed as having breast cancer, which involved a small malignant tumor in her right breast. The doctor scheduled her for a mastectomy (removal of the entire breast), and she underwent the operation. But several weeks after the operation she was talking with other women who had had breast cancer, including a friend who had been operated on in Pennsylvania for what seemed like the same type of tumor. This woman had received a lumpectomy, or the removal only of the portion of the breast that contained the malignancy.

When Lois asked her doctor about this difference in surgical procedures, he told her that it was always better to be sure you get all the cancer by taking off the entire breast.

Was he right?

FACTS: You know something is amiss on the breast cancer surgery scene when you hear a report like this: In the mid-1980s, breast cancer victims in New York, Pennsylvania, and Massachusetts were more than three times as likely to have surgery that preserved the breast (a lumpectomy) than were women in Texas, Wisconsin, Georgia, and Virginia. Even within a single city according to some studies, educated and affluent women are more likely to receive breast-conserving surgery than a complete mastectomy. In short, there has been little consistency in the way that doctors approach surgery for many breast cancers. Often, it's only *after* the operation that women patients learn that they might have had an option.

To try to resolve this issue, the National Cancer Institute convened a consensus conference of cancer experts in 1990. Their conclusion was that lumpectomy is as effective in saving lives as is a full mastectomy for most women with early breast cancer.

Furthermore, if the odds of survival are roughly equal, most women prefer to preserve their breast with a lumpectomy. A few with early cancer do still choose mastectomy, usually for one of these two basic reasons:

1. Some are unwilling or unable to take the six or seven weeks of radiation treatment that is routinely given after lumpectomy

surgery. (This regimen of radiation isn't usually required for a mastectomy.)

2. Some believe they will feel safer from cancer in the future if their entire breast has been removed. They are willing to give up the breast to achieve that sense of security.

WHAT TO DO: If you learn that you have breast cancer, one of the first things you should discuss with your doctor is the option of a mastectomy (removal of the entire breast) versus lumpectomy (removal only of the malignant tissue) plus radiation. If your surgeon indicates that he rarely does a lumpectomy, even for early tumors, seek a second opinion.

An important danger area involves special technology and testing procedures that can threaten to take the surgery decision away from you. The problem can emerge this way: When you go in for the biopsy of the suspected cancer, you may be placed under general anesthesia. *Before* this biopsy, of course, you won't know for sure whether you even have cancer. The surgeon will do the biopsy and, thanks to a speedy *frozen section* report on the suspect tissue, he will learn almost immediately whether you have cancer. But you won't be able to discuss the matter with him because you're still asleep on the operating table. So, depending on the amount of discretion you've given him in advance, he may go ahead with the operation. When you wake up, you may find not only that you had cancer, but also that you're missing a breast! Even if you are awake during the biopsy, that's not the best time to make your decision about what to do next.

Obviously, it's *essential* for you to discuss in advance with your doctor what he should do if he finds cancer. If you're not sure what you'll want to do, tell him you want to delay any operation until you've had a chance to discuss your options further in light of the facts.

If you choose a lumpectomy rather than a mastectomy, you should be sure that your physician has confirmed with the pathologist that no tumor at all has been found at the edges of the tissue that is to be taken out from your breast. The reason this information is important is that perhaps 10 percent of women with breast cancer have a microscopic unsuspected tumor at the margin of the lump to be removed. Because this can't be detected at the time of surgery, this 10 percent needs a second operation to take out all of the malignancy.

In difficult cases, it's not unusual for a hospital pathologist to send slides from a biopsy for a second opinion from a cancer pathology specialist at a cancer referral center. The pathologist's judgment is critical because the choice of cancer treatments depends on such factors as the exact type of cancer and the degree of the malignancy. So for every cancer biopsy, you should absolutely insist that your surgeon or your oncologist personally discuss the details of your biopsy slides with the hospital pathologist to be sure that she is absolutely secure in her diagnosis.

E R R O R :

Your Doctor Fails to Recommend Radiation Treatment After a Lumpectomy

After a lumpectomy, which was done in a small community hospital in the Midwest, Isabel's doctor said, "We got it all! Now you can go home and not worry about cancer of the breast anymore!"

Two years later, cancer appeared again in the breast, and Isabel had to undergo a mastectomy.

What did the doctor overlook?

FACTS: Current research indicates that women who receive radiation treatment after a lumpectomy are more likely to be disease-free after five years than are women who receive a lumpectomy alone. One study found a 16 percent relapse rate with radiation versus a 26 percent relapse rate without radiation.

As with other aspects of treatment of breast cancer, there is a wide variation in approaches throughout the country. One recent survey, for instance, indicated that about 15 percent of the women participants didn't receive radiotherapy after a lumpectomy.

WHAT TO DO: As a patient, you must recognize that radiotherapy, although no guarantee, does improve cancer-free survival after a lumpectomy. Consequently it should be done routinely after a lumpectomy unless there is a strong reason not to use it. Some reasons not to do radiotherapy are that the patient is very old or quite frail, conditions where radiation could greatly increase the risk of serious health consequences. But for the average woman of any age who is in relatively good health, combining a lumpectomy with radiotherapy is a must.

ERROR:

Your Doctor Does Not Offer You the Option of Preventive Chemotherapy After Breast Surgery

Marge had cancer, a malignant tumor about 2 centimeters (1 inch) in diameter, which was localized in her breast. There was no evidence of cancer in the lymph nodes of the armpit or elsewhere. She underwent a lumpectomy plus radiation for six to seven weeks, and her doctor pronounced her cured. He didn't recommend or even discuss any other possible treatment. But three years later, evidence of a recurring malignancy appeared.

Did the doctor overlook something?

FACTS: The absence of tumor involvement in the lymph nodes of the armpit (axilla) is a very encouraging sign for women with breast cancer. But even for those whose malignancy is apparently localized and has been treated properly with a lumpectomy or mastectomy, significant relapse rates do occur. In fact, for some of these patients, the relapse rates can be as high as 30 percent at five years after the operation and 40 percent at the ten-year point.

After a review of the evidence, the National Institutes of Health Consensus Conference concluded that the rate of recurrence of breast cancer can be decreased by a course of chemotherapy that is done after the initial breast cancer operation. The typical course of such chemotherapy would take six months.

But there's another side to this story. In fact, the majority of women with localized cancers will be cured by mastectomy *without* chemotherapy or by lumpectomy plus radiotherapy. Also, chemotherapy is often uncomfortable and sometimes causes uncomfortable or dangerous side effects, such as loss of hair, nausea, or serious infections. So routine chemotherapy shouldn't be chosen by every patient.

Here are some guidelines. About 25 percent of women with breast cancer have characteristics that predict such an excellent outlook that routine preventive chemotherapy should *not* be recommended automatically. These include the following:

- Breast cancers involving tumors that are smaller than 1 centimeter (about 0.5 inch). Marge's tumor was larger than this, and so she might have been a candidate for chemotherapy.

- Cancers where the microscopic examination of the tumor shows certain specific tumor subtypes, such as *ductal carcinoma in situ, pure tubular carcinoma,* or *papillary carcinoma.* If your tumor doesn't fall into any of these categories, you may be a candidate for chemotherapy.

On the other hand, chemotherapy is usually a better choice for women whose tumors were very large before surgery (more than 2 centimeters, or about 1 inch, in diameter). Women with these large malignancies have a high relapse rate: Cancer appears again after surgery in nearly 50 percent of them. For those who have smaller tumors or are otherwise at intermediate risk, chemotherapy is a judgment call by physician and patient.

Of course, these are only guidelines, to which there may be exceptions. Other factors that affect the choice of treatment include the microscopic appearance of the tumor, the presence or absence of certain genetic markers, and the general health and preferences of the patient.

WHAT TO DO: In a case like Marge's, where the chemotherapy issue isn't clear, the pros and cons of the treatment should at least be discussed with the patient. That's the main mistake that her doctor seems to have made.

If your main cancer physician has been a surgeon, be sure to ask for a referral to a chemotherapy expert, that is, a medical oncologist. Keep in mind that the benefits of treatment are likely to be lessened if you are old or if you suffer from other diseases.

Also, ask the oncologist for the latest update about what has been learned about the relative relapse risk for patients whose condition resembles yours. This way, you'll at least have an idea about the current odds of your getting cancer at a later date.

Finally, ask your oncologist about the results of the microscopic examination of your cancer. She will undoubtedly have evaluated those results thoroughly, but because of the volume of cases many of these doctors handle, it's wise to pose a question or two that will cause her to focus specifically on your test results. With all this information at your disposal, you'll be able to have significant input into a decision about chemotherapy.

ERROR:

Your Doctor Doesn't Measure Estrogen Hormone Receptors on Malignant Breast Tissue

Allison, who was in her midfifties, had been diagnosed as having localized breast cancer and underwent a lumpectomy plus radiation for seven weeks after the operation. After the radiation, her doctor recommended chemotherapy, and she went through the entire course of treatment even though she experienced a number of uncomfortable side effects, such as hair loss and nausea. She also developed several potentially serious infections because of the suppression of her white blood cells.

Was there a less oppressive alternative to the chemotherapy?

FACTS: There may indeed have been a better postoperative treatment option for Allison: hormone therapy with tamoxifen (Nolvadex), a drug that blocks the effects of the female hormone estrogen. Tamoxifen can be taken by mouth and is much less toxic than standard chemotherapy. This drug appears to reduce the rate of cancer recurrence by about one-fourth to one-third among women like Allison, who have localized breast cancer (that is, their axillary lymph nodes, located in the armpit, are normal). Usually, tamoxifen is administered for a period of two to five years.

To determine whether or not the tamoxifen treatment will work, however, the woman's tumors should be analyzed to see if they carry receptors for estrogen. (Also, a test is done to see if the tumor has receptors for progesterone, another hormone secreted by the ovaries.) One recent study found that between 4 and 14 percent of all breast cancer samples—and Allison's samples were in this category—had not been tested for the presence of estrogen receptors. Consequently, these women had no chance to benefit from tamoxifen treatment.

There are some potential negative side effects to tamoxifen. These include menopauselike hot flashes, menstrual abnormalities, and increased appetite. Also, concern has been raised about this drug raising the risk of osteoporosis and increased rates of cancer of the uterus. But when compared with traditional chemotherapy, tamoxifen is an attractive alternative for most women.

Actually, many oncologists have recently begun to offer tamoxifen to women whose estrogen receptors are negative—especially for women, like Allison, who are already past menopause. Tamoxifen may even have a breast-cancer prevention effect. The National Cancer Institute is now involved with a very large study in which women who are at high risk for developing breast cancer will take the drug over a period of years. You can ask your doctor about the current status of this study, or call 1-800-4-CANCER.

WHAT TO DO: If you have localized breast cancer, as Allison did, you should discuss tamoxifen with your doctor. Most experts feel that the majority of women with positive estrogen receptors on a tumor should be on tamoxifen for at least the first two years after surgery. Tamoxifen may also be given for postmenopausal women with estrogen-receptor-negative tumors. But there's not yet enough information available to decide whether or not tamoxifen can help premenopausal women if the estrogen receptor markers tested negative.

ERROR:

You Are Diagnosed with Prostate Cancer, and Your Doctor Immediately Recommends Surgery Without Exploring the Possibility of Radiation Therapy

After being diagnosed with localized prostate cancer, Jim was referred by his doctor to a urologist, who was an expert in surgery of the urinary area. Surgery was scheduled, and Jim's prostate was removed. As far as Jim could remember, no mention was ever made of any other treatment, such as radiation therapy.

Should Jim have been presented with another option?

FACTS: Most studies suggest that for localized prostate cancer of the type Jim had, the chances of long-term survival are roughly the same for surgery as for radiotherapy treatment. There are pros and cons to both approaches, and every patient should be made aware of these before a decision is made.

Serious complications tend to be less frequent after radiotherapy, though diarrhea, rectal scarring, bladder inflammation, and impotence may occur. Also, many patients who have been treated with radiotherapy do continue to harbor cancer cells in their prostates. It remains unclear whether or not those remaining malignant cells greatly increase the average patient's risk of developing cancer again later.

As for surgery, recent advances in techniques have greatly decreased the chances for impotence, but the outlook for this problem is still far from perfect. Generally, surgery appears to continue to present more problems with impotence than does radiation. But surgical treatment of the prostate does have the advantage of allowing the surgeon to check nearby lymph nodes to see if the cancer has spread. So surgery is more likely than radiation to get rid of all remaining malignant cells.

A third option has been gaining popularity as the new PSA blood test brings to light literally millions of new prostate cancer cases in apparently healthy men. This option involves just watching and waiting. Among men age 75 and older, in particular, there is an excellent argument that doing nothing is often the best approach. Those in this age range whose biopsy slides show localized, low-grade malignancy may experience no symptoms at all for ten or more years.

WHAT TO DO: If you are diagnosed as having prostate cancer, you should consult with three experts: a urologist, who will be a specialist in surgery; a radiotherapist, who will probably lean heavily toward radiation therapy; and an oncologist, a cancer specialist who can act as a referee between the other two.

The oncologist's recommendation may be influenced by the qualifications and skills of the local urologist or radiotherapist. He may also take into consideration your own willingness to have your treatment done at a center away from your home.

An oncologist will also be in the best position to apprise you of other treatment possibilities that may have become available. For example, the oncologist should know which of the urologists in your community have obtained solid training and skill in the new potency-sparing technique of prostate surgery. This approach leaves a much smaller proportion of patients suffering from postoperative impotence than does traditional surgery.

Of course, it's impossible without my knowing you and your specific health situation to say definitely that you should undergo surgery, radiation, or some other procedure. But I can say with certainty that you should explore all the possible options in depth with each of these three experts before you make your final decision.

| ERROR: |

Your Doctor Fails to Treat Advanced, Spreading Prostate Cancer Aggressively Enough

Having neglected undergoing a general health exam for several years, Todd, who was in his early sixties, scheduled an appointment with his doctor. He was particularly concerned because the force of his urine stream had declined significantly in the past couple of years. Also, he was experiencing pain in his rectal area.

A rectal exam revealed an extremely enlarged prostate, and a biopsy confirmed that the gland was malignant. Further tests showed that the cancer had spread to surrounding tissue and bone.

Surgery was performed, but it was clear that the cancer had spread beyond the prostate. After surgery, Todd's doctor prescribed relatively low doses of a painkiller, in part because he said he didn't want Todd to get "hooked" just yet on any medication. Also, he limited the treatment doses that suppress the male hormones because they triggered a loss of potency and an increase of certain feminizing traits, such as decline in muscle mass, which bothered Todd.

Were the doctor's decisions appropriate?

FACTS: I believe in treating any cancer patient, including those with prostate cancer, more aggressively than did Todd's doctor. This means that I would have considered (1) more powerful male hormone-suppressing treatments and (2) larger doses of painkillers.

Most prostate cancers decrease in size when male hormones are suppressed. In the past, this meant castration or treatment with estrogen, the female hormone. Today, there is a much wider variety of means to suppress male hormones during prostate therapy, and the feeling among oncologists is that *multiple* male hormone-suppressing measures can prolong prostate cancer survival. During this sort of therapy, blood testosterone levels have to be checked to be sure that the medicines are actually being taken and that maximal hormonal response has been achieved.

Note: In general, prostate cancers that don't respond to hormone treatments won't improve with standard chemotherapy.

When the cancer has spread, or *metastasized*, to bone, pain may result, as happened in Todd's situation. In such a case, aggressive radiation therapy can be effective in preventing fractured bones and can help relieve any pain. Also, narcotic painkillers, such as morphine, can be extremely useful, and shouldn't be withheld from a patient just because the doctor doesn't want to hook him on a drug.

WHAT TO DO: If you have advanced prostate cancer and you've been under the care of a urologist, you should be sure to consult with an oncologist as well just to be sure that you understand all your options.

Although a cure may not be possible, pain relief should be within reach through radiotherapy and aggressive pain medication. Also, there may be an excellent chance that you can prolong your life significantly by having multiple male hormone-suppressing therapies.

ERROR:

Your Doctor Fails to Refer Aggressive Lymphoma and Hodgkin's Disease to a Specialized Cancer Center

A diagnosis of early-stage Hodgkin's disease (cancer of the lymph nodes and glands) was made when Ron went in for a medical checkup. His doctor decided to treat the cancer at the local hospital. The course of the disease went on virtually unchecked, and although he was eventually transferred to a specialized cancer center, Ron died about a year and a half later.

Should Ron have received the specialized treatment at an earlier date?

FACTS: The ability to cure early-stage malignant tumors involved in lymphoma and Hodgkin's disease is still heavily dependent on the quality of the radiation therapy equipment and on the experience and skill of the radiotherapist. However, contrary to the situation twenty years ago, excellent equipment and skilled specialists are now available in many community hospitals. The latest treatments are no longer restricted to medical school–based hospitals or to nationally known cancer centers such as M. D. Anderson in Houston or Memorial Sloan-Kettering in New York.

Leukemia is another form of cancer for which initial treatment methods are well standardized and can be administered capably by an excellent local oncologist.

Unfortunately, standards of care do vary—not only among different community hospitals but also among academic centers. Some academic specialists argue that community-based oncologists are often reluctant to use the most effective high doses of chemotherapy drugs for fear of causing side effects. These experts also question whether local radiotherapy units have the technical sophistication and experience to give optimal treatment for less common tumors such as Hodgkin's disease.

Community oncologists, on the other hand, argue that local care is often superior to that at academic centers with respect to better quality nursing, the individual attention your doctor can give you, and the ease and frequency of follow-up care.

So, the challenge you face if you have a new onset lymphoma, Hodgkin's disease, or leukemia is to evaluate the advantages and disadvantages of your local oncologists and their hospital versus those at a regional referral center for cancer.

If your lymphoma, Hodgkin's disease, or leukemia is especially aggressive, of a rare type, relapsed, or not responsive to standard therapy, then the odds shift to favor the regional cancer center. Regional cancer centers typically have more experience with difficult cases. Their doctors' expertise is more highly specialized (for example, you might see an oncologist whose practice is limited to only lymphoma), and they are more likely to use advanced or experimental treatments that are not available at the community hospital.

How do you decide whether you should stay in the community or be referred to a regional cancer center? And if you have a choice of several centers, how can you choose among them?

Your most effective ally in making these key decisions has to be your oncologist. But you will certainly want to confirm his recommendations with a second or even a third consultation, at least one of which should be from a regional cancer center.

If chemotherapy is planned, then your local oncologist has a professional and financial stake in keeping you under his care. (He probably does not have this conflict of interest if radiotherapy is the choice.) However, almost every oncologist takes tremendous professional pride in acting, first and foremost, in his patient's best interest. Like most of us, oncologists might make a biased judgment about their own professional capabilities compared to that of their "competitors." Still, you should usually assume that their opinions are ethical and honest and are offered with your best interests at heart.

Of course, you should definitely ask questions to test the oncologist's opinion. For example: If it were your mother, wife, or son in my situation, which treatment would you recommend and where would you have it done? How many tumors of this type and stage have you actually treated in the last year? Is there any doubt at all about the exact diagnosis? Could this type of cancer ever be confused with a different type? Should the biopsy slides be reviewed by an outside pathologist?

There are also several independent quality checks. One clue that your community hospital is up-to-date is its participation in the Community Clinical Oncology Program (CCOP). This network, in association with the National Cancer Institute, offers patients participation in clinical trials that test new or experimental cancer treatments.

You can locate a regional cancer center by calling 1-800-4-CANCER. Sponsored by the National Cancer Institute (but usually based at a regional referral center), the non-physician advisers at this telephone number can provide detailed information about your specific kind of tumor, its prognosis, and the track record for standard treatments. They can also provide a list of regional cancer centers in your area and the names of individual physicians who are doing research or offering experimental treatments that might be relevant to your needs. However, as you can appreciate, they cannot recommend over the phone what you should do.

WHAT TO DO: If you have early-stage lymphoma, Hodgkin's, or leukemia, first discuss the advantages and disadvantages of each treatment alternative with your local oncologist. Ask specifically whether she feels that the treatments that would be recommended at a regional center would be the same or different from what she would recommend locally and whether the regional center provides any advantage for your particular type and stage of tumor. Be ready to accept a recommendation to stay with the local facility if your lymphoma, Hodgkin's, or leukemia is in an early stage, not too aggressive, and of a type that your oncologist commonly treats. Be ready to decline local treatment if your tumor is relapsed, not responding to treatment, in an advanced stage, aggressive, or of a type not often encountered locally.

With serious disease, always get a second consultation, usually at a regional medical center. (Ask your oncologist which of the regional cancer centers and which specific doctors are most highly skilled in your type of tumor.) You can expect that the regional cancer center doctors, like your local oncologist, will provide their honest opinions—although you must take into account their standard bias that what they do at the "Mecca" is usually superior.

If opinions conflict, discuss each consultant's opinion with the others and ask them to talk to each other directly about your case. Remember, unlike car salesmen, whom you expect to be "selling," physicians, by and large, take very seriously their responsibility to act in your best interest, not in their own. The several physicians you consult should not be reluctant to work together to evaluate the pros and cons for each of your options.

Of course, you or a family member should also educate yourself about your disease, starting with the excellent information which is available from 1-800-4-CANCER and also from the American Cancer Society.

How to Distinguish Between Lymphoma, Hodgkin's Disease, and Leukemia

It's easy to mix up certain types of cancer, even when you've been diagnosed with one of them, because in some ways they seem quite similar. Lymphoma, Hodgkin's disease, and leukemia are easily confused with one another even though they are quite different and require different types of treatment.

As medical residents at Mount Sinai Hospital in New York City, which both then and now is a great cancer treatment center, my colleagues and I used to refer to these cancers as "liquid" tumors to distinguish them from the hard, "solid" tumors that plagued other organs. The reason they were described as liquid is that they are associated with the blood or lymph gland fluids.

Both *lymphoma* and *Hodgkin's disease*, which is a special type of lymphoma, are cancers of certain lymph nodes and glands. High doses of radiotherapy may either cure lymphoma or cause a remission. Some of the remissions are long-term, sometimes lasting for years. Other relapses occur rather quickly, and subsequent relapses become increasingly difficult to treat. But various combinations of new or experimental drugs—available in many special cancer centers around the country—hold some hope of longer remission.

Many forms of *leukemia*, which is a cancer derived from certain immune system cells in the blood, can be treated with chemotherapy. Advanced leukemia and lymphomas can often be put into remission by chemotherapy.

$$\boxed{\text{E R R O R :}}$$

Your Doctor Doesn't Tell You That Your Cancer Doesn't Respond Well to Chemotherapy

Greg, who was suffering from advanced lung cancer, had been undergoing chemotherapy treatments, which were making him miserable with side effects, including nausea. He asked his doctor if there was anything that could be done to relieve the discomfort, but the doctor replied, "It depends on whether you want to live longer and maybe have a chance to improve or whether you just want to give up."

Was the doctor correct to say this?

FACTS: No, the real issue here was Greg's quality of life. Cancer chemotherapy is very effective for many forms of cancer. However, with advanced lung cancer—as well as advanced cancer of the pancreas, kidney cancer, liver cancer, and stomach cancer—standard chemotherapy is not likely to cure or provide any benefits other than short-term remissions. Furthermore, "chemo" treatments often have so many negative side effects that many physicians recommend that in the later stages of many cancers, they should be discontinued.

WHAT TO DO: If your cancer has spread and you are experiencing pain or discomfort as a result of chemotherapy, be sure that your cancer specialist is very clear and specific about what your prognosis would be without any treatment at all.

Also, question your doctor about the expected quality of life both with and without treatment. If, for example, you're experiencing substantial nausea with chemotherapy, as Greg was, you should know whether it's likely that nausea will decrease or disappear without the treatment.

If you're being treated at a special cancer center, you may be receiving experimental treatments. But you should be just as aggressive in asking about these as about standard chemotherapy. You should know the track record for remission or cure with the particular treatment you're getting and also how you'll feel if it's discontinued.

As you talk with your doctors, don't allow yourself to be satisfied with such clichés as "We see lots of remissions." That's great, but how long do they last? And don't be put off with the response "It's hard to say because every person is an individual." It's obvious that each of us is an individual, but you still have a right to know what percentage of people improve and how long those improvements last. It's only with this specific information that you can weigh the odds, compare possible benefits with known discomforts and side effects, and come to an intelligent decision that's right for you.

Every cancer patient should know the telephone hot line for the National Cancer Institute: 1-800-4-CANCER. Through this number, you or your physician can talk to knowledgeable cancer experts and receive specific information about your type of cancer. You can also obtain a listing of hospitals that have been endorsed by the National Cancer Institute for their work with cancer.

ERROR:

Your Doctor Fails to Educate You About Signs of Chemotherapy Toxicity

A friend of mine who had pancreatic cancer had left his suburban home for treatment at one of the five most prestigious regional cancer centers in the country. I'm sure he received excellent technical care, but none of the four highly skilled specialists who treated him really adopted my friend as his own "special" patient.

At discharge, this man was told to follow up with his local oncologist, but he did not remember being told how quickly he should do this. He did recall his last discussion with his doctor as being fairly rushed. The physician had to leave early, and my friend didn't receive any written instructions. Also, he was told something about side effects from the medications, but he couldn't recall precisely what they were. Neither he nor his family realized that the chemotherapy he was taking might destroy enough of his white blood cells (which fight infection) to cause a serious infection in the next few days.

My friend developed a severe sore throat three days after his discharge, but not recognizing the importance of this condition, he didn't call his local physician immediately. By the time he did call—after three more days had elapsed—his white blood cell count had plummeted, and he became critically ill from a spreading infection.

FACTS: The error here was not rooted in a lack of medical knowledge, but rather in a failure of the doctors to communicate effectively with the patient and his family. Certainly, all the doctors understood the potential for chemotherapy side effects. But even if anyone had explained in detail to the patient how those side effects should be managed after he left the hospital, it wouldn't have been surprising if the instructions didn't sink in, given the severity of the illness. So a key error by the doctor was in failing to provide clear explanations not only to the patient, but also to members of the family, who were fully able and willing to watch over the patient, if they had been taught how to do this.

WHAT TO DO: If you're undergoing chemotherapy, don't leave the hospital or doctor's office without either you or your family asking and getting adequate answers to these questions:

1. What chemotherapy or other drugs am I taking? Why have you chosen these particular drugs for me? How do they work inside my body?

2. What are the potential short-term side effects of the chemotherapy? Ask specifically about the effect on your white blood cells, which can result in susceptibility to infections; on platelets, which can result in bruising or bleeding; and on red blood cells, which can trigger anemia. Also, ask about possible loss of hair, diarrhea, nausea, headache, lung damage, and heart problems.

3. What schedule should I be on for routine monitoring for chemotherapy side effects? In between visits, what signs should I look for, and how urgent is it that I contact you if these signs occur?

4. What are the long-term risks of my treatment, including possible sterility, vulnerability to new cancers, or nerve damage?

5. How soon should we start chemotherapy? How and where will it be given? How long will each treatment take? How long will the whole series last? Do I need a friend or relative to accompany me for each treatment? Do I need to see my dentist first to check for gum or tooth infections that might flare up with the chemotherapy?

6. Can I continue to work during chemotherapy?

7. Are there special precautions I should take while I'm on chemotherapy or afterward? For example, should I avoid people who have infectious diseases?

8. Will my treatments be covered by insurance?

(I've adapted these questions from a National Cancer Institute paper entitled "Questions to Ask Your Doctor.")

ERROR:

Your Doctor Doesn't Suggest Behavioral Techniques to Overcome Side Effects of Chemotherapy

Ned experienced frequent headaches, nausea, and diarrhea from his chemotherapy treatments. When he complained to his doctor, the physician said, "Sometimes these side effects get better, so let's give the treatments a little more time. At some point I may reduce the amounts of the drugs you're getting, but remember: We're doing our best to knock this cancer out."

FACTS: Nausea, headaches, and other unpleasant side effects do occur often with chemotherapy. But there are techniques experienced oncologists can use to reduce the discomforts.

For one thing, certain medicines given just before chemotherapy can be quite helpful in preventing or treating the side effects. A new class of drugs, the serotonin antagonists (e.g., Zofran), has improved our ability to prevent nausea as a reaction to chemotherapy. Ned should ask his doctor about these.

In addition to such medicines, there has recently been an increasing interest in and use of behavioral techniques for countering pain and other discomforts associated with chemotherapy. These include guided visual imagery, self-hypnosis, and various meditation and relaxation techniques. Some chemotherapists actively recommend these approaches for management of side effects, but most ignore them. It's not that these specialists object to behavioral techniques; it's just that they lie outside the routines of treatment with which most doctors are familiar.

WHAT TO DO: If you're undergoing chemotherapy and are experiencing unpleasant side effects, ask your doctor for a referral to a stress management specialist or hypnotist who has had experience treating cancer side effects. For that matter, even if you're just starting these treatments, you might ask for a referral. Having a name and telephone number at your fingertips can be very reassuring if you suddenly are overwhelmed by nausea, headaches, or some similar problem.

If your doctor doesn't know of such a specialist, check with your local chapter of the American Cancer Society or a cancer patient support group. Many hospitals in larger cities or medical teaching centers have pain centers that offer the latest instruction in how to employ behavioral techniques to reduce the discomfort you're experiencing from your chemo treatments. Whichever specialist you choose, she should have extensive experience with cancer patients and be willing and able to communicate regularly with your oncologist.

ERROR:

Your Doctor Doesn't Explain the Hospice Option

After struggling with chemotherapy for six months in and out of the hospital, Peter and his family realized that further aggressive treatment for his widespread stomach cancer would be pointless. Still, he wasn't ready to die. He wanted to live out his last remaining months in as comfortable a way as possible—close to his family, preferably at home.

What Peter and his family didn't realize—and what was never explained to them in any detail at the small hospital where he was being treated—was that there might be an alternative to the incredible drain that Peter's medical routine threatened to impose on his wife at home. She tried taking care of him after he left the hospital, but she couldn't keep up the pace. Finally, she seriously considered moving him to a nursing home, but she worried about the institutional setting of those in their community.

Only a chance remark by a neighbor brought the best treatment into focus: What about a hospice?

FACTS: Most people have heard of hospices, but few really understand how valuable this type of care can be until they experience it. During the last twenty years, the hospice movement has greatly improved the quality of life for patients who are dying of cancer or other diseases. Hospice is the choice when the treatment goal is comfort rather than cure.

When a patient enters a hospice, she receives emotional and spiritual support as well as pain medication, nursing care, and other routine treatment. Typically, hospice care can be provided at home, in certain hospitals, or at a related facility. Most private insurance, Medicare, and in some states Medicaid will cover hospice care, and the cost is consistently less than is hospital treatment.

In Peter's case, there was a hospice serving his town, which was able to send a visiting nurse to his home three times a week. Also, a nurse's aide was available on two other days. Psychological counseling and emotional support were extremely helpful for both Peter and his wife.

Peter lived another three months and died with dignity at home. A hospice doctor even made house calls during the last, difficult week. After Peter's death, his wife joined the hospice's self-help bereavement group.

WHAT TO DO: Hospice aid is appropriate for people with cancer or other terminal diseases if they are expected to live only six months or less. There are more than 1,800 hospice programs in the country. Your doctor, local hospital, or American Cancer Society chapter should be able to direct you to a hospice program in your area. Or you can call the Hospice Helpline at 1-800-658-8898 for a free booklet: "The Basics of Hospice." You can also ask for a referral to a hospice in your area. You can also write to the National Hospice Organization, 1901 North Moore Street, Suite 901, Arlington, VA 22209.

ERROR:

Not Confronting the Insurance Implications of Your Treatment Early Enough to Take Assertive Action

Helen was doing well recovering from a bone marrow transplant operation—a desperate and successful attempt to achieve remission from the breast cancer that had spread throughout her body. That's when her husband brought the news that her health insurance plan had decided not to pay for the bone marrow transplant's $80,000 cost.

FACTS: In recent years health insurance plans and HMOs have increasingly resisted paying for certain expensive cancer treatments such as bone marrow transplants on the grounds that they are un-proven or experimental treatments—and are therefore not covered by their health insurance contract.

I'm not talking about "coffee enemas," apricot-pit extracts or other alternative cancer treatments such as one finds in Mexican cancer clinics. The insurance controversy concerns the cutting edge treatments being recommended and performed by our most re-spected cancer specialists.

To make matters worse, most insurance companies and HMOs who deny cancer treatment benefits have no clearly written internal guidelines for doing so. They appear to vary their decisions from case to case in an arbitrary manner, and have been shown to be much more likely to change their minds and pay up when a smart, aggressive lawyer takes up the patient's case.

The insurance companies, of course, do have a point. A few pa-tients with hugely expensive treatments can raise the health insur-ance premiums for everyone else. And often these treatments are truly long shots—failing to help most patients for long. Still, patients do often benefit, as in the case of bone marrow transplant for breast cancer where an extra year in remission might be a typical result. And of course, your job at this stage is to take care of your health, not to worry about its effect on the national deficit.

WHAT TO DO: Ask your doctor at the start whether the treatment being proposed will likely be covered by insurance. If the doctor indicates that the other patients have had problems, do not balk at the treatments on these grounds alone. Get your second opinion on the medical merits of the treatment just as you would if no insur-ance question were involved.

Often, the problem is solved simply. Your doctor contacts your insurance plan requesting a "predetermination" that authorizes you to go ahead with the treatment. However, if discussions with the insurance company suggest that there is likely to be a problem, you should start gathering the information you will need to persuade your health plan's chief executives to accept your point of view.

If your doctor has dealt with this problem before, he may be able to refer you to an attorney with relevant experience. You should seek information from patients in the cancer support groups spon-sored by the local hospital or American Cancer Society chapter.

The National Coalition for Cancer Survivorship is an organization with information on and interest in the practical aspects of insurance as it pertains to cancer patients (1010 Wayne Ave., Silver Springs, MD 20910; tel.: 301-585-2626).

My best advice is for you to pursue the course that you and your doctors believe is the best for you medically. If your doctors and your lawyers can make a good case for that, then the chances are very good that your health insurance plan will eventually come around—voluntarily or on the order of a court.

PART THREE

What's Going On with My Gut?

Special Alerts:
The Digestive System

- Your doctor diagnoses your abdominal pain over the telephone. As a result, you delay going in for a critical emergency procedure. (See error, p. 205.)

- You have pain in the right shoulder, but your doctor misses the fact that the true cause of the pain is in your abdomen—signaling a gallbladder condition. (See error, p. 209.)

- You are suffering from chronic pain in the upper abdomen. Your doctor is concerned that your problem might be an ulcer, gastritis, or even intestinal gas. But he fails to check for the real cause: the extremely serious condition inflammation of the pancreas. (See error, p. 213.)

- A quite painful stomachache has caused you to make an appointment to see your family doctor, but she delays treatment with the explanation, "I'm sure it's not appendicitis or food poisoning or something serious like that. It's usually a good idea to watch this sort of thing for a day or so to see if it goes away." Fortunately, you go to the emergency room that night. There, you learn you have a potentially fatal problem, a leaking aneurysm of the aorta, the main artery from the heart to the chest and abdomen. (See error, p. 218.)

- You've had a problem with constipation for more than a year. At your annual physical, your doctor says, "This has gone on for too long. We've got to get to the bottom of this." With that, he orders a battery of complex tests, including a colonoscopy and a barium enema. (See error, p. 223.)

- An enzyme deficiency, which your doctor has overlooked, is contributing substantially to your irritable bowel syndrome. (See error, p. 238.)

- Your teenager is injected with the hepatitis B immunization shots in the buttock rather than in the deltoid muscle of the upper arm. (See error, p. 245.)

- Your elderly father, who is a heavy drinker (more than three alcoholic drinks per day), is brought to the hospital for an unrelated illness. He is placed on an intravenous line that feeds the sugar glucose into his body, but the hospital fails to begin the treatment with a shot of vitamin B_1 (thiamine). (See error, p. 253.)

- Your aunt is on a low-calorie weight loss diet, but her doctor neglects to warn her about her increased risk for developing gallstones. (See error, p. 260.)

- Your doctor assumes too quickly that a burning sensation in the upper abdominal area is a result of your ulcer rather than your heart. (See error, p. 214.)

Abdominal Pain

Your Doctor Tries to Diagnose Your Abdominal Pain over the Telephone

Helen was smart enough to realize that many factors can contribute to a queasy stomach and general abdominal discomfort. So when she telephoned her doctor, she made every effort to give a calm, accurate, and precise description of her symptoms. Even so, she was somewhat uneasy requesting a diagnosis over the telephone.

But her doctor reassured her that he could tell from what she had related to him that she almost certainly was at the beginning of a viral illness, because, among other things, she had told him she had been exposed to the flu by her children.

But Helen's symptoms grew worse, with fever and increasing pain that began to localize to her lower right abdomen. She wound up in the hospital with a burst appendix, which required two surgical procedures. Now, a year after these operations, she still suffers from abdominal discomfort, which results from scar tissue that formed as a result of her infection.

FACTS: You simply can't diagnose abdominal distress over the telephone. Much abdominal pain or distress has a tendency to evolve or change into something else. So physicians should make it clear to patients that they can't make a final decision after one phone call, even if they choose to offer some initial telephone advice.

There are at least two key questions that a doctor must answer about a patient who is experiencing serious abdominal pain—questions that can't be dealt with adequately over the phone:

1. Does she require a consultation with a surgeon?
2. Is there any likelihood that she will have to be referred to an emergency room or hospital?

Delays in answering either of these questions may create tremendous danger for a patient. And hazardous delays become more likely if the patient is dismissed too early and removed from the doctor's regular observation. Early on, it's hard to distinguish a developing surgical emergency from more common, but less serious nonsurgical illness, such as an intestinal virus or excess stomach acid. The difficulty is that when an abdominal organ becomes inflamed, the patient may at first suffer only a vague, dull distress in the midline of the abdomen, sometimes with accompanying nausea.

Some specific developments related to abdominal pain should alert you to contact your physician immediately and should also warn your doctor that further action is required. These include intensification of the pain (as Helen experienced); fever (as with Helen); nausea (as with Helen); vomiting; swelling of the abdomen; or shifting of the pain to a specific section of the abdomen (as with Helen).

Of course, *most* abdominal distress results from viral illness, indigestion, constipation, or some other benign, self-limited cause. So it's wasteful and inappropriate to see the doctor every time you have a stomachache. But if you are experiencing more than one symptom or if somehow the pain seems unusual, there's no way any physician can get the "feel" of your problem without seeing your face and physically touching your abdomen.

Another conservative rule of thumb that I follow in a case like Helen's goes like this: If a patient is sufficiently concerned about abdominal distress to call the physician, then the patient should usually be seen in person.

The biggest error made by Helen's physician may have been that he gave her a false certainty that his telephone "diagnosis" was definite. A better response might have gone like this: "This may be a virus, but we can't know yet for sure. Call me back in a few hours if things get worse and especially if you develop a fever, nausea, vomiting, or pain that becomes localized in a specific part of your abdomen."

Approximately two-thirds of emergency room malpractice suits involve an incorrect diagnosis of abdominal ailments. The most commonly missed serious abdominal complaints that lead to lawsuits include abdominal aortic aneurysm, appendicitis, ectopic pregnancy, ruptured or perforated intestine, gastrointestinal bleeding, acute pancreatitis, diverticulitis, and intestinal obstruction. (See the accompanying box, Organs That May Cause Abdominal Pain.)

WHAT TO DO: If you develop abdominal distress that seems different from what you've experienced before, you should usually insist on seeing your doctor. If the abdominal discomfort is rather mild and you seem to have no other symptoms, you may be able to get some instructions over the phone, but be sure that you understand how to proceed after you hang up.

If symptoms related to your abdominal pain change or increase, don't hesitate to have the doctor's nurse call him out of a consultation so that you can talk with him and make an appointment. You're facing a potential emergency, and you have to be *persistent* and *vigilant* in getting that point across. Otherwise you may find yourself in the midst of a serious health crisis.

Once you've seen your doctor about your abdominal distress, if you seem to have something more than a benign, garden-variety stomachache, insist on one of these four options:

1. You may be kept under continuous observation. This usually means checking into a hospital.

2. You may be sent home, with the understanding that your doctor should recheck on you within a few hours. If you choose this option, you should set a specific time for your next appointment and go over important new symptoms to watch for most closely. The new symptoms that your doctor is most likely to mention are the ones listed above: intensifying pain, fever, nausea, vomiting, swelling of the abdomen, or change in location of the pain.

3. You may be sent home, with the understanding that you'll be provided with precise instructions to report in by telephone at frequent, designated intervals. With this option, you must be ready to seek medical care promptly if any alarming changes occur, as described earlier in this error. Again watch for the appearance of the new symptoms summarized in option 2.

4. You may obtain a consultation with a surgeon. If your pain is continuing at the same level or growing worse, this step must be taken immediately.

Organs That May Cause Abdominal Pain

Site of Pain	Possible Abdominal Organs Involved	Other Possible Causes
Right upper abdomen	Liver, gallbladder, duodenum, small intestine, pancreas, large intestine, kidney	Backup of fluid from the heart and lung into the liver, early shingles (before rash appears), muscle sprain, pneumonia, pleurisy
Left upper abdomen	Spleen, large intestine, stomach, esophagus, pancreas, kidney	Early shingles, muscle sprain, gas, pneumonia, pleurisy
Right lower abdomen	Appendix, small intestine, large intestine, kidney	Disc disease of spine, ovaries/fallopian tubes (cysts, infections, ectopic pregnancy), endometriosis, early shingles
Left lower abdomen	Appendix, small intestine, large intestine (especially diverticulitis)	Same as right lower abdomen
Upper midline (epigastric area)	Esophagus, stomach, duodenum, pancreas	Heart or lung inflammation, aortic aneurysm
Lower midline	Large intestine, rectum, kidney	Bladder, prostate, abdominal aortic aneurysm, ovaries, uterus, fallopian tubes, endometriosis
Flank (back and to the sides)	Kidney	Spinal arthritis or disc disorder, shingles, muscle spasm
Rectum	Hemorrhoids, rectum, large intestine, appendix	Ovaries, fallopian tubes, uterus, prostate
Groin (where leg connects to abdomen)	Hernia (abdominal wall protruding), kidney, prostate	Swollen lymph glands, spinal arthritis or disc disorder, muscle sprain
Testicles	Testicular infection/inflammation or twisting of testicle (an urgent emergency), hernia, kidney	

ERROR:

You Have Pain in Your Right Shoulder, but Your Doctor Misses the Real *Source of the Pain—Your Gallbladder*

Bob, who was being treated for heart disease, began to feel pain in his right shoulder and on the right side of his back around his shoulder blade. Understandably, the first thing his doctor thought of was that Bob might be having a flare-up of his arthritis. So, without considering any other possible sources of the pain, he suggested that Bob see an orthopedist.

Fortunately, the orthopedist realized that Bob's arthritis was not the real problem, in part because moving the muscles of his shoulder, back, and arms had no noticeable effect. But pressing on the right upper sector of his abdomen did seem to make the pain worse. The specialist returned Bob promptly to his regular doctor with the recommendation that an evaluation be done for gallbladder disease.

FACTS: A common error doctors make is to mistake the main site of pain for the *real* source of the problem, which actually lies some distance away in the body. This separation of pain from source of the pain is known as the *referred pain* phenomenon.

One of the odd facts about our internal organs is that the pain they trigger can be at some location fairly far away from the site of the organ that's in trouble. The best known example of this may be cardiac chest pain, which is often felt in the left arm or shoulder. Cardiac pain can also be felt in the upper abdomen, neck, jaw, teeth or right arm—sometimes without any distress at all in the chest area near the heart.

In fact, any inflammation in the chest can be felt as mainly in the upper abdomen, regardless of the true source organ. Such upper abdominal pains can arise from the heart, the pericardium (the sac surrounding the heart), the lungs, the pleura (the sac surrounding the lungs), the esophagus (the tube running from throat to stomach), or major blood vessels in the chest. A physician will fail to identify the chest source of these cases of abdominal pain unless she is alert to the possibility of referred pain from the chest to the abdomen.

This trap can also work the other way, as Bob's doctor discovered. Pain in the chest, back, or elsewhere can have an abdominal source

that won't be detected unless the physician focuses in on the abdomen. Gallbladder pain, of the type that Bob suffered, is often perceived in the right shoulder or right scapula area whether or not
there is much pain in the true gallbladder area, which lies in the
right upper portion of the abdomen.

Here are some other referred pain mistakes:

- An abscess in the upper abdomen under the diaphragm, the
  large muscles separating the abdomen from the lungs and heart,
  may be felt as a pain in the shoulder or upper back.

- Pain arising from the kidneys, which are located just behind the
  abdominal lining in the right and left flank, may be felt in the
  lower abdomen or in the groin area.

- Pain arising in the testicles may be noticed in the flank area (on
  the side of the hip) or in the lower abdomen.

WHAT TO DO: If your main complaint is abdominal distress, you
should expect that your doctor will also examine your chest and
back. If your main complaint seems to center in your chest or shoulders, expect that she will also examine your abdomen.

In most cases of abdominal distress, especially lower abdominal
pain, a thorough examination should also include the following:

- A rectal exam.

- An examination of the groin area, especially for hernias.

- A checkup of the male genital organs, particularly in children
  and young men, for whom a twisted testicle can be a major
  emergency.

- A urinalysis.

- An evaluation of the female genital and reproductive area with
  special attention to the time of the woman's last period, possible
  pregnancy, and possible infection in the pelvic region.

ERROR:

Your Doctor Fails to Do a Rectal Exam When You Complain About Abdominal Distress and Misses Your Appendicitis, Diverticulitis, or Another Serious Condition

Kirk had been feeling vague, generalized abdominal distress for a couple of days, and the mild pains seemed to be getting worse. He went in for an exam by his doctor but was told after a quick checkup that he was probably suffering from an intestinal virus that was going around. The next day, Kirk was admitted to the hospital with acute appendicitis.

FACTS: Failing to do a rectal examination is a frequent reason for missing or delaying the diagnosis of acute appendicitis. Most patients with appendicitis eventually develop pain in the right lower abdominal area after initial, vague upper abdominal discomfort of the type Kirk felt.

But some patients have an appendix that is not in the usual position. Their pain and tenderness may only be localized when pressure is applied up and toward the right during the course of a rectal exam. In this exam, the doctor puts on a rubber glove and inserts a finger into the rectum.

The rectal exam may also be useful with many patients who have abdominal distress because they are in the process of bleeding slowly into their gastrointestinal tract. The cause may be gastritis (inflammation of the stomach lining), an ulcer, bowel cancer, or divticular disease (which involves an outpouching and inflammation of sections of the colon, or large intestine).

This internal bleeding can often be detected by a rectal exam because there is usually some blood-containing stool in the rectum. A routine part of rectal exams should include a chemical test for blood in the bowels.

Of course, many cases of abdominal pain are due to nothing more than severe constipation, especially in patients who are old or infirm. In men, prostate inflammation may cause lower abdominal distress. Again, a rectal exam is the quickest way to detect both of these conditions.

WHAT TO DO: If you are experiencing serious abdominal discomfort, expect a rectal examination to be part of your checkup. If your doctor fails to give you this test, don't automatically let out a sigh of relief for "letting you off the hook." Granted, a rectal exam can be a little uncomfortable. But properly executed, it's one of the fastest and most efficient exams, and it's one of the most important in checking for potentially serious problems that may be causing your abdominal discomforts.

ERROR:

Your Doctor Fails to Do a Pelvic Exam and Evaluate Your Menstrual and Pregnancy Status When You Complain of Lower Abdominal Distress

Georgia complained to her doctor about pains she was feeling on the lower right side of her abdomen. She also was running a low-grade fever. The doctor immediately assumed that she had appendicitis and had her hospitalized.

Her problem? A particularly intense bout with menstrual cramps plus an upper respiratory virus.

FACTS: With all female patients having lower abdominal distress, a doctor should at the outset check three possibilities:

1. An infection or other problem related to the reproductive organs, which must be checked with an internal pelvic exam.

2. The woman's menstrual cycle.

3. Her pregnancy status.

Infection or inflammation of the ovaries, fallopian tubes, or uterus can be confused with a host of other problems, including diverticulitis (inflammation of outpouchings of the large intestine) or appendicitis. A missed or abnormal recent period could mean that nausea or abdominal distress is from a normal pregnancy. Or these symptoms could indicate a misplaced, or *ectopic*, pregnancy—a potentially life-threatening emergency.

Abdominal pain developing during the menstrual period could result from more intense than usual menstrual cramps, as happened with Georgia, endometriosis (a condition where cells that normally line the uterus grow in unusual places, such as the lining of the abdomen), various pelvic bacterial infections, or the life-threatening syndrome known as toxic shock.

WHAT TO DO: If you are a woman who is experiencing acute lower abdominal distress or pain, you should expect an internal pelvic examination as part of your checkup. Also, be prepared to answer questions about your sexual, menstrual, and contraceptive history. If your doctor doesn't raise any of the pertinent issues described under Facts, be sure to bring them up yourself.

> E R R O R :

You Have Steady Pain in the Upper Abdomen, Which Your Doctor Misdiagnoses as Gastritis Instead of Pancreatitis

Edward called his doctor late one afternoon to complain of a steady pain in his upper abdomen that had been bothering him for a couple of days. The doctor, who was eager to head for home, examined Edward briefly in his office. He diagnosed the problem as either intestinal gas or perhaps gastritis, an inflammation of the lining of the stomach that could arise from such easily correctable factors as too much aspirin or excess acidity in the stomach.

"This will keep until tomorrow," the doctor said. "Give me a call if you're still having trouble."

The pain intensified that evening, and Edward had to be admitted to the emergency room, where he was diagnosed after a blood test with the extremely dangerous condition pancreatitis (inflammation of the pancreas).

FACTS: The pancreas lies deep in the upper abdomen, behind the stomach and small intestines, and stretches out almost far enough to touch the gallbladder and liver on the right and the spleen on the left. This organ has several digestive functions, including the secretion of enzymes that break down fats and starches. When the pancreas is not working properly, the digestive system doesn't work properly either. The end result over time may be significant weight loss and other serious health consequences.

When the pancreas is inflamed (pancreatitis), pain can be acute and overwhelming or relatively mild and chronic. It can be felt in the upper middle part of the abdomen, where Edward experienced his discomfort, and may radiate through to the back or toward the right or left side. Pancreatitis can be mistaken for gallbladder or liver inflammation, an ulcer, a rupturing spleen, gastritis, or even intestinal gas. As you can see, Edward's doctor, in his hurried diagnosis, was focusing on the last two possibilities. Patients with gallstones or with stomach pain due to excess alcohol may have pancreatitis at the same time, because these two factors can themselves trigger pancreatitis.

When the pancreas is inflamed, a high level of pancreatic enzyme called *amylase* can usually be found in the blood. It was this test for amylase that was performed on Edward in the emergency room—a test that his own doctor should have performed.

WHAT TO DO: If you have substantial upper abdominal distress, a blood amylase level should be obtained even if your doctor is already confident of another diagnosis, such as an ulcer, gastritis, hepatitis, or gallbladder disease. Ask your doctor about this test if you have upper middle abdominal pain, especially pain that has radiated out into your back or to one side.

ERROR:

Assuming Too Quickly That the Burning in Your Upper Abdomen Is from Your Ulcer Rather Than Your Heart

Dwight, who was in his late fifties, had suffered from an ulcer off and on for several years. Usually antacid prescriptions and a strict diet worked well enough, but this approach hadn't worked in recent weeks, and Dwight was feeling frequent discomfort in his upper abdomen. The pain became so bad one night that he started sweating. That's when his wife checked him into the local emergency room—where he was diagnosed as being in the midst of a heart attack.

FACTS: Many people immediately associate pain in the upper center of the chest, around the sternum, with a possible heart attack.

But it's easy for anyone—even a well-meaning physician—to be thrown off the track in making a diagnosis when a patient, such as Dwight, is known to suffer from another problem that causes similar symptoms.

Pain from the heart due to chronic angina or an actual heart attack can sometimes be felt mainly in the stomach. Or it may be felt in the chest but be confused with your usual abdominal distress. Even when the pain actually feels different, the thought of having a heart attack is so frightening, and the thought of calling 911 for an ambulance so embarrassing, that it's psychologically hard to shift focus.

WHAT TO DO: If your distress in the mid-upper abdominal region is relatively recent, or if the pain has changed from its usual character, notify your doctor promptly that you think something else is going on besides acid indigestion. Have your doctor run down the alternatives, even if your distress seems to improve when you take antacids. If you are over 50 or if you have heart-disease risk factors, be sure your doctor thinks systematically about whether the problem could be your heart. In most cases, he should perform a resting electrocardiogram (EKG). He may also order an exercise stress test or even check you into a hospital for closer observation.

The key to identifying less-than-obvious alternatives to indigestion or ulcers is to get your doctor to ask himself this question: "Is there anything else these symptoms are likely to point to?" Once the question is asked, most doctors will be motivated and able to find out the answer.

ERROR:

In Diagnosing Your Abdominal Pain, Your Doctor Fails to Check Your Medication Schedule or Exposure to Toxic Substances

Harriet was feeling quite fatigued, and she suspected that the problem was loss of iron as a result of blood loss during her menstrual periods. So she started taking large doses of iron supplements.

She began to experience severe abdominal pain, but after ordering a battery of expensive and time-consuming tests, her doctor couldn't discover the cause. A brief period of hospitalization seemed to relieve the problem, but a couple of weeks after she was released, Harriet started having the pains again.

Suspecting that her problem might be psychological, her physician referred her to a psychiatrist. But the pains continued to plague her.

What was the doctor's mistake?

FACTS: In evaluating a patient's abdominal pain, a doctor should always take into account medications, including over-the-counter drugs and supplements, and exposure to toxic substances. In Harriet's case, a gastroenterologist finally determined that the problem was the iron supplements she was taking. When she stopped them, the pains ceased.

The following medications and toxic exposures are a few of the common culprits that can cause severe abdominal pain, and a doctor should always ask about their presence in making a diagnosis:

- Alcohol (including regular alcoholic beverages as well as alcohol-type products not meant for consumption, such as isopropyl alcohol and methanol).
- Aspirin and related nonsteroidal antiinflammatory drugs.
- Acetaminophen (Tylenol), but only in overdoses.
- Amphetamines (used as stimulants or appetite suppressors).
- Chlorinated chemicals (such as cleaning fluids and carbon tetrachloride).
- Cocaine.
- Digitalis (Lanoxin) in excess.
- Iron tablets.
- Arsenic, lead, mercury, pesticide, or phosphorus poisoning.
- Asthma (theophylline) medications.
- Zinc tablets.

WHAT TO DO: If you contact your doctor about abdominal pains, he may identify the problem quickly and correct it without your having to go into your medications or a discussion of your exposure to possible poisons. But it's always best to be prepared.

I recommend that my patients always collect all their medications, including supplements and over-the-counter drugs, together in one bag, which they carry to my office when they see me. This approach may be a little cumbersome, but it's effective. The next best way is to keep a written list of your medications and supplements, with all doses indicated.

On your way to your doctor's office, you should also go over in your mind what you've been doing during the past few days. In particular, try to remember unusual activities or situations that may have exposed you to substances that could be causing your problem. For example, recall if you've been exposed to cleaning fluids around the house or pesticides out in the yard. You have to be able to help your doctor zero in on your precise problem and prescribe proper treatment without delay.

ERROR:

Failing to Do a Urinalysis and Blood Count in Evaluating Lower Abdominal Distress

Frank began to suffer from a lower abdominal pain, which intensified to some degree and spread out to his right flank or hip. At this point, the pain could best be described as moderate rather than severe. His doctor thought the problem was appendicitis and without any further tests, he immediately had Frank admitted to the hospital. Frank's pain increased to the point that he worried he might pass out. After a urine test that showed red blood cells in the urine, and a blood count, which was normal, his condition was diagnosed not as appendicitis but as a kidney stone.

Did the doctor make the right decision?

FACTS: Without being on the spot, I could never say that what Frank's doctor did in this case was wrong. A sharp pain on the lower right side can definitely signal appendicitis, and in such a situation, it's important to get the best, most comprehensive treatment, which would normally be available only in a hospital.

But this physician did neglect an important test, which could have been initiated immediately before Frank left his office, especially since Frank wasn't yet debilitated by the pain. That was to take a sample of urine for a urinalysis and to draw blood for a complete blood test.

A urinalysis will usually be abnormal if there is a problem with the kidneys (such as Frank's kidney stones), the prostate, or the bladder. Red blood cells in the urine may signal irritation of the lining of these organs or internal bleeding. White blood cells in the urine may indicate infection. This test may also signal certain cases of appendicitis or a leaking aortic aneurysm (involving the main artery leading from the heart to the chest and abdomen).

A blood test that shows an elevated white blood cell count will increase the doctor's concern that there may be a serious internal infection or actual damage to the tissue of an internal organ. (On the other hand, a normal white blood cell count doesn't necessarily mean that everything is okay.)

WHAT TO DO: Expect a urinalysis if you have any flank or lower abdominal pain, even a moderate pain of the type that was initially bothering Frank. Your doctor should order a white blood cell count if your abdominal symptoms are severe or if the cause of your problem isn't certain.

In Frank's case, the urinalysis and blood test were eventually performed in the hospital. But if his doctor had started the ball rolling in his office by taking the urine and blood samples there, the tests might have been completed much more quickly, and treatment for the kidney stones could have begun sooner.

ERROR:

Your Doctor Tells You to Wait a Day for Treatment for a Painful Stomachache, but an Emergency Room Doctor Identifies a Potentially Fatal Blood Vessel Problem

Will's stomachache started late one morning and continued through the afternoon. Finally, just before he went home from work, he called his doctor, who told him to come over for a checkup.

The doctor noted that Will, who was 56, had eaten a heavy Mexican dinner the previous night and also that he had not yet had a bowel movement. Will's abdomen seemed full, and Will said he could feel his heart beating in the fullness. But the doctor decided to have him wait until the next day—"after you've had a bowel movement"—to see if the discomfort continued.

Early the following morning, Will's wife drove him to the emergency room, where a quick abdominal ultrasound test showed that he was suffering from a leaking aneurysm of the aorta, the main artery that leads from the heart to the chest and abdomen. He was rushed into surgery.

Should Will's family doctor have discovered this problem?

FACTS: Abdominal pains of the kind that Will was feeling may result from two serious blood vessel disorders. First, the source of the difficulty may be a leaking or rupturing aneurysm of the aorta. Second, the problem can stem from an ischemic bowel—a kind of "heart attack of the bowel," where the intestinal tissue begins to die because it's not getting enough blood.

Both a leaking (or rupturing) aneurysm of the aorta and ischemic bowel can be fatal if they are not operated on within hours. These problems are rare in people under 50, but they account for an estimated 2 percent of emergency room visits for abdominal pain among people older than 50.

A pulsating mass in the abdomen, of the type that was bothering Will, suggests the likelihood of an aortic aneurysm. Abdominal X rays, ultrasound and an emergency computed tomography (CT) scan of the abdomen are quick, noninvasive ways to evaluate this possibility. Most hospital emergency rooms should be able to provide one or more of these tests on a twenty-four-hour-a-day basis.

In addition to abdominal pain, an ischemic bowel can cause occult blood in the stool—usually indicated by black or tarry-colored stool or, rarely, by gross bleeding. Your doctor will also have to rule out other possible causes. Tests that often help include abdominal X ray, CT scan, blood tests such as white blood cell count and lactic acid levels, and angiography—an X ray in which dye is injected into the arteries of the abdomen. The blood amylase level, usually used to diagnose pancreatitis, may also be high in ischemic bowel disease.

Experience has taught most emergency room physicians and surgeons to think automatically of the possibility of an aortic aneurysm or ischemic bowel. But many times, family physicians and internists, who may see abdominal emergencies infrequently, might omit checking for these serious problems until it's too late.

WHAT TO DO: If you're over 50 and if you have your wits about you, ask your doctor, Could my pain be due to a rupturing aortic aneurysm or a blockage in blood flow to my bowels?

If she gives you a thoughtful response and yet rejects either of these diagnoses, you can at least be assured that she has thought seriously about the possibility. If she acknowledges that you may be suffering from either the aneurysm or the ischemic bowel, then she'll probably refer you to the local hospital or to a specialist for further tests. The specialists who could provide the soundest evaluation of your condition include a general surgeon, a gastroenterologist, a cardiologist, or a vascular surgeon. Sometimes, you'll need to be treated at an emergency room and then examined by a specialist.

Here are some guidelines on when to seek out the opinion of a specialist. You should insist on a consultation with a surgeon or gastroenterologist in any of these circumstances:

- The abdominal pain has lasted six hours or more. (Will was in this position.)

- Nausea or vomiting is present and persistent.

- A formal, highly credible nonsurgical diagnosis hasn't been made. If you personally lack confidence in your personal physician's evaluation—if you just don't quite believe her—you should definitely seek the opinion of a specialist. By the way, good doctors understand and usually don't feel offended if you seek a second opinion.

- Your symptoms return or worsen after you've been seen once and then sent home either by your family doctor or by a hospital.

- The treating physician at an emergency room or hospital is a resident-in-training. In this case, insist on being examined by the attending physician, who is legally responsible for your care.

- The physician who treats you in an emergency room is a "moonlighting" physician whose regular work is not in emergency room care.

ERROR:

*You Are Placed "Under Observation"
in an Emergency Room as a Result
of Abdominal Pain, but More than
Thirty Minutes Elapse Before
You Are Checked by a Physician or Nurse*

Nora was admitted to the local hospital emergency room after complaining about severe abdominal pains. She was told by a nurse that she had been placed "under observation," but forty-five minutes went by during which she wasn't checked by any member of the medical staff.

Before long, she began to feel feverish and sensed her heartbeat was becoming irregular, but she was having trouble getting the attention of a doctor or nurse. Nora was afraid that if she got up from the examining table where they had told her to lie, she might faint.

What exactly was happening here?

FACTS: During the hours or even minutes that it takes for an abdominal problem to evolve, many things may change. Blood pressure may fall or rise; heartbeats may become irregular; and body temperature may rise, suggesting inflammation of some internal organ. In Nora's case, a later checkup confirmed that she was wrestling with an internal infection.

On the other hand, body temperature may fall—a signal of possible sepsis (a diffuse infection throughout the blood). In addition to these changes, the intensity or position of the pain may shift, or internal bleeding may occur.

Because things usually don't remain stable with a serious abdominal problem, patients who are placed "under observation" should be checked at least every thirty minutes by a doctor or nurse. Furthermore, they should be within visual view of a health professional at all times.

It's also advisable for patients in this situation to have a family member or friend on hand in the emergency room. This companion can serve as an advocate who can get the attention of the professional staff in the event that the patient is too weak or disoriented to communicate forcefully.

WHAT TO DO: If you're alone and sick in an emergency room, have the medical staff call a family member or friend to stay with you. Their function will be not just to provide emotional support, but also to help you negotiate your way through the maze of the medical care system.

This friend—or you yourself if you must operate on your own—should be polite but assertive in letting nurses or doctors know if your symptoms have changed and particularly if they have grown worse or if you've developed new symptoms. If no one has been by for more than a half hour, you or your advocate should ask for a progress report. Just posing a question or two will remind them of your presence, and that reminder will help you get better care and treatment.

ERROR:

Your Doctor Does Not Treat Your Chronic "Acid" Problems with Antibiotics

Helen was a five-year veteran of a battle against a duodenal ulcer. She did reasonably well on Zantac, a powerful acid-blocking medicine, while abstaining from alcohol, coffee, and spices. But whenever she would stop the medicine for a few weeks, her symptoms returned.

Helen's doctor's working hypothesis was that too much stress was the key to her problem. Helen didn't feel very stressed—except when her stomach pain drove her "nuts," but, lacking any other alternative, she assumed that her doctor must be right.

FACTS: Stress certainly can cause or worsen ulcers and other conditions that trigger excess stomach acid. However, specialists have now come to accept that many ulcer patients and also some without ulcers but with chronic "acid" complaints actually suffer from a bacterial infection that weakens the resistance of the lining of the upper digestive track.

This bacteria is called *Helicobacter* (or *H.* for short) *pylorus*. The most accurate way to diagnose it is to take a biopsy through a long tube inserted through the mouth into the stomach (gastroscopy). Fortunately, a more convenient blood test is now available to diagnose whether you have been exposed to *H. pylorus*.

Ironically, plain old Pepto-Bismol acts like an antibiotic against *H. pylorus*, but *H. pylorus* usually becomes resistant to Pepto-Bismol after a period of treatment. So Pepto-Bismol is typically not effective for more than short-term relief.

Long-term cure usually requires a fairly long course with Pepto-Bismol, together with at least two other antibiotics. The treatment itself can cause considerable gastrointestinal distress, but when it works, most ulcer patients would agree, the cure is quite worth it.

WHAT TO DO: If you have ulcers or other recurring upper digestive symptoms (e.g., gastritis, esophagitis, heartburn), be sure your doctor addresses the possibility of an *H. pylorus* infection. But do not try to treat yourself with Pepto-Bismol or leftover antibiotics. Partial treatment may help for a while, but when antibiotic resistance develops—as it usually does—your symptoms will return. After that your *H. pylorus* will be even more difficult to treat.

Constipation and Diarrhea

E R R O R :

Your Doctor Orders Many Fancy Tests for Ordinary Constipation

Flora had been plagued by periodic constipation for more than two years, and she complained a couple of times about it to her doctor. Finally, at her annual physical, the physician said, "This has gone on for too long. We've got to get to the bottom of this."

So he ordered a battery of sophisticated tests, including a colonoscopy (an inspection of the entire colon, or large intestine, with a special instrument) and an upper gastrointestinal (GI) series (which involves swallowing a barium solution and then having an X ray made of the upper intestinal tract).

These tests revealed nothing unusual.

FACTS: Many doctors will order a series of fancy tests on a patient who is constipated, primarily to screen for intestinal cancer. But bowel cancer that is severe enough to cause constipation isn't likely to sit stable for more than two years. So the fact that Flora had been wrestling with constipation for well over two years was actually a *good* sign, at least as far as the possibility of cancer was concerned.

I encourage my patients to have regular cancer detection examinations, including chemical checks of the stool for hidden blood and flexible sigmoidoscopy (the inspection of about one-third of the lower colon with a flexible tube equipped with a viewing device). But long-term, stable constipation isn't usually a reason for doing these tests more often. Nor is constipation alone sufficient justification for doing a full colonoscopy or a GI X ray, such as Flora was given.

People who have a strong family history of colon cancer or other risk factors for colon cancer (for example, a history of colon polyps or ulcerative colitis) should be especially alert to *changes* in their bowel habits or the appearance of blood or black, tarry stools. Many gastroenterologists argue that this small group of patients should be examined more aggressively, such as with a full colonoscopy to increase the odds of detecting cancer at its earliest stage.

WHAT TO DO: Keep up with your regular early cancer detection checkups, such as the chemical stool test for hidden blood and the flexible sigmoidoscopy. Any chronic, stable constipation you are experiencing shouldn't affect this schedule.

During your basic physical, your doctor should focus on your constipation problem by going over the issues discussed in the accompanying box, The Basics of Promoting Regular Bowel Movements. Among other things, he should know the type of foods you eat, the fluids you drink, and your medication schedule. He should also ask you for a description of the frequency, size, and consistency of your bowel movements and whether pain is associated with them. During your actual exam, he should check your abdomen and rectum thoroughly and should order lab tests that measure your blood count and thyroid levels.

E R R O R :

Ignoring Significant Worsening of Your Constipation

Bud, who was 68 years old, had been suffering with constipation for a couple of years, and he regularly took a laxative recommended by his doctor. He was also a very sedentary person, whose main walking was for a short distance from his office to his car and then from his car into his home and the television set. His main liquid intake was a little wine at dinner, and he never had water with his meals.

When Bud was having particular difficulty with his bowel movements during one two-day period, he increased the dose of his laxative, but he found that his symptoms worsened. At the same time, he was taking fairly large doses of an over-the-counter antihistamine for a cold. His stomach began to hurt, his abdomen seemed to be

The Basics of Promoting Regular Bowel Movements

Many doctors neglect to teach their patients the fundamental truth that the bowel is a creature of habit. Most people can count on their bowel movements coming every day at about the same time, just like clockwork. That's why most laxative advertisers proclaim that their products promote "regularity."

I define constipation as any inability to have a bowel movement with the frequency that best fits the rhythm of your life. Some people may have bowel movements more than once a day; most go at least once a day; yet others may have bowel movements as infrequently as about three times a week. If you are less regular than this, the chances are you may develop symptoms like abdominal discomfort, abdominal pain, vague headaches, or a feeling of being "logy" or "slow."

A variety of unusual events is capable of upsetting this regularity and causing constipation. For example, you may become constipated after a painful bout of hemorrhoids, a spell of bed rest during an illness, decreased food intake while you're on a weight loss diet, or having to stay for a while in a place where the bathroom hygiene is repulsive.

If you're lucky, your bowel movements will return to normal once the disturbing event is over. If you're not lucky, your bowel may begin to "forget" its natural rhythm, and a vicious cycle, which ends in constipation, may begin.

A simple antidote to constipation, which many physicians, including gastroenterologists, may forget to explain, is just to sit on the toilet at the same time every day. Then *gently* try to move your bowels at that time whether you feel an urge to do so or not. Don't strain excessively, however, because this habit can irritate your rectum and even damage nerves, which, in turn, may lead to a loss of bowel control.

The best times to reinforce bowel regularity are after meals or the first thing in the morning. It may take a while, even eight to ten weeks of this kind of "bowel retraining," to reestablish a pattern of regularity. So don't become impatient if this approach doesn't work immediately.

At the same time you're following this regular bathroom ritual, you should also pay close attention to your diet. A common cause of constipation is not taking in enough fluids. The old homespun advice of drinking at least eight glasses of water a day—or the equivalent in clear juices—applies here. Also, you should take in plenty of fiber in your daily meals, including at least four or five servings of fruits and vegetables and high-fiber cereals like All-Bran.

Your doctor should also evaluate the medications you're taking, because one or more of them could be causing your constipation. (See the box, Drugs That Often Cause Constipation, p. 228.)

Finally, an alert doctor will advise those with constipation problems to be sure that they are getting regular exercise. Just walking two or three miles a day, three or four days a week, is often enough to induce regularity.

bloated, and he was puzzled because he wasn't even able to pass gas.

When he notified his physician of these symptoms, the doctor, apparently suspecting this was just more of the same constipation problem that had been plaguing Bud, told him over the phone to "sleep on it." But early the next morning, the pain had become so excruciating that Bud checked in to his local hospital, where an operation was performed for a dangerous bowel blockage.

What had happened?

FACTS: People who have previously been constipated can develop new diseases, such as low thyroid or bowel cancer, which can alter the bowel pattern. People over age 60 are at a higher risk for developing these diseases. They are also more likely to have other health factors that can worsen constipation, such as an increase in drug intake, a lack of exercise, dehydration, loss of appetite, or hemorrhoids. In any event, it's the *change*, not the previous character of the bowel movements, that should cause both the doctor and the patient to search for an explanation.

Constipation accompanied by a long, narrow stool should suggest the possibility of bowel cancer, though other noncancerous conditions can also create this appearance in bowel movements.

If the constipation seems to be getting worse, that is always a cause for a thorough checkup by your doctor. You may find you go to the toilet even less frequently than before. Or there may be abdominal pain, as Bud had, which is more severe than what you've experienced before. Or you may notice that your abdomen seems distended (again, Bud), or you're nauseated, or you begin vomiting. Pain and distension, along with a failure to pass gas for a day, may mean that your bowel is completely obstructed, a condition that should be treated as an emergency.

WHAT TO DO: If the nature of your constipation changes, contact your doctor. Be prepared to give her a precise, detailed list of all the symptoms you're experiencing, particularly the new ones.

Also, you should be ready to give your doctor the specific schedule you've been following for medications, including over-the-counter drugs and supplements that she may not have prescribed. Some of these can actually cause or worsen constipation.

As you can see from the above account, Bud was taking large quantities of a laxative, which can actually backfire by *causing* constipation in some situations. He was also taking an antihistamine, another type of drug that can impede regularity. (See the accompanying box, Drugs That Often Cause Constipation.) His lack of exercise would have contributed further to the constipation, and his failure to drink enough liquids probably left him in a partially dehydrated condition. Together, these factors seem to have contributed to the extreme case of constipation and blockage in his bowels, which required surgery.

What might Bud's doctor have done differently? A major mistake he made was not having Bud come in for a complete physical and especially a rectal exam. This test involves the doctor's donning a rubber glove and then inserting a finger up into the rectum.

This simple procedure would probably have revealed Bud's problem as fecal impaction, where hard, dry bowel movements completely blocked up the rectum. This is fairly common among people who are elderly, ill, or dehydrated (as Bud most likely was). Increasing fiber or prescribing laxatives not only won't help, it can easily make things worse. That's why Bud made a mistake increasing his laxative intake.

Much less frequently, bowel movements will stop because of a tumor in the rectum, very enlarged hemorrhoids, or a collapse of the lower large bowel into the rectum (known as a *rectal prolapse*). A simple rectal exam would usually alert the doctor to these problems as well.

ERROR:

Your Doctor Fails to Recognize That Your Constipation Is a Symptom of Anxiety or Depression

Arlene, who was going through a divorce, felt constantly on edge. She worried about her children, her finances, and her future after

Drugs That Often Cause Constipation

The *Physician's Desk Reference* lists about 500 medicines that can cause constipation. Here are a few of the most common:

• Laxatives that are used in excess. The irritant type are the most frequently abused. These include bisacodyl (Dulcolax); casanthranol (Peri-colace) (not to be confused with Colace, which is not an irritant); castor oil (Neoloid Purge); Agoral, Correctol, Ex-Lax, and Feen-a-Mint (all of which contain phenolphthalein); and Fletcher's Castoria, Perdiem, and Senokot (all of which contain senna).

• Narcotic-type pain or cough medicines, including codeine, Demerol, Hycodan, and Robitussin-DM.

• Calcium or iron nutritional supplements.

• Aluminum-containing antacids.

• Calcium channel blockers.

• Aspirinlike nonsteroidal antiinflammatory medicines.

• Anticholinergic-type irritable bowel medicines, such as Donnatal and Levsin, and antipsychotic major tranquilizers (e.g., Thorazine).

• Antidepressants.

• Antihistamines, commonly used to treat both colds and allergies.

the divorce was finalized. She began to experience frequent constipation. The doctor she consulted prescribed a laxative.

Was this the right treatment?

FACTS: Emotional upset can cause diarrhea, gas, constipation, or a combination of these problems. Your doctor, like Arlene's, isn't likely to think of this unless she has reason to suspect that you are upset or asks questions about your emotional state. Unfortunately, many physicians these days focus only on physical problems, not on mental concerns. If this doctor had probed a little or if he had known her longer, he might have learned about the turmoil in Arlene's family life and might have made the connection between that and her constipation.

WHAT TO DO: If you're experiencing constipation and you are also going through some unusual emotional stress, including anxiety or depression, be sure to disclose these facts to your doctor. Also, if you know that you're inclined to become constipated when you're upset or otherwise confronting emotional problems, tell your physician about this characteristic as well.

The best antidote to Arlene's constipation would probably not have been the laxatives that were prescribed, but rather, a psychotherapist. Those who are able to lower their stress levels, either through professional counseling or simply by "talking the problem through" with friends or family members, are much less likely to experience emotion-triggered constipation. (Of course, it would also have been important for her to focus on the practical advice described in the box The Basics of Promoting Regular Bowel Movements, pp. 225–226.)

One great advantage of developing a long-term relationship with a personal physician is that you will probably be more comfortable discussing emotional issues. Also, the doctor is more likely to recognize, without being told, when you are having emotionally related distress.

E R R O R :

Not Recognizing Diarrhea Caused by Antibiotics as a Potentially Life-Threatening Emergency

I had been treating Ann, the mother of a local psychiatrist, with heavy doses of antibiotics for a difficult case of chronic sinusitis. After about a week, her stool became loose. I had told her this might happen and asked her to give me a call if it did. But with so much else going on in her care, I had not specifically warned her that this side effect might actually be dangerous.

Over the weekend, her diarrhea worsened, but because she was mostly concerned about her sinuses, she decided to keep taking the antibiotic. To control the loose stool, she took Imodium, an anti-diarrhea medicine recently made available without prescription. That choice, though it seemed logical, might have actually proven fatal, but fortunately, she was taken off of the Imodium in time.

What Kind of Laxative Should You Take?

If your doctor feels you need a laxative, here are some of the considerations that you should keep in mind and that he should discuss with you in choosing a drug:

- *Irritant-type laxatives.* These are listed in the box Drugs That Often Cause Constipation, p. 228. Although these are popular because your doctor wants you to experience quick results, they can be habit-forming and tend to worsen constipation by reducing the ability of your bowel to move on its own.

- *Lubricant-type laxatives.* These include mineral oil and related medications and are popular and effective for short-run relief. Unlike the irritant laxatives, the lubricants are not habit-forming. But chronic reliance on them can inhibit absorption of vitamins and minerals by your body. Also, older people may breathe (aspirate) mineral oil into their lungs and, as a result, get pneumonia.

- *Stool softeners.* These include docusate sodium (Colace), docusate potassium (Dialose), and docusate calcium (Surfak). They are detergents that soften the stool by dispersing the feces in water. This process helps in the short run but is much less helpful when the medications are used for a long time.

- *Fiber or bulk-type laxatives.* Most physicians properly place a high priority on bulk-forming laxatives, such as psyllium (Metamucil, Naturacil), methylcellulose (Citrucell), malt extract (Maltsupex), and polycarbophil (FiberCon). These act by increasing the stool's water and bulk. This action usually stimulates the intestines to contract and thus moves the feces toward and then out of the rectum. The resulting soft, bulkier stools are easier to pass than hard, dehydrated ones.
  Caution: Bulk-forming laxatives *must* be taken with large amounts of fluid, or they may actually make constipation worse.

- *Osmotic-type laxatives.* These can be quite effective and are acceptable for longer-term use. They stimulate the bowel with a large number of nonabsorbable particles. ("Gas" is a common side effect.) Examples are Chronulac, Duphalac, CoLyte, and GoLyteley.

Another group of much more potent osmotic laxatives contain magnesium (Milk of Magnesia, Haley's M-O) or sodium phosphate (Phospho Soda, Fleet enema). These work very quickly and are effective for severe constipation. But they can cause dehydration and may upset the balance of mineral levels in the blood, so they aren't recommended for regular use.

- *Enemas and suppositories.* Tap water enemas and glycerine suppositories act by distending the rectum and lower bowel, an action that stimulates their contraction. Some people find them to be quite useful on occasion, either by themselves or in addition to other types of laxatives. But don't routinely add irritating agents, such as a soap suds enema or Dulcolax, to these locally acting laxatives. Irritant suppositories can damage the rectum.

FACTS: Many people suffer intestinal irritation with loose stools and mild diarrhea from taking antibiotics. Mixed in among these cases, like a deadly needle in a haystack, is a potentially life-threatening form of diarrhea caused by an intestinal bacteria known as *Clostridium difficile* or *C. difficile.* When antibiotics kill off large numbers of the normal intestinal bacteria, *C. difficile* ''bugs'' may take advantage of the opportunity to increase their normally tiny share of intestinal living space. *C. difficile* produces a toxin that, when present in large enough amounts, attacks intestinal tissue to cause diarrhea. The severity of this condition can range from very mild to massive and bloody.

The three worst things you can do for antibiotic-induced diarrhea that is caused by *C. difficile* are: (1) keep taking the antibiotic, (2) take an antidiarrhea medicine (which will prevent your body from expelling the toxin), and (3) fail to tell your doctor *immediately* so that he can start treating the problem.

Ann, unfortunately, wasn't aware of these three points—and she had decided not to bother her ''busy'' psychiatrist daughter. She made all three mistakes and suffered three days in the hospital with severe dehydration before we got her back under control.

Is it realistic to expect every doctor to review what to do about possible diarrhea every time he prescribes an antibiotic? Perhaps not, but I've certainly redoubled my effort to be vigilant since this incident occurred—and I would advise other physicians to do the same. In any event, you should be aware of the dangers and alert your physician if you sense there is a problem with your antibiotic.

WHAT TO DO: Notify your doctor if you develop loose, frequent stools while taking an antibiotic, especially if you have previously taken that drug with no problem. This is an especially urgent concern if the diarrhea is severe, if there is any blood in your stool or if you develop fever. *Do not* take any medicine to stop the diarrhea or keep taking the antibiotic unless you are specifically told to do so by your doctor. If he does suggest that you continue with the antibiotic, be sure to raise the question of *C. difficile* just to be sure that he has considered this possibility.

Some physicians feel that patients who must take long courses of antibiotics should also take live yogurt cultures or acidophilus capsules, which are available in most health food stores. This step, which should at least do no harm, may increase your supply of the "friendly" bacteria that normally live in the gut and that act as natural competitors to *C. difficile* and other such invaders.

Irritable Bowel Syndrome

ERROR:

*Your Doctor Overtests You for Irritable Bowel
Syndrome*

Mary was a 42-year-old with a fifteen-year history of abdominal cramps; bloating; and loose, frequent bowel movements alternating with constipation. In being evaluated for her problems, she had consulted with two general practitioners, three gastroenterologists, one psychiatrist, and one parasitologist (an expert in treating parasites).

The tests performed on her included one gastroscopy (using a fiber-optic tube to look down into the stomach), one upper gastrointestinal (GI) series X ray, one barium enema X ray; two flexible sigmoidoscopies (using a 2-foot-long tube to look into the large intestine from the rectum), and two colonoscopies (using a 5-foot-long tube inserted through the rectum so that the entire length of the large intestine can be viewed). Total charges for the doctors and use of a hospital's outpatient procedure room were in excess of $4,000.

Mary's doctors said they wanted to be sure that "nothing important is being missed." After the first evaluation, her family doctor said, "I think it's just an irritable bowel. But it won't hurt to do some further tests."

But the "further tests" seemed to go on endlessly. Although Mary had felt reassured after the first examination, she had become frustrated at hearing the same thing—"It's probably just irritable bowel"—after each subsequent procedure. At the end of all the tests, they seemed pleased that they could assure her once more, "There's nothing really wrong. Just a case of irritable bowel."

At that point, Mary exploded. "I *know* I have irritable bowel, but what I want is *treatment!*"

Who was right here: Mary or her doctors?

FACTS: Mary was right for a number of reasons. I hope my gastroenterology colleagues will forgive me because I do respect and value their sophisticated technical skills. But many, if not most of them, view irritable bowel patients as a necessary evil that helps them pay the rent so that they focus their attention on what they feel they were best trained to do. And that means to diagnose and treat "real" GI diseases, such as ulcerative colitis, cancer of the bowel, bleeding ulcers, and Crohn's disease.

Irritable bowel syndrome (IBS), which affects 10 to 20 percent of the adult population in the United States, can be frustrating for patients and physicians. Patients' symptoms wax and wane but rarely ever go away. Because of the "slippery" nature of the symptoms, many doctors, deep down in their guts, view IBS as mainly psychological and hence not quite legitimate. Certainly, they don't feel it's the kind of a problem that a highly trained doctor oriented toward the latest high-tech procedures is supposed to be treating.

As a result, the typical gastroenterologist or other specialist will tend to order a wide battery of tests to exhaust every possible alternative to IBS. When this has been done, the doctor often shows a marked lack of enthusiasm for the slow, detailed, and unexciting work of modifying the dietary or psychological factors that may be triggering the IBS.

The fact is that most IBS patients don't need any more GI procedures than the rest of us, especially if, like Mary, they are under 50 and have had a stable pattern of symptoms for more than five years. (See the accompanying box for typical signs and symptoms of IBS.) One flexible sigmoidoscopy and perhaps a stool test will usually do nicely, and some authorities even question whether these procedures are necessary.

WHAT TO DO: If your problem involves a stable, long-term pattern of recurring symptoms like abdominal pain, gas, diarrhea, or constipation, be skeptical of the need for a battery of expensive high-tech tests. You probably don't need to undergo GI X rays or fiber-optic procedures to evaluate your large bowel or stomach. Be particularly gun-shy if you've had these procedures before and your doctor wants to repeat them "just to be sure nothing has been missed."

Of course, there are good reasons for doing extensive GI procedures, such as situations where your stool turns dark black (a sign of blood), you begin to lose weight even though you aren't on a diet, or your pattern of symptoms changes. Also, like everyone else, IBS patients need periodic cancer detection exams.

Still, your time and money and your doctor's energies are usually best served by first making a tentative diagnosis of IBS from your symptoms. Then, the bulk of your time and effort can be spent looking for factors that can be corrected so as to relieve your IBS discomfort.

ERROR:

Insisting That You Continue a High-Fiber Diet Even Though Your IBS Seems to Be Getting Worse

In response to a diagnosis of IBS, Stan dutifully followed his doctor's instructions to increase the fiber in his diet. He added several extra helpings of fruits and vegetables and also increased the amount of

Typical Signs and Symptoms of IBS

Some leading gastroenterologists have recently proposed simple criteria for diagnosing IBS—criteria that don't require extensive GI tests. According to these standards, you have IBS if you have certain continuous or recurrent symptoms for at least three months:

1. Abdominal pain or discomfort relieved by moving your bowels or associated with a change in frequency or consistency of your stool AND

2. An irregular or varying pattern of bowel movements at least 25 percent of the time, which includes three or more of the following:

- Altered stool frequency.

- Altered stool form (hard or loose, watery stool).

- Altered stool passage (straining or urgency, feeling of complete evacuation).

- Passage of mucus.

- Bloating or feeling of abdominal distension.

insoluble wheat bran he was consuming every day. But his intestinal gas and abdominal distress grew worse.

The doctor said, "I wonder if you're really eating as much fiber as you say. High fiber usually takes care of this."

Was the doctor right?

FACTS: No, in this case, the doctor was wrong. Many IBS patients do improve when they increase their intake of high-fiber foods, such as fruits, vegetables, whole grains, or psyllium-containing supplements, including Metamucil. This approach is particularly effective when constipation is a major symptom.

But there are also many IBS patients who actually get *worse* after increasing their fiber, especially those like Stan, whose dominant symptoms include gas and abdominal distress. The reason for this problem is that bacteria in the gut digest the high-fiber foods and release gas as a by-product.

Many IBS patients find that a relatively new synthetic form of fiber—calcium polycarbophil—provides better relief with fewer gas problems. Gut bacteria are less able to digest this product, as they digest natural fibers. Polycarbophil is available as a tablet under the brand names Fiberall Chewable Tablets Lemon Flavored, FiberCon, and Mitrolan.

Caution: You must take these and all fiber supplements with a large glass of water.

WHAT TO DO: If you have IBS and especially if constipation is one of your main symptoms, you should increase your intake of high-fiber foods for a trial period of two weeks or so. If you find that increased intestinal gas becomes a problem, back off until you feel better. Then try increasing doses of a polycarbophil formula.

If high fiber still does not help, discuss alternatives with your doctor. Some possibilities include an elimination diet, enzyme supplements, or behavioral approaches. (See the next three error discussions.)

ERROR:

Your Doctor Lacks the Patience to Help You Identify a Particular Food That May Be Causing IBS

Thomas continued to suffer from regular bouts of diarrhea, pain in the abdomen, and gas, even though he was following closely the general high-fiber dietary recommendations of his doctor. Thomas suspected that something in his lifestyle might be contributing to the IBS, because usually when he went on a vacation or business trip, the condition got better. His doctor had no comment when Thomas reported these variations in his symptoms. Finally Thomas figured out the answer. At home his wife included garlic or onions in almost every evening meal. Away from home, Tom omitted these irritating foods, which turned out to be a major cause of his IBS symptoms.

FACTS: Except for the importance of consuming fiber, many doctors underestimate the significance of *specific* foods in setting off IBS. Even allergists often abandon the search for specific foods that may cause vague or hard-to-evaluate symptoms, such as abdominal distress. It's quite difficult to identify a response to a single food, which may take two to three days to pass through your gut.

Still, many foods that we eat all the time are potential triggers for IBS symptoms, the ones that Thomas was experiencing—gas, abdominal pain, and diarrhea. In many IBS patients—about 40 percent in my practice—eliminating trigger foods can make a big difference in the way the people feel. Here are some of the foods that have been found in certain individuals to make IBS worse:

- Milk, including hidden milk in breads and cakes.

- "Gassy" foods, such as beans, cabbage, and cauliflower.

- Fruits and vegetables, especially if they are eaten raw.

- Caffeine and also, in some situations, decaffeinated coffee.

- Spices and flavor enhancers, especially garlic, onion, and hot pepper.

- Sorbitol, a carbohydrate added to gums, diet sodas, and some other foods.

- Wheat.

- Sugars.

- Yeast.

WHAT TO DO: If you have IBS and you and your doctor can't seem to find and eliminate the cause, focus on specific foods you're eating. Begin with a diary, in which you should list everything you eat and also the variations in your symptoms. See if you can spot which foods are suspect.

If keeping a food diary doesn't help, take the next essential step: Ask a physician who is interested in nutrition or a registered dietitian to supervise you in an *elimination diet*. The health professional you select should have had some experience working with patients on elimination diets.

Note: Allergy blood and skin tests are notoriously inaccurate for identifying most food triggers of irritable bowel. The reason is that most reactive foods act by irritating the bowel, not by a true allergic reaction, which is all that allergy tests are designed to detect.

An ideal elimination diet will allow you to eat only foods that you usually eat fewer than two times a week and that don't seem to worsen your symptoms. Also, these foods should rank low on the list of usual IBS triggers. Typically, you'll be limited to three to ten foods for a one- to two-week period. If reaction to a specific food is the cause of your IBS, you should improve dramatically while you're on this diet.

At the end of the two weeks, begin to reintroduce your regular foods one at a time. As a general rule, you should reintroduce each new food for three to six consecutive meals and then watch for any symptoms so that you can be sure to identify those factors that are giving you problems. When you find the offending food or foods, they should be eliminated from your diet for at least a few months before trying them again.

Caution: Reintroducing a "sensitive" or allergic food after several days absence can trigger a more intense reaction than occurs when the same food is eaten every day. So definitely consult with a physician, preferably an allergist, before doing an elimination diet—especially if the reactions you might get are potentially dangerous (e.g., asthma, hives, anaphylaxis, or severe migraine).

ERROR:

An Enzyme Deficiency, Which Your Doctor Has Overlooked, Is Contributing to Your IBS

Andrea, a great salad lover, has been experiencing symptoms of IBS for several years. These symptoms included excessive gas and abdominal discomfort. Her doctor had ordered a number of medical procedures and was now emphasizing Andrea's need to increase the fiber in her diet, including her vegetable and fruit consumption. But if anything, her symptoms seemed to get worse.

What was the doctor's mistake?

FACTS: At least 5 percent of the patients I see for IBS have unrecognized deficiencies of certain digestive enzymes that are contributing substantially to their symptoms. Often, other physicians they have seen have overlooked the enzyme connection.

By far, the most frequent enzyme problem involves lactase, the enzyme that normally digests milk sugar (lactose). In the United States, about 10 percent of white people and about 40 percent of African-Americans have a limited ability to make lactase. When their intake of milk products gets too high, they begin to suffer from gas, bloating, abdominal pain, or diarrhea.

Fortunately, there's often an easy solution to this problem. You can buy lactose-free milk or take a lactase enzyme supplement just before eating dairy foods.

Other enzymes help digest starch in beans and leafy vegetables—and that is where Andrea's problem comes to the fore. But like those with milk sugar intolerance, these patients also have a possible solution: They can use Beano, a recently introduced supplement with the appropriate enzymes, which is available in drug and health food stores. (Note: some experts question Beano's effectiveness. It's still new enough that I don't yet have a firm opinion on its general use, but it certainly seems to work well with some people.)

Although most IBS patients have nothing wrong with their pancreas, every so often I meet someone who shows dramatic improvement after taking a low-dose supplement of pancreatic digestive enzymes. Other people, especially senior citizens, may suffer from poor digestion because of inadequate acid in the stomach. This lack can be helped with an acidic supplement, betaine hydrochloride.

Swallowing too much air can also cause IBS-like symptoms. The excess air may result from talking while you eat or from drinking too much carbonated beverage. Poor chewing due to missing teeth or painful gums can also disturb digestion.

WHAT TO DO: For most enzyme-related IBS problems, you don't even have to see your doctor at first. For a week or so, you should try experimenting with eliminating milk products or taking a lactase enzyme supplement, which you can buy over the counter. If that doesn't work, try taking Beano with beans or vegetables. Finally, if you're still having IBS symptoms, you might see what happens when you use an over-the-counter pancreatic digestive supplement for just a few days.

If none of these works, you may have a problem with inadequate acid in your stomach—a situation that can be trickier. Taking acid supplements can irritate the esophagus or stomach. So it's important to use this approach only after consulting with your doctor.

ERROR:

Your Doctor Overlooks a Possible Psychological Component to Your IBS

Donald, a 48-year-old advertising executive, was constantly under stress, so much so that he usually felt at loose ends when he tried to take a holiday or vacation. He felt he needed the steady pressure to make life fulfilling and exciting.

However, the chronic stress was taking its toll. He began to suffer from borderline high blood pressure, and he also developed classic IBS symptoms, such as diarrhea, excessive gas, and abdominal discomfort.

In trying to treat his IBS, Donald's doctor downplayed the possible psychological component and focused more on medications and diet.

Was the doctor right?

FACTS: Popular impressions notwithstanding, most IBS patients are no more neurotic than anyone else. Still, it's a generally accepted medical fact that stress usually makes IBS symptoms worse. Furthermore, in some patients—though certainly not all—chronic exposure to stress can be a dominant trigger for IBS symptoms.

Unfortunately, many people who are suffering from chronic stress don't recognize its importance because they have become so accustomed to the pressure that it almost seems normal. That was the situation in which Donald found himself.

Donald's doctor mentioned that stress might contribute to Don's symptoms. But, pressured for time, he was reluctant to trigger a long, intimate discussion of the issue, and so he allowed the discussion to drift on to other matters. Some doctors do discuss stress but convey a judgmental attitude that in effect says, "Stress may be a factor, but you're the one who has to take care of that. If you allow stress to take over your life, that's your fault, not mine." Or a doctor may somehow suggest that the stress is "all in the mind" of the patient and should somehow just be made to disappear.

Such an approach is obviously unhelpful. If you are experiencing IBS, if you and your doctor can't find the source of the problem, and if you are also under a great deal of stress, then your doctor should either work with you to clarify the role of the stress or refer you to a professional who is able to help you.

WHAT TO DO: If dietary manipulation or other measures don't give you relief from IBS, you and your doctor should evaluate how important stress may be as an IBS trigger.

One approach you might take is for your doctor to refer you for a two- or three-session evaluation with a psychologist or psychiatrist. The purpose of these consultations is to decide whether stress is really a problem. Psychotherapy makes the most sense if anxiety or depression is affecting your life severely. If emotions pose such a problem, meeting with a mental health specialist will place you in a position to evaluate just how significant a problem you have and also the best way to treat it.

Warning: Do *not* enter into open-ended, long-term psychotherapy unless you agree after your initial evaluation that such extensive treatment really makes sense.

Another stress-reducing strategy that I have found to be quite helpful for many IBS patients is to seek training in simple relaxation techniques. These might include self-hypnosis, visual imagery, deep muscle relaxation, meditation, biofeedback, or regular endurance exercise, such as fast walking or jogging. Recent research indicates that for people with IBS who don't improve much through dietary manipulation, relaxation training is often very helpful—considerably more so, in many cases, than traditional "talk" psychotherapy.

ERROR:

Your Doctor Diagnoses You as Having IBS When You Really Have Parasites

When I was 12 years old, I developed severe abdominal pain, gas, and diarrhea. Life was misery. Six doctors I saw said, "Too much stress." My mother replied, "Nonsense."

Finally, a parasite specialist, whom I'll never forget, took a swab from my stool, looked at it under the microscope, and said my real problem was amoebas. After being treated with one medicine for six weeks, my "irritable bowel syndrome" was gone for good.

FACTS: There's no question that amoebas, *Giardia,* and other intestinal parasites can mimic IBS and cause symptoms for months or even years. But many doctors dismiss these possibilities as not "middle-class" diseases. Not so! These conditions are easily transmitted and not at all rare among those in every socioeconomic group. Ironically, supposedly "clear" mountain rivers and lakes and wells are often infested with *Giardia,* which may be the most common intestinal parasite in the United States.

A big problem, however, is that a single stool test for parasites can often miss a particular parasite despite the presence of that creature in your intestines. You need a minimum of three stool samples, and even then, the parasite might be missed. Even multiple stool samples may miss *Giardia,* for instance. A gastroenterologist may have to pass a long tube into the duodenum to obtain an adequate sample for examination.

Of course, everyone agrees that parasites can masquerade as IBS. But a few doctors, mainly those of a holistic or nutritional orientation, feel that much, if not most, IBS is due to overlooked parasite infections. They argue that symptoms can be triggered by a common variant of amoeba or by an overgrowth of intestinal yeast. Most physicians disagree with this position, however; they feel that the amoeba or intestinal yeast found in these tests is relatively harmless.

WHAT TO DO: If your IBS symptoms don't respond to diet or to relaxation training, be sure you have been checked for intestinal parasites and other intestinal infections. Be especially persistent if your IBS symptoms are predominantly gas, bloating, abdominal discomfort, or diarrhea and if these symptoms are relatively recent. Also, be particularly persistent if your symptoms began after a period out of the country or after a hiking or camping trip.

Hepatitis

Although You Are Sexually Active, You Haven't Been Immunized Against Hepatitis

Beth, a 23-year-old, broke up with her fiancé after an engagement that lasted for six months. Within a few weeks, she began a very serious relationship with a new companion. In both cases, she engaged regularly in sexual intercourse, and she didn't consider her sexual behavior in any way unusual for a single woman of her generation.

Beth saw no reason to discuss her personal romantic life with her doctor, nor did her doctor make any inquiries. So understandably, she was shocked when she was diagnosed a few months later with hepatitis. The question of whether she had needed a hepatitis immunization shot had simply never come up.

What was the problem here?

FACTS: Most people who need immunization against hepatitis are not receiving it. In fact, hepatitis B increased by more than a third during the 1980s to more than 300,000 new cases and 5,000 deaths per year. Fortunately, we now have vaccines that are highly effective for preventing hepatitis B, the most common serious type of the disease. But unfortunately, many high-risk patients do not know about the vaccine, and physicians are lax in recommending it.

Yet ultimately, as the public health situation grows worse, I predict that we'll try to give *everyone* the three-shot vaccination series against hepatitis B, just as we do for polio and whooping cough. Whether you're an ordinary junior high school student or a grandmother in a nursing home, it will be a medical error for you not to get the vaccination.

Current guidelines recommend vaccinating all infants and people in high-risk groups, a definition that's broad enough to include at least half the population. Here are groups that are considered at high risk:

- Sexually active heterosexual men and women who have acquired other sexually transmitted diseases or who have had more than one sexual partner in the previous six months. (Beth was in this latter category.) Given prevailing social mores, it may be medical error not to give this shot to most junior high and high school students.

- Health workers and others who have contact with blood.

- Clients and staff of institutions for the developmentally disabled.

- Household contacts and sexual partners of persons who are carriers of hepatitis B.

- Sexually active homosexual and bisexual men.

- Kidney dialysis patients and staff.

- Adoptees from countries with a high rate of hepatitis B.

- International travelers who plan to spend more than six months in areas with high rates of hepatitis B or who are likely to have sexual contact or contact with blood in those areas.

- Intravenous drug users.

- Inmates of long-term prisons.

- Infants born to women who are carriers of hepatitis B.

WHAT TO DO: Regardless of your social, economic, or occupational status, you should seek a hepatitis B vaccination from a public health clinic (where it may be offered free or at low cost) or from your private doctor. Don't wait to be invited!

If you do become infected with hepatitis, you will probably develop lifelong antibodies against the particular type of hepatitis virus that infected you. Unfortunately, this immunity does not extend to other kinds of hepatitis virus.

As you begin to feel better, it remains important that your blood be monitored by a physician. Some people do not develop protective antibodies. Even though they may feel perfectly well, they still carry the hepatitis virus and might infect others. Blood tests can tell whether your antibodies have developed. You should also have periodic liver function tests since a certain proportion of hepatitis victims continue to undergo low-grade inflammation, which can damage the liver. Newer treatments, such as interferon, can be used in such cases.

ERROR:

Your Teenager Receives a Hepatitis Shot but in the Wrong Part of the Body

Mark, a 14-year-old boy who was scheduled to visit a Latin American country with a relatively high incidence of hepatitis B, was given a hepatitis immunization shot in the buttock.

What was wrong with this?

FACTS: Mark was clearly in one of the high-risk groups listed under the previous error, and he should have received the shot. But for reasons that we don't completely understand, the hepatitis B vaccine is much more likely to provide protection if you get it in the deltoid muscle of the upper arm and shoulder rather than in the traditional shot site, the buttock.

WHAT TO DO: Except for infants and young children, who may receive it in the upper leg, be sure that any hepatitis shots you get are given in the upper arm.

ERROR:

Your Doctor Forgets That Hepatitis May Be Involved When You Have Flulike Symptoms

Cora suffered from weakness and fatigue and a feverish feeling for nearly two weeks before she went to see her doctor. He diagnosed her as having one of the flu viruses that was going around and told her to wait and come back to see him in a week or two if she didn't feel better.

The symptoms continued for another ten days, and Cora made another doctor's appointment. At that time, the doctor performed a complete series of blood tests, which he hadn't done before, and discovered that Cora's basic liver chemistries were abnormal. She was diagnosed with hepatitis B.

FACTS: A common mistake doctors make is not to think of hepatitis when a viral illness, "mono," or the flu becomes more severe or lasts longer than expected. You don't have to have the more common symptoms, such as skin that turns yellow or urine that turns dark, to have severe hepatitis. Furthermore, hepatitis can follow many kinds of viral illness, some bacterial infections, all kinds of chemical toxins, and, of course, alcohol abuse.

WHAT TO DO: If you develop a virusllike illness, fever, weakness, or fatigue and the cause can't be identified within two weeks, you may have hepatitis. Remind your doctor, in case he forgets, that you should receive a complete set of blood tests that include an evaluation of your basic liver chemistries. The technical name for one type of such blood test is the *SMA panel*.

ERROR:

Failing to Monitor Your Liver Inflammation

Hal was diagnosed as having hepatitis B, and he was placed on a schedule for regular blood tests to check his liver function. Because he felt extremely tired from a business trip the day he was due to return for his blood test, he decided to skip it to stay home and rest. His doctor's office failed to remind him that he had missed an important checkup.

FACTS: About 1 percent of infectious hepatitis victims have an extremely rocky course of treatment, where liver inflammation may careen out of control. That's why it's extremely important for liver function to be monitored regularly, especially during the first few weeks of the illness, just to see how well the patient's condition is stabilizing.

Liver failure can quickly stop the manufacture of key chemicals needed for the normal clotting of blood, and internal bleeding may result. Also, continued liver failure can result in coma and in the most severe cases an early death rate of 70 to 90 percent of patients.

The tragedy is that with meticulous medical support and care, many of these patients could have been saved. The liver has an immense power to regenerate its cells—if it's given the opportunity and time to do so.

Also, failing to follow up on hepatitis patients will place those people with whom they come in contact at risk. People who seem to recover from hepatitis B and C often still carry the virus in their blood. They can infect others through sexual relations, blood contamination, or mother-to-fetus contact during pregnancy. There are an estimated two million hepatitis B carriers in the United States and an unknown but probably large number of infectious carriers of hepatitis C.

WHAT TO DO: If you're diagnosed with hepatitis, you can't assume that your real health status is reflected by how well you feel. Many hepatitis victims are absolutely miserable, yet most of them won't become dangerously ill. On the other hand, some who have only mild or moderate symptoms may still be in an extremely dangerous position.

So it's essential to keep tracking liver function tests during the first weeks of the illness. This way, a doctor can separate out those whose inflammation is leveling off and focus treatment on the small minority who have what doctors call *fulminant,* or very serious, hepatitis.

If liver inflammation continues or grows worse, the doctor should also track blood clotting through prothrombin time (PT) and partial thromboplastin time (PTT). If these indicators begin to weaken, your doctor will have to intensify her monitoring of your condition, probably by referring you to a gastroenterologist or a liver specialist.

For hepatitis B, simple blood tests are available to determine whether a recovering patient is still infectious. We don't yet have such a test for hepatitis C, but we probably will within a few years. Even without these special tests, routine liver function tests, which measure inflammation, can provide a fairly good idea of who might still be infected and contagious. If blood test results show that inflammation is still present, continued surveillance is necessary, even if the patient feels well. This monitoring is required to limit the possibility of infecting others and to treat potential late-stage complications in the patient himself.

Alpha-interferon, a natural body hormone now available through biotechnology production, has greatly increased our ability to treat people who develop chronic or progressive hepatitis.

ERROR:

Your Doctor Prescribes Standard Doses of Medicine Despite Your Having Liver Disease

Paul, who was in his midseventies, had been diagnosed with an early case of cirrhosis (chronic scarring) of the liver and was placed on a medication at what was usually considered a normal, or standard, dosage. His condition worsened.

What went wrong?

FACTS: Typically, medicines are metabolically processed, deactivated, or excreted from the body by the action of chemical pathways in the liver. Liver damage may reduce the effectiveness of these pathways and allow the levels of medicine to accumulate to dangerous levels in the body. This means that what is an average or even a low dose for someone with a healthy liver could be a severe or even deadly overdose for someone whose liver isn't well.

WHAT TO DO: If you have a liver disease like cirrhosis or hepatitis and especially if your SMA blood profile suggests continuing liver inflammation, don't count on your doctor to remember this fact! Remind him *every time* he suggests or prescribes a new medicine or increases the dose of an old one. It's advisable to ask him specifically if the medicine involved is one whose dose should be lowered for patients who have liver problems such as yours.

Always inspect the package insert or look up each new medicine in the *Physician's Desk Reference* (*PDR*), which should be available in your local library. The manufacturer usually makes a specific statement if the dose of that medicine should be reduced for people with liver disease.

ERROR:

Your Doctor Prescribes a Drug That Makes Your Liver Damage Worse

Herbert was placed on a popular cholesterol-lowering medication and was told in general terms that he should "come back for a checkup in a few months." Nothing was said about the importance of a follow-up liver function blood test. He continued on the medication faithfully for more than a year but never found time to return for an interim checkup. When he did have his annual physical, a blood test revealed that his liver functions were impaired.

What went wrong?

FACTS: Almost every drug can trigger liver inflammation in a rare susceptible person, and we have to live with this uncertainty whenever we prescribe or use drugs. But certain drugs are more likely than others to irritate the liver. These should be watched closely in people who have had a recent case of hepatitis, who have ongoing diseases of the liver, or who turn out to be especially sensitive to certain medications.

You should be particularly alert to the potential liver toxicity of two very popular over-the-counter medicines: acetaminophen (Tylenol), which is a painkiller; and niacin (vitamin B$_3$), which is used to control cholesterol.

Tylenol in high doses damages the liver, particularly if you also drink alcohol. Niacin is safe in the low doses contained in most multivitamins. But in the high doses that are used to lower blood cholesterol—and especially above 3,000 milligrams per day—niacin can cause liver inflammation in many people. In a March 1994 issue of *The Journal of the American Medical Association,* researchers from the Medical College of Virginia confirmed earlier findings and concluded that the sustained-release niacin (which many patients prefer because it causes less flushing) was more toxic to the liver than the standard non-sustained-release type.

If you already have liver damage or disease, the risk of problems from these two drugs increases significantly. Here's a list of a few drugs that are most likely to harm a patient with a damaged liver: acetaminophen (Tylenol), Accutane, alcohol, Aldomet, anabolic steroids, Antabuse, Bactrim, Capoten, Dilantin, Fansidar, Elavil, Floxin, Mevacor, niacin, Normodyne, Pravachol, Prinivil, Prozac, Quinaglute, Septra, testosterone, Vasotec, Zestril, Zocor.

WHAT TO DO: If you have liver disease, ask your doctor *and* pharmacist about the potential effect on the liver of any new drug you may be considering. To be doubly sure, ask your pharmacist for a copy of the package insert, or look up the new medicine in the *PDR* or a similar drug reference book, which you should be able to find in your library or doctor's office.

Even if you don't have liver disease, check to see if you are taking or are scheduled to take any of the medications listed under the Facts section. If you're on any of these drugs or another drug that your doctor confirms may have a negative impact on your liver, be sure to take regular blood tests (initially after a month or two and then at least every three to four months) to check your liver function.

Again, most standard drug references such as the *PDR* and also the package insert, which your pharmacist will give you if you ask for it, should state very clearly if there is a significant risk of a medicine's tendency to cause liver damage.

ERROR:

You Are Infected with Hepatitis Through Contaminated Medical or Dental Instruments

Lon noticed that his wife, Jean, seemed to be unusually tired, and her skin took on a yellowish cast. A diabetic, Jean had just had her glucose checked at a hospital about eight weeks before these symptoms appeared. When she went in for a checkup, her doctor diagnosed her as having hepatitis B.

What happened?

FACTS: Although it doesn't happen often, hepatitis may be transmitted accidentally through contaminated medical or dental instruments. In most medical facilities, simple instruments such as needles are thrown away rather than reused. Still, many instruments are reused, and if they aren't cleaned thoroughly, they may transmit diseases like hepatitis from one patient to another.

For example, in one California hospital, during a nine-month period, twenty-six patients contracted hepatitis after having their blood sugar checked with a portable blood glucose testing meter. The needle used to prick the finger had been changed. It was apparently the permanent plastic base that holds the needles that was contaminated. (That may have been what happened to Jean.)

Another offending instrument is the sigmoidoscope, which is used to examine the rectum and colon (large intestine). This device contains tiny channels through which the doctor can inject fluids, air, or biopsy clippers. These instruments are notoriously difficult to clean, particularly with the hand-scrubbing methods used by many individual doctors.

How can patients protect themselves? More expensive and effective cleaning machines are used in most hospitals. Also, a new type of sigmoidoscope, with a throwaway outer sheath, might help solve the problem of contamination, but this device is only now becoming available to doctors.

Finally, inadequately sterilized dental instruments are a dangerous channel for transferring contagious diseases like hepatitis from one patient to another.

WHAT TO DO: Much of this problem is beyond your control because you're not the one in charge of cleaning the instruments that are to be used on you. But it's still wise to ask your doctor and dentist how their instruments are cleaned to prevent cross-contamination. Just letting them know you're concerned will make them more alert to cleaning the devices they use more thoroughly. You want to do your best to make them *compulsive* about cleaning things!

Do not allow reuse of instruments when disposables are available. I know at least one allergist who, when I last checked about three years ago, was still washing and reusing needles and syringes instead of switching to throwaways. Make it clear to your doctor that such a practice is not acceptable to you.

ERROR:

After You Are Exposed to Hepatitis, You Are Given the Wrong Kind of Gamma Globulin

Richard was exposed to hepatitis B through sexual contact. When he went in to see his doctor, he was given a standard gamma globulin shot as a preventive measure. This was the wrong shot in this situation.

FACTS: The preventive vaccination for hepatitis B stimulates your immune system so that you can fight off the hepatitis B virus if you encounter it at some future date. But you may be exposed to hepatitis *before* you are immunized, such as through work you do in the health care industry or through sexual contact, as occurred with Richard.

To counter the threat from exposure to hepatitis, we used to give a shot of standard gamma globulin, which contains a broad spectrum of antibodies derived from the blood of human donors. This procedure is still often used preventively by people who will be traveling in areas with poor sanitation, where hepatitis A may be a threat.

But the standard type of gamma globulin isn't very effective against hepatitis B. Fortunately, we now have a product called *hepatitis B immune globulin* (HBIG), which provides a high concentration of antibodies specifically directed against hepatitis B.

WHAT TO DO: Find out the precise type of hepatitis that you've most likely been exposed to. If the disease is hepatitis B and you haven't already been immunized with the hepatitis B vaccine, you should receive the HBIG and *not* standard gamma globulin. The HBIG shot should be given as soon as possible and certainly within seven days of exposure. The standard course of a hepatitis B preventive vaccine should also be started.

ERROR:

Failing to Take an Accurate Alcohol History from Patients with Hepatitis

I remember once that I was completely fooled by a patient who fell sick with symptoms that suggested a liver problem. In response to my questions, he told me he drank two alcoholic drinks a day, and that was truthful, as far as it went. Two drinks a day was all he'd had for the two days since he had fallen sick.

But the full story came out after I checked him into the local hospital. While there, he became very agitated, and after twenty-four hours, he had a seizure. Although he recovered quickly, he began to sweat and hallucinate. These were classic indications of withdrawal from alcohol addiction, or the condition known as *delirium tremens* (the DTs). It turned out that as a general practice, he drank a fifth of whiskey every day.

FACTS: Overdoing alcohol is an extremely common cause of hepatitis. Also, some patients with viral hepatitis who drink alcohol are placed in increased jeopardy of liver problems once they get sick. But physicians don't always obtain a realistic picture of a patient's alcohol intake, in part because patients, like mine described above, may be reluctant to admit how much they are drinking.

People who do drink are at risk for severe, even fatal symptoms of withdrawal from their addiction if their alcohol intake is decreased rapidly without any backup from drugs or medications. Yet it's essential that they cut back, especially if they are suffering from a liver problem like hepatitis. Your doctor must understand your drinking pattern correctly because withdrawal symptoms can easily be prevented if certain medications are begun along with your stopping alcohol consumption.

WHAT TO DO: Whether you have hepatitis or any other health problem, you should be sure to explain to your physician both your usual drinking habits and also your recent alcohol consumption. Being open about your drinking is especially important if you are ill or about to enter the hospital, where alcoholic drinks won't be available.

ERROR:

Your Elderly Father, a Heavy Drinker, Is Placed on an Intravenous Feeding Line, but He Is Not Given a Shot of Thiamine (Vitamin B_1)

An elderly man, a heavy drinker, had to check into the hospital with a variety of health problems, including symptoms indicating a liver problem. He was placed on an intravenous feeding line that fed glucose, a sugar, into his body. He began to experience irregular heartbeats and shortness of breath. It took considerable work on the part of the medical staff to stabilize his condition.

What happened?

FACTS: People who drink heavily or don't eat well or have both of these problems are often marginally deficient in thiamine (vitamin B_1). Infusing glucose intravenously can cause metabolic changes that further drain the body's supply of vitamin B_1. The resulting deficiency can be catastrophic, causing psychosis, heart failure, or even sudden death.

WHAT TO DO: If you drink three or more alcoholic drinks daily on a regular basis, you should play it safe. If you're scheduled for treatment in the hospital, ask your doctor to give you a shot of vitamin B_1 plus a general multivitamin supplement before she hooks you up to an intravenous glucose solution.

For more information on these and other liver problems, contact the American Liver Foundation, Cedar Grove, NJ 07009, phone 1-800-223-0179.

Gallbladder Complaints

ERROR:

Your Doctor Immediately Suggests Surgery When He Finds You Have Gallstones

Pamela's doctor discovered that she had gallstones and immediately suggested that she undergo surgery.

Was this necessary?

FACTS: About 20 million Americans have gallstones, but most authorities agree that just having gallstones is not a sufficient reason for taking out the gallbladder. In fact, studies have shown that if you have a "silent" gallstone, which isn't giving you any problems, your risk of developing symptoms from gallbladder inflammation (cholecystitis) is only about 2 percent per year.

Diabetics with gallstones are at a higher risk for problems and do less well with emergency operations. As a result, some experts have also argued for the preventive removal of gallstones and the gallbladder in diabetics, but again, most doctors disagree with this position.

A stronger, but still controversial case can be made for removing the gallbladder in people who have very large gallstones, in those whose entire gallbladder shows diffuse calcium deposits (a rare condition called *porcelain gallbladder*), and in women from certain Native American tribes who have a very high risk of cholecystitis and gallbladder cancer.

Most people who develop specific gallbladder symptoms should be treated with either medicines or surgery. Although many—

probably a majority—of those who recover completely from their first gallbladder attack never develop a serious second attack, a large minority do. The justification for treating people with even mild gallbladder symptoms is that when future attacks do occur, the risk of serious illness, emergency surgery, or death is unacceptably high.

The real problem with gallbladder surgery is not in operating too aggressively on those with true gallbladder symptoms, but in deciding which symptoms are really caused by an inflamed gallbladder and which—despite the presence of gallstones—are really due to nongallbladder causes. Too often, people receive gallbladder surgery as treatment for vague abdominal symptoms only to find after surgery that their problem remains.

Dr. Howard Spiro, chief of gastroenterology at Yale Medical School and author of a prestigious textbook on gastroenterology, puts it well: "The only two symptoms of gallstones are biliary colic and jaundice." Biliary colic is a very specific episodic pain that occurs in the right upper or middle abdomen, lasts one to five hours, and often awakens the patient at night. Jaundice, of course, turns people yellow.

Other common symptoms—such as nausea, abdominal pain after eating, heartburn, bloating, steady abdominal pain, belching, fatty food intolerance, abdominal cramps, or gas—can be triggered by gallstones, but can also be the result of many other conditions. Unless there is typical biliary colic, jaundice, or other good reason to believe that gallstones are the real problem, operating on the gallbladder exposes the patient to unnecessary risks and usually doesn't make him or her feel better.

The advent of laparoscopic surgery has changed the equation somewhat. This procedure—where the surgeon looks at and manipulates the gallbladder using tools that are passed into the abdomen through a small puncture in the abdominal wall—is much less traumatic than traditional surgery. Still, there are risks to laparoscopic surgery, especially when a surgeon is doing his first cases with the newer technique.

Because gallbladder surgery is now easier, the number of people having their gallbladder removed is rising, approaching the point where gallbladder surgery threatens to nose out hysterectomy as the most common operation. Although the risk for *each* operation is lower than with traditional surgery, the number of surgeries has so increased that the *total* number of deaths each year due to gallbladder surgery has hardly decreased at all. The moral: even with recent advances, you don't want your gallbladder taken out unless there's very good reason to believe that disease of the gallbladder is the real cause of your symptoms.

WHAT TO DO: If you feel well but your doctor, in the course of an exam, finds that you have gallstones, be skeptical of suggestions that your gallbladder should be removed. Obtain a second opinion. If the first and second opinions conflict, it usually makes sense to give the opinion of a gastroenterologist priority over that of a surgeon.

If your symptoms are mild, ask your surgeon and your gastroenterologist to explain the probable benefits and risks of operating now versus waiting to see if your symptoms disappear. Also, ask whether a nonsurgical alternative, such as dissolving the gallstones with medication or breaking them up with sound waves (lithotripsy), would be appropriate.

On the other hand, if your gallbladder symptoms are severe or worsening, you will probably require surgery to prevent your problem from turning into an emergency.

ERROR:

You Are Given an X Ray Instead of an Ultrasound Test of Your Gallbladder

Allen was diagnosed as having probable gallbladder disease and was scheduled for an X ray of the gallbladder. The test came back negative. A few weeks later, he learned that many doctors use an ultrasound test instead of X rays to prevent their patients from being exposed to unnecessary radiation. He raised this question with his doctor, who replied, "There's no problem with an X ray, and that was the best thing to do in your case."

Who was right?

FACTS: An ultrasound test of the gallbladder is usually preferred to the traditional gallbladder X ray. Gallbladder X rays (known as *oral cholecystograms*) are still a useful test, but they require an inconvenient, uncomfortable swallowing of an iodinated contrast agent the day before the exam. Furthermore, most experts these days feel that ultrasound (a kind of radar) provides a somewhat better picture without the need for exposure to X rays.

Like most medical tests, of course, ultrasound isn't infallible. It may miss as many as 15 percent of all stones. So if the ultrasound is not conclusive or if no stones are seen but gallbladder disease is still suspected, then a gallbladder X ray, or a high-tech nuclear scan of the gallbladder, should be considered.

WHAT TO DO: If your doctor leads off by recommending a gall-bladder X ray, ask why not perform an ultrasound test instead. The doctor may have a good reason for preferring the X ray, or he may just be out of date.

In any event, it's worth asking him about the ultrasound option and then seeing if his response makes sense. If he doesn't convince you, you might seek a second opinion.

E R R O R :

You Are Assigned an Inexperienced Surgeon for Your Gallbladder Operation

Michael was told he needed to have his gallbladder removed, and he was assigned a surgeon who used the new laparoscopic technique. This involves taking out the gallbladder without cutting open the abdomen, by inserting a slim instrument with a camera through a small hole in the abdomen.

During the operation, the surgeon severed an artery, and Michael's abdomen had to be opened up to repair the damage. Although he recovered completely, the healing process took three times as long as it should have.

How could this mistake have been prevented?

FACTS: About 600,000 gallbladder operations are performed each year in the United States, and about five to six years ago, most were done by standard surgical procedures, which involved cutting open the abdomen. All this changed after 1987, when surgeons in France introduced laparoscopic surgery. Now, the insertion of the slim lap-aroscope into the abdomen is the preferred method of gallbladder removal in 80 percent of operations. In using this technique, sur-geons insert cutting instruments and a small camera through small holes in the abdomen and manipulate these devices while they observe the action on a video screen.

The benefits of this kind of surgery, when it's done correctly, are that there is minimal pain after the operation, and the patient can be discharged and sent home in one to two days instead of one to two weeks.

But there are also some problems, as Michael found out. Even experienced, capable surgeons don't become expert at this radically different way of operating after just a weekend or even week of training. The field of vision provided by a laparoscope is narrow and two-dimensional (rather than three-dimensional). One expert has likened the feel of this type of surgery to picking up beans with chopsticks instead of with your fingers.

There is also a real risk of nicking nearby anatomical structures, including arteries and bile ducts. This problem almost never arises with traditional surgery, but it does happen with the laparoscope—and it did happen with Michael. For this reason, a significant number of operations that start out as laparoscopic have to be converted promptly to traditional open abdominal surgery.

There is a real learning curve with this type of surgery, with the large majority of complications seeming to occur in the surgeon's first dozen cases. The challenge is to find a surgeon who is experienced in this technique before you go under her knife.

WHAT TO DO: Ask your surgeon how many laparoscopic gallbladder operations she has done. One expert in this procedure told me that he'd prefer a minimum of forty successful cases before he would consider allowing a surgeon to operate on his own family member.

In addition, you have to consider the quality of the surgeon's experience. Learning by trial and error on your own is a much less reliable route than a formally supervised course of training. So ask the surgeon whether or not she has taken a course in laparoscopic surgery which required that she assist experienced laparoscopic surgeons in their operations. Also, ask how many cases she did under the supervision of a teacher before she left to practice on her own.

New surgeons learn laparoscopic training during their residencies. Everyone else should have enrolled in a formal training course, such as those sponsored by the Society of American Gastrointestinal Endoscopic Surgeons. Other courses, which may involve doing cases in the morning and then skiing in the afternoon, aren't the same as the SAGES program.

Your main defense against a less competent surgeon is your relationship with your family physician, internist, or gastroenterologist. Part of their job is to evaluate the reputation and skills of their surgical colleagues so as to be able to make wise referrals.

ERROR:

Your Aunt Is on a Low-Calorie Weight Loss Diet, but the Doctor Doesn't Warn Her About an Increased Risk for Gallstones

Aunt Edna was placed on a low-calorie weight loss diet, which involved about 600 calories a day of liquid protein, and she lost nearly 50 pounds in only about nine weeks. But then she started to experience classic gallstone symptoms—a pain radiating from the upper right abdomen into the right shoulder.

What could her doctor have done to prevent this result?

FACTS: Heavy people are much more likely to develop gallstones than people who are thin or normal weight. But ironically, when you go on a diet to decrease that extra weight—and especially if you lose the weight rapidly, as Aunt Edna did—your risk of developing gallstones and gallbladder inflammation increases.

Some studies suggest that as many as 1 to 2 percent of people on a 500- to 600-calorie liquid protein diet will develop new gallstones while on the diet or shortly thereafter. The added risk is probably less, but still significant, on a standard 1,200-calorie weight loss program.

Of course, the possibility of developing a gallbladder problem is no reason to stay heavy. But many people, even those in organized weight loss programs, have not been informed of their gallbladder risk or monitored for this complication.

WHAT TO DO: If you start a diet on your own or with an organized program, inform your physician. According to the calorie count of your diet and your own personal gallbladder risk, your physician should advise you about whether you should be consuming more calories. He may suggest a baseline ultrasound exam of the gallbladder as well as periodic physical examinations of your abdomen. He should also instruct you about which symptoms to report to him and whether or not a gallstone preventive medicine, such as Actigall, should be prescribed.

PART FOUR

When Your Problems Are Respiratory

Special Alerts: Respiratory Problems

- Your doctor assumes you have the flu when you really have a potentially deadly inflammation of a heart valve. (See error, p. 266.)

- You're given the wrong antibiotic for a case of "atypical" pneumonia, which has subtle symptoms that have escaped your doctor's notice. (See error, p. 268.)

- Your doctor thinks you have an ordinary cough when you really have congestive heart failure. (See error, p. 269.)

- Because of the absence of wheezing, your doctor fails to link your shortness of breath to an impending asthma attack. Instead, he attributes it to deep anxiety. (See error, p. 275.)

- A pulmonary (lung) specialist misses the fact that your asthma attacks, which have been getting worse, are being triggered by a simple allergy. (See error, p. 277.)

- Your child's pediatrician fails to give her a spacer to use with her asthma inhaler. As a result, her asthma symptoms are approaching emergency status. (See error, p. 281.)

- Your doctor prescribes theophylline for your asthma but doesn't measure your blood levels of the drug—and you end up in the emergency room. (See error, p. 282.)

- The doctor recommends a dangerous overdose of oxygen for your father, who has chronic bronchitis. (See error, p. 284.)

E R R O R :

Your Doctor Prescribes Antibiotics for Your Upper Respiratory Viral Infection

Laura saw Dr. Smith whenever she had a particularly bad cold. These visits usually ended with a shot of penicillin. Another doctor had told Laura that antibiotics don't help colds. But she was grateful that Dr. Smith always made an effort to help her. Why pay good money, she often said, if the doctor isn't going to treat you?

Then, after several injections of penicillin, Laura had an allergic reaction. Her face became swollen, her throat tightened, and she was rushed to the emergency room about an hour after a penicillin shot.

FACTS: Many doctors unnecessarily prescribe antibiotics for upper respiratory viral infections. Some doctors, like Dr. Smith, still start their treatments with an antibiotic shot, even though this practice is now generally frowned upon.

The problem is that at least nine out of ten upper respiratory infections are triggered by viruses rather than bacteria. Antibiotics have no effect on viruses. Also, overuse of antibiotics is costly and encourages the development of antibiotic-resistant bacteria.

Unfortunately, it's difficult to tell which upper respiratory infections are bacterial from the start or to distinguish colds that will be over in three to five days from those that will be prolonged by bacterial involvement. So some doctors and patients prefer to "play it safe" by taking antibiotics early, even though they aren't usually needed.

Antibiotic shots make sense only in a few special situations and should certainly not be used on a routine basis. Oral antibiotics are usually just as effective as shots and may be less likely to cause severe allergic reactions.

WHAT TO DO: If you are in the first days of something that feels like a cold and are offered an antibiotic, question whether the medication is really desirable or necessary. Nine times out of ten, it will do little to help you through what is most likely a viral illness. But early antibiotics might make sense for a few people who are ultra-vulnerable to bacterial superinfection after each viral illness.

One useful tactic is to ask your doctor for an antibiotic prescription that you can hold but don't have to fill immediately. Then, call your doctor after a few days to discuss whether or not the prescription is really needed.

With certain exceptions, it's always advisable to take any antibiotics orally rather than by injection. Your doctor should provide a very good reason if she is recommending a shot.

ERROR:

Failing to Link Your Sore Throat to Strep Throat

Allen, a 19-year-old college student, developed a nagging sore throat and finally went to have it checked by the physician on duty at the student health service. He was told to take some pain and cold pills and to gargle regularly with an over-the-counter solution.

Two weeks later, the throat condition had grown worse. Allen was diagnosed as having an advanced strep throat, which had now turned into an early case of rheumatic fever accompanied by joint pains and presenting a possibility of damage to the valves of his heart.

FACTS: When I was a medical student, doctors and patients both feared rheumatic fever, a heart inflammation mysteriously triggered in young people whose throat, nose, or skin has been infected with the streptococcus bacteria. Partly because of alert diagnosis and treatment of sore throats, rheumatic fever decreased dramatically during the 1970s and early 1980s even though strep throat and other strep infections continued to be common.

Unfortunately, many doctors have lost the habit of taking throat cultures in search of "strep." That's one reason that rheumatic fever is now making a comeback. Another may be a change in the streptococcus bacteria itself toward a more virulent form.

WHAT TO DO: Ask your doctor about taking a throat swab for strep with any upper respiratory infection—especially when accompanied by a sore throat—if you fall into one of these categories:

- You are 21 years old or younger.
- You have had rheumatic fever or a heart murmur in the past.
- You are in close contact with children or teenagers.

ERROR:

Your Doctor Assumes You Have the Flu When You Really Are Suffering from Endocarditis

Natalie made an appointment with her doctor in the middle of flu season, with fever and chills, which had been continuing for about five days. Her doctor decided that she probably had a bacterial infection along with the flu, and he put her on a round of antibiotics. The doctor had not taken into account that she had just had a dental procedure. Still, with the treatment, the condition got better, and both Natalie and her doctor assumed that she was on the road to recovery.

But then Natalie took a turn for the worse. She was hospitalized with a serious bacterial infection of a heart valve (endocarditis)—a potentially deadly illness.

What did the doctor do wrong?

FACTS: When it's the middle of flu season and your doctor is seeing ten patients a day who really do have the flu, he may let down his guard in identifying other diseases that may mimic the flu.

First of all, it's important to understand what the flu really is. Two kinds of flu may make your life miserable. First, there is the influenza virus, which becomes epidemic every year in the winter or early spring and for which we can take the flu vaccine. Other illnesses that we call the flu may arise from a number of viruses other than influenza. Regardless of the type of flu you get, you're likely to have symptoms that include but go beyond those of the common cold: fever, chills, muscle aches, swollen glands, sore throat, joint aches, nausea, diarrhea, abdominal pain, light-headedness, and even fainting.

Unfortunately, the symptoms accompanying a number of very serious nonflu conditions may look like the flu. These include

- Bacterial infections of a heart valve (endocarditis), the type that Natalie confronted. Though relatively uncommon, this is a deadly illness that is accompanied by fevers and chills that don't quiet down as quickly as those of the ordinary flu. Furthermore, adding antibiotics for a short time can give the doctor and patient a sense of false security, which may look like recovery but is really a prelude to serious complications.

- Appendicitis, which often begins with nausea and fever just before the classic right lower abdominal pain begins.

- Certain types of pneumonia, called *atypical pneumonia*. With this condition, mucus or phlegm production is less, and flulike symptoms of headache, muscle ache, and joint pain are more frequent than with typical pneumonia.

- Food poisoning, kidney infections, hepatitis, or withdrawal from addictive drugs, including caffeine and barbiturates.

WHAT TO DO: If you have flulike symptoms, try to associate them with other aspects of your health history. Also, be sure to inform your doctor if you develop symptoms that seem unlike what you should be suffering from the flu.

For example, it's possible that you may really have a heart valve infection if you've just had a dental procedure (because dental work often lets bacteria from the mouth enter the blood), if you have a history of a heart murmur, if you take intravenous drugs, or if your fever and chills have gone on for more than three days.

Rather than flu, your problem may be the appendix if pain in your abdomen is localized on the lower right side. Or you may have a kidney condition if the pain is on your flank or midway up your back.

Because pneumonia can also mimic the flu, be alert for unusual coughing, phlegm coming up from the chest, or shortness of breath.

Most important of all, speak to your doctor every day until you begin to improve. If you don't really have the flu, telltale clues will begin to appear. But your doctor can't make sense from those clues unless you let her know precisely how you feel.

ERROR:

Not Recommending an Influenza Vaccination If You Are at High Risk

Marty, who had adult-onset diabetes, came down with such a serious case of the flu that she had to be hospitalized. Her doctor had never recommended that she have an annual flu vaccine or that there were steps she could take to prevent the flu in case she felt she had been exposed to the virus.

FACTS: Influenza vaccine for the next season's flu strain usually becomes available in October or November. The main epidemic can begin by midwinter and increase through early spring. Those at high risk should be sure to take the shot. These include people who are old or weak or who are suffering from diseases that could be made worse by severe influenza, such as asthma, emphysema, heart disease, or diabetes. Also, those who feel they are at particularly high risk because of their work, such as medical personnel, should take the shot.

It's even possible to take steps to prevent the onset of flu if you haven't had the shot but suspect you've been exposed. The drug amantadine hydrochloride (Symmetrel), which is used to treat Parkinson's disease, is fairly effective in preventing one common form of influenza or at least reducing its seriousness. But doses of the drug must be started before you become ill. Rimantadine, which is related to amantadine, is a recently introduced drug that also has antiflu effects.

WHAT TO DO: If you're in one of the above-mentioned high-risk groups, you should definitely ask your doctor for the flu vaccine. Also, consider having it if you live or work in a high-risk environment, such as a densely populated urban environment with a high incidence of flu cases. There is a small risk of side effects from the vaccination itself, but these are usually much less of a danger than a bad case of the flu.

If you're a candidate for an annual flu shot, you should also consider getting a vaccination against pneumococcus, the most serious cause of bacterial pneumonia. Unlike the flu shot, which must be given repeatedly, the pneumococcus vaccination (Pneumovax) keeps working for many years.

Caution: Although the flu vaccine is derived from eggs, most, but not all, people who are allergic to eggs can safely take the vaccine. If you are allergic to eggs, raise this issue with your doctor.

ERROR:

Your Doctor Chooses the Wrong Antibiotic for Pneumonia

Stanley suffered from a mild cough and low-grade fever for several days and then went in to see his doctor. The doctor did a series of tests, suspected pneumonia, and confirmed the diagnosis with a chest X ray. He then prescribed a powerful new antibiotic, but Stanley's symptoms persisted and the pneumonia grew worse.

FACTS: When I first started medical practice, a wide range of inexpensive antibiotics, such as erythromycin, penicillin, ampicillin, amoxicillin, tetracycline, and doxycycline, worked well against most respiratory infections, including pneumonia. These still frequently do a good job, but resistance to them among bacteria is increasing alarmingly. So we can no longer assume that the traditional antibiotics will work every time.

On the other hand, even the newer, expensive antibiotics don't always work, especially with a condition known as *atypical pneumonia,* which was Stanley's problem. In recent years, a growing minority of pneumonia cases are being caused by this atypical bacterial disease, which does *not* display classic pneumonia symptoms, such as high fever, chills, green-yellow chest phlegm, or loud noises in the chest. Instead, atypical pneumonia has less dramatic signs and often masquerades as the flu or an upper respiratory illness with a mild cough.

With atypical pneumonia, a number of powerful antibiotics that are usually chosen to treat typical pneumonia don't work well. These include penicillin, amoxicillin, Augmentin, Ceclor, and Ceftin. Ironically, the older less-expensive drugs, erythromycin and tetracycline, often do a better job. Two newer, more expensive antibiotics, clarithromycin (Biaxin) and azithromycin (Zithromax) also do a good job for atypical pneumonia.

WHAT TO DO: It's reasonable to give your doctor two chances at hitting the right antibiotic. One question your doctor should consider if you remain ill with a cough is whether you might have an atypical pneumonia, which may be treated most effectively with one of the older drugs.

If two different antibiotics fail, further consultation should be done with a specialist in infectious diseases or pulmonary problems.

ERROR:

Your Doctor Mistakes the Serious Nature of Your Cough

Paula found herself coughing fairly regularly over a period of several days. She couldn't even get a good night's sleep. She called her doctor, who, after a quick examination, prescribed a cough suppressant and noted that her problem was probably related to a long-standing allergy that hit her about this time every year.

But the cough suppressant didn't work very well. She did have periods of relief, but the condition kept on recurring. Finally, the doctor put her through an extensive battery of tests, including a chest X ray and an electrocardiogram. The actual diagnosis: congestive heart failure.

FACTS: A common error is for the doctor to assume automatically that a cough is due to an upper respiratory inflammation, such as an infection, allergy, or other irritation. But a key clue that this is the wrong diagnostic track is that traditional cough medicines don't seem to be working. When coughing is from inflammation in the nose or throat, standard over-the-counter cough medicines, including derivatives of codeine or dextromethorphan, usually work well.

But if the source of the cough lies elsewhere, these cough medicines won't do the job as well. The most frequent alternative reasons for a cough are diseases in the chest, some of which can be serious. For example, the patient may be suffering from unsuspected asthma, bronchitis, or congestive heart failure (a condition where fluid backs up from the heart into the lungs). With these diseases, codeine-type cough suppressants may even make things worse since they prevent the natural removal of irritants from the lungs.

WHAT TO DO: Don't let your doctor forget about your cough, even if it seems to get temporarily better while you're actually in his office. Also, make sure that your physician is aware if these conditions exist:

- Your cough doesn't seem clearly related to a stuffy nose or postnasal drip.

- It doesn't respond well to standard cough suppressant medicines.

- It seems to come partly from your chest.

A cough *may* indicate an ordinary respiratory infection. But it may also be a signal of much more serious illness, such as asthma, bronchitis, pneumonia, tuberculosis, congestive heart failure, a tumor in the lungs, or a pulmonary embolism (a blood clot in the lungs). Also, the cough may stem from other sources, such as certain medicines (including angiotensin-converting enzyme inhibitor medicines or beta-blocker drugs, which are used to control blood pressure or, in the case of beta-blockers, as an eye drop for treating glaucoma).

ERROR:

Your Doctor Overlooks Sinusitis as the Cause of Your Lingering "Cold" or Postnasal Drip

A number of years ago, a patient, Sally, used to ask me, "Why do my colds always linger for months?"

She wasn't allergic, didn't smoke, and had none of the classic signs of acute sinus infections, which involve green or yellow mucus, or sinus area headaches. Her main symptoms were a postnasal drip and a vague sense of "fullness" in her head. Her routine sinus X rays were normal on three different occasions.

I was stumped. But then, in the early 1980s, a newfangled form of X ray called *computed tomography* (or a CT or CAT scan) became available. The problem was the cost—about $500 per exam. I stalled for two years, not wanting to recommend such an expensive procedure without being certain we were going to find an answer.

Then, we took the plunge. And sure enough, Sally was diagnosed as having a full-blown infection in the small sinuses (ethmoid sinuses) that run between the eyes. It was a chronic infection that she had probably had for years and was clearly the source of her "colds." After vigorous treatment with antibiotics, the change in Sally was amazing. As her postnasal drip and head pressure improved, so did her overall energy and sense of well-being.

FACTS: Acute sinusitis is hard to miss. There's almost always yellow or green mucus and also sinus area pain or pressure. But chronic, low-grade sinus infection of the type that Sally had is subtler. The doctor must stay alert or this diagnosis will be overlooked.

Nearly everyone with chronic infection in the sinuses will have a postnasal drip and nasal congestion. In fact, some people are so used to this condition that they consider it "normal," rarely complain, and would never think of seeing a doctor. But some symptoms can be much more serious. Here is the possible array of signs and symptoms associated with sinusitis:

- Postnasal drip.
- Nasal congestion.

- Clear, yellow, or green nasal mucus.

- Head pressure or headache, usually between, above, or below the eyes but rarely radiating to the ears or top of the head.

- Pain in the gums or teeth.

- Swollen eyelids.

- Loss of the sense of smell.

- Worsening of prior allergies or extension of allergies to other seasons.

- "Winter" allergies, which clear up in the summer.

- Snoring or poor, nonrestorative sleep.

- Bad breath.

- Hard-to-treat asthma.

- Nausea due to excessive postnasal drip.

- Chronic fatigue.

WHAT TO DO: If you have a chronic postnasal drip and any of the symptoms listed above, ask your doctor, Could this be due to sinusitis?

If he agrees that could be the cause and gives you tests, even including an X ray, but *fails* to order a CT scan, insist on this procedure. The CT is the gold standard for identifying sinusitis and should be conducted when this condition is suspected yet can't be identified in any other way.

Traditional sinus X rays miss about half the cases of chronic sinusitis. Other tests, such as examining the front of the nose, pressing over the sinus area for tenderness, shining a bright light into the mouth, or imaging the sinuses with an ultrasound machine, may pick up some cases of acute sinus inflammation. But they are inaccurate procedures for detecting the subtler chronic form of sinusitis.

If you're worried about the cost of a regular CT scan, you might ask about a less expensive measure: A few radiology centers do what's called a *limited* or *screening* CT scan, which involves less radiation and can be done for less than half the cost of a normal CT. Unfortunately, most CT centers around the country don't offer this option. Also, to limit your costs, you should compare CT scan prices at different centers and be sure to check whether the center will accept your form of insurance.

If you do have sinusitis, you'll be placed on high doses of strong antibiotics along with decongestant medicines for at least two to three weeks and in some cases for four weeks. Don't be discouraged by slow improvement because it often takes a great deal of drug treatment to knock out a sinus infection.

ERROR:

Your Doctor Overtests for Allergies

For several weeks, Margot had periodically experienced allergic symptoms, including watery eyes and sneezing. Thoroughly miserable, she went in to see her doctor, who referred her to an allergy specialist.

The specialist conducted a wide battery of tests, which included an evaluation of many different types of foods, inhalants, and other substances, at a cost of more than $600. In the end, this specialist found that the problem was the hair of Margot's cat. The doctor recommended that because she was so allergic, she should get rid of the cat.

Did anybody make a mistake here?

FACTS: Some allergists test more than necessary and may quickly run up an excessive bill. It rarely makes sense to test initially for more than fifteen to twenty allergens in the effort to identify the cause of your symptoms.

An allergist usually does a much better job than most internists or family physicians in the detective work of sorting out the multiple factors that can affect chronic nasal congestion, asthma, hives, or other allergic disorders. These include allergy, infection, and various environmental pollutants and irritants. But if the main question you want answered is simply, Am I allergic? your family doctor can probably give you the answer at much less expense.

She can order a blood radioallergosorbent (RAST) allergy test for the most common allergens, such as dust, dust mite, a few common molds, and your household pets. If your symptoms flare up in spring and in fall, she will also screen for the most common trees such as oak and maple, a grass mix, and ragweed. A negative or low-level result on all these tests usually means that inhalant allergens—by far the most common cause of allergies—are *not* a key cause of your problem.

Broad testing for unknown food allergies is almost always a waste unless you already know which foods to suspect. The most effective test for unknown food allergies is the old-fashioned elimination diet. With this approach, you eat only a few specially designated foods, such as rice, lamb, or pear, for a week or two before you begin adding your regular foods back one at a time.

Caution: If your allergy symptoms are potentially serious (for example, if they are linked to asthma, throat swelling, or the shock reaction known as anaphylaxis), never do an elimination diet without expert supervision. Reintroducing an allergic food in these circumstances has the potential for triggering a life-threatening reaction.

As for allergy shots, they are inconvenient because they require weekly visits to the physician, but they certainly can help when used correctly. Unfortunately, certain specialists, including surprisingly some pulmonary physicians, tend to underestimate the importance of allergy treatment. On the other hand, a few unethical allergists put almost everyone on shots, even if the allergy test results are only minimally positive. People who have very strong allergies, for example, class III or higher on the RAST test or large reactions on skin tests, usually will benefit from allergy shots. Those with class I RASTs or lower reactions to skin tests are much less likely to improve with a shot program.

WHAT TO DO: Ask for a referral to an allergist if you have poorly controlled asthma, chronic nasal congestion, or hives or if your treatment requires the regular use of high doses of medication. Be especially assertive if you note a relationship between the ups and downs of your symptoms and when you are exposed to allergens.

Either skin tests or RAST blood tests are acceptable as a starter, but always obtain a written copy of your tests, and be sure your family doctor gets a copy. Be open to allergy shots if your symptoms seem to be related to allergy exposures and if your allergy test reactions are pronounced. Be skeptical if you can't link allergy exposures to your symptoms or if your allergy tests are only mildly positive. Your family physician should be able to help you decide whether your allergist's recommendations are leading you down the right or wrong path.

Caution: If you do get allergy shots, always wait in the doctor's office for *at least* thirty minutes. Allergy shots, while usually safe, can sometimes trigger potentially dangerous reactions. About 90 percent of these reactions begin within thirty minutes after the shot, but on rare occasions the first symptoms—hives, wheezing, shortness of breath, or low blood pressure—might not appear for an hour or more.

If you have ever had a potentially life-threatening allergic reaction, such as to a food or an insect sting, you should wear a Medic-Alert bracelet, which you can order by calling 1-800-432-5378. You should also carry an explanation card in your wallet and an up-to-date adrenaline injection kit, such as an Epipen. (Antihistamines, such as Benadryl, are helpful against mild allergies but aren't nearly strong enough to counter serious reactions.)

ERROR:

Assuming That an Anxious Patient's Shortness of Breath Is Caused by Anxiety Rather Than by a Serious Physical Problem

A doctor I know recently misdiagnosed a very breathless, anxious 50-year-old woman as having panic disorder. After listening to her lungs with his stethoscope, he prescribed a tranquilizer.

Later that night, however, an ambulance rushed her to the emergency room, where her lung (pulmonary) function test confirmed severe, obvious asthma. This doctor knew very well that there is sometimes no wheezing in very severe asthma because so little air is being moved with each breath. But he didn't take a lung test because he subconsciously had made the mental equation that anxiety symptoms equal psychological cause. In this case, her anxiety was justified. She wasn't getting enough air.

The consequences could well have been tragic if the patient had reached the emergency room any later.

FACTS: There are a number of causes for shortness of breath, which may easily be mistaken for psychological disturbance or illness. For a list of these causes, possible clues that can help you identify the cause, and ways to check the problem, see the accompanying box, Causes of Shortness of Breath.

WHAT TO DO: If you develop severe shortness of breath that's different from symptoms you've previously experienced, don't automatically accept anxiety as the diagnosis. Instead, be sure that your doctor looks thoroughly for other causes, including those listed in the accompanying box.

An essential, minimum medical work-up should include a careful

Causes of Shortness of Breath		
Causes of Shortness of Breath	*Possible Clues*	*How the Clue Can Be Checked*
Asthma	Cough and wheezing are usually but not always present; suspect if ever had previous asthma or if episode began with an infection, allergic reaction, or pollution exposure	Lung function test
Congestive heart failure, abnormal heart rhythm, "silent" angina, heart valve abnormality, low blood pressure, pneumothorax (torn lung)	Noise (rales) in lung; ankle swelling; history of high blood pressure or heart disease; chest tightness, pain, or pressure; slow, rapid, or irregular heartbeat	Listen to heart, lungs, and blood pressure, chest X ray, electrocardiogram, echocardiogram
Pulmonary embolism or blood clot in lungs	May appear normal or breathless; suspect if history of leg or pelvic inflammation (phlebitis), taking birth control pills, cancer, or prolonged bed rest or inactivity	Chest X ray, electrocardiogram, measure blood oxygen level, lung scan, arteriogram, Doppler study of legs
Allergic or anaphylactic reaction	Swelling especially of face; might have itching; diarrhea; hives can start with insect sting, new medicine, or eating specific food	Careful history, check blood pressure, emergency trial shot of adrenaline
Sepsis (severe infection) or toxic shock syndrome	Fever might or might not be present, began with infection, vaginal tampon use or began with menstrual period, red or mottled skin, low blood pressure	White blood cell count, check blood pressure and temperature, blood culture, pelvic exam

Causes of Short- ness of Breath	Possible Clues	How the Clue Can Be Checked
Overdose of stimulants, e.g., caffeine, cocaine, amphetamine, theophylline, or aspirin poisoning	Careful history is necessary	Careful history, drug screen, measure blood acid–base balance
Other physical disorders, e.g., low blood sugar in diabetics; internal bleeding or severe anemia; low blood oxygen due to emphysema, lung infections, or toxins such as carbon monoxide	History of preexisting disease	Check blood count, sugar, blood oxygen level, blood carbon monoxide level

personal and family medical history, a physical examination, lung function tests, chest X ray, and basic laboratory blood tests.

Of course, you may agree with your doctor that anxiety may be a factor in your shortness of breath. But if treatment for anxiety doesn't bring improvement or if things start to get worse, contact your doctor immediately or go to the emergency room. It's better to be a pest than to be the victim of a serious misdiagnosis.

ERROR:

Your Doctor Treats the Allergy While Ignoring the Trigger

Larry had been suffering from asthma for several years, with symptoms that included wheezing (a high-pitched sound in the chest), coughing, chest tightness, and shortness of breath. The internist who was treating him had employed a number of medications to control the symptoms, but Larry felt he was getting worse.

So he sought out another doctor, an allergy specialist, who determined that the asthma was probably being aggravated by two triggers—his pets and a chronic sinus infection. When these problems were cleared up, the asthma symptoms improved dramatically.

FACTS: About one American in twenty has asthma, and most lead normal lives. When the condition seems to be getting worse, there's usually a reason—a "trigger" that is exacerbating the problem. Unfortunately, many doctors try to treat asthma symptoms with medication alone while ignoring triggers, which, if removed, can actually effect an almost miraculous cure!

What sort of doctor is best able to recognize a trigger? Allergists and pulmonary (lung) specialists both treat asthma. Pulmonary specialists are usually the most skilled at treating very severe asthma cases, particularly when hospital intensive care is required. But allergists, who are also skilled in the use of asthma medicines, tend to be better at searching out environmental and allergic triggers.

Here are some of the most commonly overlooked asthma triggers:

- *Allergies.* One-third to one-half of asthmatics have significant allergies. But many doctors underrate the importance of allergy as a trigger for asthma. If you're asthmatic, *always* insist that your physician determine whether you have allergies!

- *Tobacco and other pollutants.* Everyone knows that smoking makes asthma worse—and that includes secondhand smoke from household members or colleagues at work. Also, exposure to fumes or other pollutants, whether at work or around home, can increase problems with asthma. I have one patient who breathes auto exhaust fumes all day as toll-taker at New York City's Lincoln Tunnel. Small wonder his asthma has been difficult to control!

- *Sinus infections.* I find that at least 10 percent of my "difficult" asthmatics have completely unsuspected chronic sinusitis, which shows up on CT scans. Often, the asthma improves when the sinus infection is treated.

- *Viral infections.* Certain viral infections exacerbate asthma over a period of days or weeks. Other viruses, by triggering an allergylike reaction, can create an almost instant asthma emergency within hours or even minutes.

- *Heartburn, hiatal hernia, or gastroesophageal reflux (backing up of stomach acid into the esophagus).* These conditions may be made worse by asthma, or they can aggravate an asthmatic condition.

- *Medicines.* A number of drugs may cause or worsen asthma: Beta-blockers (Inderal, Corgard, Lopressor) increase the tendency of lung muscles to spasm; eye drops used to treat glaucoma may contain these offending beta-blockers (e.g., Timoptic); and about 10 percent of asthmatics get worse when they take aspirin or related nonsteroidal antiinflammatory medicines (such as Advil, Voltaren, Naprosyn, and Clinoril). If you have asthma, avoid any medicine to which you are allergic.

- *Stress.* Any stress that is not managed well may trigger asthmatic symptoms.

- *Exercise.* Vigorous physical activity, especially in cold, dry air, will make asthma worse.

If you notice that your asthma symptoms seem to bother you more in the presence of one or more of the triggers described above, alert your doctor to these observations. If your doctor does not follow up with appropriate explanations, tests, or treatment, ask for a referral to an allergy or a pulmonary (lung) specialist. You may find you have a quick cure for your problem.

ERROR:

Your Doctor Allows You to Overuse Quick-Relief Asthma Drugs and Neglect Slower-Acting Antiinflammatory Preventive Drugs

Amy, a 36-year-old advertising executive, had mild asthma for years, which she kept under control with a prescription for Ventolin, an asthma inhaler spray.

Amy needed her asthma spray only once or twice a day until a severe viral illness triggered worsening asthma. Over the next few weeks, she increased her medicine use to four and then six times a day. But each day, the medicine seemed to provide shorter and shorter periods of relief.

Did Amy or her doctor make a mistake in her treatment?

FACTS: Many asthma patients don't realize it, but there are two very different types of asthma medicines: the quick-relief type, which relaxes the tight muscles of the bronchial airways, and the preventive type, which slowly quells inflammation.

The quick-relief medicines include the bronchodilators (Proventil, Ventolin, Alupent) and also the less rapidly acting theophylline medicines (Theo-Dur, Slo-bid, Slo-Phyllin, Uniphyl). These offer great short-term relief, but they do little to reduce ongoing inflammation in the airways. That's all right if your asthma is mild, as Amy's was originally. But these drugs are not good enough when asthma grows worse. The reason is that inflammation in the airways—whether from allergies, infection, air pollution, or other causes—is the trigger that makes asthmatic bronchial muscles go into spasm. So if you don't treat the inflammation and it gets out of hand, your asthma may worsen to the point where your quick-relief medicines fail to work.

The main antiinflammatory medicines are the cromolyn (Intal) inhaler, Tilade inhaler, cortisone-based inhalers (Vanceril, Beclovent, Azmacort, Aerobid), and oral cortisone (prednisone, Medrol). Intal, Tilade, and the cortisone inhalers are relatively safe for long-term use, but they take a week or more of regular use before you can begin to see their effect. Oral cortisone provides much quicker relief, but usually it causes side effects if used for more than a few weeks at a time.

People like Amy, whose asthma worsens, usually need an antiinflammatory medicine added to their acute-relief medicine. Most people who regularly need quick-relief medicine more than twice a day should also take an inhaled antiinflammatory medicine regularly—whether they feel sick or not. Taking the antiinflammatory type cuts down on the need for the acute-relief medicines, but more important, this approach increases the resistance against acute asthma attacks.

The error in Amy's case was that her doctor had not made sure that she understood what to do if her asthma became worse. She should have been taught that just increasing her Ventolin was not the right action. She should have understood that she needed to see her doctor when she began to have trouble, thus giving her doctor the opportunity to interrupt her vicious cycle by adding an antiinflammatory medicine.

WHAT TO DO: If you need asthma-relief-type medicine every day, discuss with your doctor the option of starting or increasing your use of inhaled cortisone spray, Tilade, or cromolyn. If you need acute-relief medicine twice a day or more or if your asthma symptoms interfere with normal activity or sleep, you would probably benefit from an antiinflammatory medicine. Your family physician or internist should certainly be familiar with these drugs. But if he seems unsure or reluctant, then don't hesitate to seek a second opinion from an allergist or a lung (pulmonary) specialist.

ERROR:

Your Doctor Fails to Instruct You in the Proper Use of Your Asthma Inhaler

A local physician referred an asthma patient, an 11-year-old girl, to me because her condition seemed to be deteriorating. He said that her asthma inhalers weren't helping her at all. As a result, she needed continuous, potentially toxic high doses of cortisone pills to keep her asthma in check.

I wasn't optimistic as I took note of her medical history, but then I asked her to show me how she used her inhaler spray. It immediately became obvious that her timing was off. Each puff of the spray hit the back of her throat *after* she had finished taking a breath. As a result, the spray never reached her lungs. It was wasted.

To help out, I gave Sarah a small plastic tube commonly known as a *spacer*, which she attached to her asthma spray. Within three weeks of starting the spacer, Sarah was completely off the cortisone. In the five years since I first saw her, she has needed cortisone for flare-ups only about two weeks a year—quite an improvement over the fifty-two weeks of cortisone she needed before.

FACTS: Most asthma patients get less than the full dose from their asthma inhalers because of mechanical mistakes in how they use the spray. They don't realize they are operating the device incorrectly, in part because their doctors and nurses have never checked them to be certain they were doing it right.

Even with teaching, it takes a fair amount of coordination to work most inhalers properly. That's why a spacer of the type I recommended for Sarah can be so useful. This device has a one-way valve, which traps the medicine that is sprayed into it. This way, when you inhale, the medicine automatically flows into your lung, thus eliminating the need for perfect timing.

Most people can double the medicine that reaches their lungs by using a spacer. Also, they can cut in half the medicine deposits that may irritate the throat. The result is better asthma control with less throat irritation and medicinal taste.

WHAT TO DO: Insist that your doctor or a member of her staff show you how to spray your metered-dose inhaler. Have her watch you do it to be sure you are operating the device correctly.

If you still have trouble or if for any reason your asthma continues to be uncontrolled, ask for a spacing device to attach to your asthma spray. These are available at most drugstores, or your doctor may be able to sell you one. The cost should be under $30.

ERROR:

Your Doctor Prescribes Theophylline for Your Asthma but Fails to Measure Your Blood Levels of the Drug

An experienced nurse was taking theophylline for her asthma. Her doctor also added an antiulcer drug to her medication—one that can affect the body's metabolism of theophylline.

The main mistake the doctor made was not following up on the nurse's condition by checking the levels of theophylline in her blood. He missed the fact that her theophylline level soared, causing extreme nervousness, nausea, vomiting, and an abnormal heart rhythm. The nurse almost died, but fast emergency room procedures saved her.

FACTS: Theophylline (Theo-Dur, Slo-bid, Slo-Phyllin, Uniphyl) is a useful antiasthma drug. But it's also a drug that is hard to monitor. The toxic dose of this medication isn't that much higher than what is appropriate for its therapeutic use. What's worse, since people metabolize theophylline differently, a dose that is not enough for one person may be too high for another.

Blood theophylline levels may change even for the same individual when a doctor prescribes other medicines, when the patient has a flu vaccination, or when food is eaten or not eaten in conjunction with the pill.

Some of the medicines that may increase the blood theophylline level, as happened with the nurse, are troleandomycin (TAO), cimetidine (Tagamet), and possibly other acid-blocking drugs. Beta-blocker drugs, such as propranolol, and the antibiotics erythromycin and ciprofloxacin may also raise the blood theophylline level.

WHAT TO DO: If you are taking theophylline regularly at any but very low doses, ask your doctor if you need to check your theophylline level whenever you alter any medication. Also, he should test you if you develop nervousness, nausea, or a rapid or irregular heartbeat.

ERROR:

Your Doctor Fails to Recognize a Bacterial Infection as the Cause of Worsening Chronic Lung Disease

Jo, who had emphysema, noticed a gradual increase in shortness of breath accompanied by greater amounts of yellow mucus. Her doctor assumed this intensification of her symptoms was just the inevitable deterioration of her condition. In fact, she was suffering from a bacterial infection, which was finally corrected by antibiotics.

FACTS: Unlike those with colds or asthma, who mostly have respiratory infections that are initially viral, people with chronic bronchitis and emphysema are very vulnerable to worsening of what may be an underlying low-grade bacterial infection.

Remember: Bacterial infections *can* be treated with antibiotics, whereas viral infections cannot.

The signs of bacterial infection in those with emphysema or chronic bronchitis can be subtle, as was the case with Jo. It's easy for a doctor to misread, as hers did, the significance of a gradual worsening of shortness of breath, an increasing volume of mucus, or a deepening of its yellow or green color. In fact, many times these symptoms do indicate a bacterial infection that can be overcome by aggressive treatment with antibiotics.

WHAT TO DO: If you have chronic bronchitis or emphysema and if your breathing becomes worse or if the phlegm from your lungs increases in volume or color, see your doctor. Ask her to consider a course of antibiotics. If your physician doesn't usually treat additional symptoms with antibiotics, seek consultation with a pulmonary or infectious disease specialist.

ERROR:

You Have Emphysema or Chronic Bronchitis, and You Overdose on Oxygen

Nat, who was in his seventies, had developed chronic bronchitis, probably from a lifetime of cigarette smoking. He regularly used oxygen at home to relieve his symptoms, but one night, when he was experiencing particularly serious respiratory difficulties, he increased the flow rate from his oxygen tank, temporarily stopped breathing, and had to be rushed to the hospital. An examination revealed that the carbon dioxide level in his blood was exceptionally high.

What had happened?

FACTS: Many people with chronic bronchitis or emphysema have a low blood oxygen level, which is a major factor in their discomfort and disability. Using oxygen intermittently or even continuously can make a big difference in how they feel and what they can do.

For many patients with chronic lung disease, oxygen levels fall dangerously low at night. This condition can make a person feel tired and achy the next morning and can also lead to serious heart complications. To avoid this problem, blood oxygen levels can be measured in the blood directly or by high-tech sensors attached to the finger or the ear lobe. This allows easy monitoring of blood oxygen while you sleep through the night.

But some people, such as Nat, may have low blood oxygen levels and yet be *harmed* by extra oxygen. They may even stop breathing or die. These patients can be identified by measuring the carbon dioxide levels in the blood. If the carbon dioxide levels are high, great care must be taken in administering oxygen. Most patients, like Nat, can benefit from low-flow oxygen, usually at a rate of one or two liters per minute. But higher rates of oxygen can suppress the breathing center of the brain, and thereby pose a life-threatening hazard.

WHAT TO DO: If your chronic bronchitis or emphysema limits your daily activities, ask your doctor to measure your blood oxygen level either randomly during the day or continuously over-night.

At the same time you have your blood oxygen checked, you should also have a test to determine your blood carbon dioxide level. If this measurement is high, adding too much oxygen can turn off the centers in the brain that maintain normal breathing. Those with high carbon dioxide levels *can* receive oxygen, but they *must* be monitored very carefully.

Without both of these tests—the blood oxygen level and carbon dioxide level—you may get temporary relief. But at the same time, you could be subjecting yourself to tremendous danger—as Nat learned, almost too late.

E R R O R :

Your Doctor Fails to Order a Tuberculosis Test

Ron, a corporate executive, was physically fit and seemingly com-pletely healthy. He hadn't missed a day of work for years until he developed a serious case of influenza. After the normal time for recovery from the flu had passed, Ron noticed that he retained a debilitating cough and persistent fever.

A battery of tests by his doctor finally revealed the problem: Ron had tuberculosis (TB). Apparently, he had caught the disease years before from his brother, who as a doctor had been regularly exposed to TB patients in a hospital.

Why hadn't this problem been identified earlier?

FACTS: Tuberculosis, once the leading killer in the United States, became a minor health problem for a long time but is now increas-ing rapidly among many high-risk groups. These include people with the human immunodeficiency virus, racial minorities, immi-grants, poor people, and alcohol and drug abusers. Also at risk are those like Ron and his brother, who live or work with these high-risk groups.

Middle-class white Americans, though in a low-risk category for TB right now, should not be complacent. Many TB cases are resis-tant to some or all TB treatment drugs, thus making TB ultimately a threat to everyone.

Most TB involves fever and symptoms related to the lungs, such as coughing or coughing up blood. But TB can affect any part of the body—the blood, heart, bones, brain, or immune cells—sometimes without causing any lung symptoms or even an abnormal chest X ray.

TB can persist for years, decades, or a lifetime in an inactive state, held in check by the body's immune system defenses. But if the immune system slips due to an illness, stress, or old age, the latent TB could turn into an active infection. In the example above, Ron's flu apparently was instrumental in triggering the TB that he had harbored for years.

WHAT TO DO: Anyone who has even a remote contact with TB should have a safe, simple, inexpensive TB skin test as part of a regular medical checkup. Also, if you develop any symptoms of chronic illness that can't be explained, you should have the test.

If you're a member of one of the above-mentioned high-risk groups, you should also have a chest X ray, which should show any scarring or indications of previously healed TB. I prefer the very slightly more painful under-the-skin "PPD" TB test to the less-reliable prick, or tine-test, version.

A positive TB skin test means you have been exposed to TB and you harbor it in your body, but it doesn't mean that you are ill or that you'll necessarily develop active TB. Nor does the test tell you when the exposure occurred—recently or years ago—unless you have kept up with regular TB tests, as I recommend. If you do have the tests regularly, you can identify the precise time period when the exposure occurred.

If you are found to have a newly positive TB skin test but the disease hasn't yet surfaced in the form of any symptoms, later activation can often be prevented by treating the condition preventively with anti-TB drugs for six to twelve months. But even though these drugs are relatively safe, they have some toxicity, particularly for those who are middle-aged or older, have liver disease, or suffer from other health problems.

The decision whether or not to treat latent TB is a judgment call, depending on your age, health, and other factors. If your doctor doesn't see TB patients very frequently—at least a few cases each year—then you should enlist the help of a pulmonary or infectious disease specialist in making this decision. In Ron's case, being tested regularly for TB and then taking preventive steps before the disease became active might have prevented his developing active TB.

PART FIVE

Checking Out Your Bones and Joints

Special Alerts: Bones and Joints

- You're poisoned by having too many cortisone injections in an arthritic joint. (See error, p. 292.)

- Your doctor uses one right drug—estrogen—along with one wrong drug to treat your advanced osteoporosis. (See error, p. 296.)

- Your doctor is too quick to recommend surgery for your carpal tunnel syndrome (wrist and hand pain from overuse, such as too much typing). (See error, p. 297.)

- When your backache symptoms change to a feeling of numbness or weakness in a leg, your doctor fails to identify your condition as a potentially dangerous emergency. (See error, p. 300.)

- Your doctor thinks you have arthritis and treats you with a painkiller when you really have fibromyalgia, which requires a different drug regimen. (See error, p. 306.)

Your Doctor Treats You for Osteoarthritis When You Really Have Another Disease

Abe, who was 62, was suffering from regular joint pains in his hands and shoulders. His doctor concluded, "You just have what we all get as we grow older—osteoarthritis. This involves inflammation of the joints as a result of wear and tear over the years."

The doctor prescribed an antiinflammatory medication and went on to the next phase of Abe's exam. Over the next year, however, Abe's condition deteriorated substantially, with the pains intensifying and moving to other joints. A more thorough exam led to a diagnosis of rheumatoid arthritis.

Where did the doctor go wrong?

FACTS: As Abe's doctor indicated, osteoarthritis—the roughening and inflammation of joints that occurs over the years with the wear and tear of daily physical activity—*is* extremely common. X rays of almost everyone over age 40 show some degree of osteoarthritis. But this great likelihood that a complaint like Abe's will result from osteoarthritis makes many doctors complacent.

In fact, a number of other diseases, which require very different treatment, may display symptoms like those of osteoarthritis. These include

- *Rheumatoid arthritis.* Rheumatoid arthritis is far more likely to be seriously disabling than osteoarthritis. This disease requires quite different treatment from osteoarthritis and may be countered with medicines called *disease-modifying antirheumatic drugs* (DMARDs). These drugs, which decrease pain *and*, more importantly, may actually slow the advancement of the disease, include gold, hydroxychloroquine (Plaquenil), sulfasalazine (Azulfidine), and methotrexate.

- *Lyme disease.* This infection, which is commonly picked up by a bite from a deer tick, causes arthritis, skin rash, and heart and neurological symptoms. Special treatments, including certain antibiotics, are required, and if they aren't begun early enough, the long-term damage to joints and other organs can be permanent and progressive. (See error, p. 308.)

- *Fibromyalgia.* With this condition, you may ache all over from sore and tender muscles and joints. This disease responds poorly to the traditional painkillers and antiinflammatory drugs used for osteoarthritis. But it sometimes responds well to low doses of antidepressant medicines, physical therapy, and, sometimes, nutritional supplements.

- *A variety of other diseases, including gout, systemic lupus, psoriasis, ulcerative colitis, tuberculosis, or bacterial infections.*

WHAT TO DO: Remember this principle when you go in to complain about an aching joint: The most important issue is *not* just how to control your pain, but, rather, how to prevent progressive damage to your joints or other parts of your body. In other words, you must press your doctor to be sure to find the true underlying cause of your symptoms.

Family physicians and internists, such as the one who treated Abe, are most likely to take a narrow view of treating your problem by focusing on prescribing medication to control pain. In contrast, arthritis specialists (rheumatologists) are more likely to take a more comprehensive and effective approach to treatment.

A basic arthritis evaluation, which should take into account all of the possible *other* diseases listed under Facts, should cover the following laboratory tests: CBC (a composite blood count, which among other things helps identify anemia); SMA (a broad screening test for liver function, kidneys, blood sugar, various blood minerals, and uric acid); urinalysis (a test of the urine for sugar, proteins, and white and red blood cells); sedimentation rate (measure of inflammation in the blood); antinuclear antibody (ANA) (a measure of antibodies that attack the nuclei of cells—a condition found in certain types of arthritis); rheumatoid factor or latex fixation (a blood test for rheumatoid arthritis); and a Lyme antibody test if you live in an area where Lyme disease is common. Also, you should receive an X ray of the involved joints. If there is substantial swelling in a joint, it's often useful for the doctor to insert a needle in to drain out the fluid for laboratory examination.

If you have questions about any treatment you may be getting from an internist or family practitioner—and certainly, if your condition begins to get worse—insist on an evaluation by a rheumatologist. He should place you on a long-term treatment plan that encompasses special medication, including painkillers; physical therapy; fitness training; a nutritional evaluation; and a regular schedule for monitoring your progress.

E R R O R :

Your Doctor Prescribes Powerful Drugs for Treatment of Rheumatoid Arthritis, Without Explaining Their Poisonous Potential

Jake, a 49-year-old who had been treated several years for rheumatoid arthritis, was being given cortisone injections every few months. He had been injected in one particular joint seven times during the past year, but the pain in that location had grown steadily worse.

What was his doctor doing wrong?

FACTS: All the main arthritis drugs, including cortisone, aspirin, and the increasingly popular "disease-modifying anti-rheumatic drugs" (DMARDs), are moderately to highly toxic medicines. They can be used safely but only with frequent, meticulous monitoring by the physician. Also, the patient must be educated so that he knows what problems to look for in case the drug begins to poison his system.

Most people are able to stay on these drugs for a few years at the most—and at relatively moderate doses—before the toxicity levels begin to rise too high. With cortisone, for example, most orthopedists will not usually inject the same joint more than several times a year for fear of damaging tissue in the area or introducing an infection along with the needle. In the above case, Jake's doctor was overrelying on the "magic" of cortisone. He clearly needed an alternative approach.

WHAT TO DO: The decision to begin DMARD medications should be made in consultation with an arthritis specialist. If your arthritis isn't severe or disabling, but your physician still recommends DMARDs, then you should get a second opinion from another rheumatologist. If your arthritis is severe and progressing, as Jake's was, then the burden of proof shifts. You should demand the reason why DMARDs are not being used.

Ongoing treatment with DMARDs can be monitored by a rheumatologist or by a primary care physician if she has experience with these drugs *and* she regularly consults with a rheumatologist. (See the accompanying box, DMARDs: Their Major Adverse Reactions and Recommended Monitoring by Your Physician.)

Disease-Modifying Anti-Rheumatic Drugs (DMARDs): Their Major Adverse Reactions and Recommended Monitoring by Your Physician		
Drug	*Major Adverse Reactions*	*Recommended Monitoring*
Antimalarials, e.g., hydroxy-chloroquine (Paquenil)	Vision disturbance, rash	Regular exam by eye doctor, e.g., every six months
Sulfasalazine (Azul-fidine)	Liver inflammation, rash, nausea, dizziness, discolored urine, sweats	CBC, liver function tests frequently
Gold, injection and oral	Rashes, low blood counts, kidney damage, diarrhea (oral)	Urinalysis and CBC before each injection
Penicillamine	Rashes, kidney damage, low blood counts, taste disturbances	CBC, urinalysis frequently
Cortisone-type drugs	Weight gain, bone thinning, bruising, fluid retention, cataracts, vulnerability to infections	Use lowest effective dose
Methotrexate	Liver damage, nausea, low blood counts	CBC, SMA frequently; avoid alcohol
Azathioprine, cyclo-phosphamide, chlorambucil	Cancer, low blood counts, kidney damage	CBC, urinalysis frequently
Cyclosporine	Kidney damage, high blood pressure	CBC, SMA, blood pressure frequently

In any event, if you begin DMARD treatment, always obtain the package insert for your medicine, which you can get from the pharmacist. Read the insert carefully, jot down questions or issues that may come to mind, and schedule a full fifteen-minute visit to discuss the drug with your physician. In the end, you should have a written list of side effects to look for, actions to take if they occur, and a never-miss schedule for medical visits and laboratory testing.

ERROR:

Your Doctor Fails to Recommend a Bone Density Measurement to Detect Osteoporosis at the Time You Go Through Menopause

Sheila, a naturally thin, small 62-year-old, had gone through menopause when she was 52, and now she was beginning to suffer from frequent fractures, including a recently broken wrist. Her doctor diagnosed her as having osteoporosis, the disease involving loss of bone mass that results in a high incidence of fractures, and sent her to a specialist for treatment. During one consultation, the specialist measured her bone density by using a dual-photon absorptiometry (DPA) machine and found that her bone mass was significantly lower than for the average woman her age.

As Sheila was being tested, the specialist remarked, "It's too bad you weren't sent in for a bone density measurement test years ago. We could have taken steps to prevent your bone loss."

Did her regular doctor make a mistake?

FACTS: Yes, most women should have a bone density measurement at the time of menopause. With this reading, a specialist can tell whether or not you are at risk for osteoporosis and can take countermeasures while there is still time to preserve the bone mass that remains.

Regular X rays are too insensitive to indicate your bone mass status, and blood calcium levels are irrelevant to this issue. The best tests involve DPA and dual X-ray absorptiometry (DXA), which should be conducted around the time of menopause. These are excellent for determining the status of bone in your hip and spine, sites that tend to be vulnerable to osteoporosis.

Another test, which uses single-photon absorptiometry, is less expensive but it's also less accurate. This test does allow measurement of the wrist and can be a good predictor of wrist fractures, but it's not good for forecasting what's likely to happen with your hip or spine.

The reason that menopause is such an important time is that this watershed in a woman's development marks a major decrease in her manufacture of estrogen, an extremely important hormone in stimulating the buildup of the body's bone tissue. When natural estrogen dries up, it can be replaced by a combination of estrogen and progesterone therapy in order to retard the natural loss of bone mass.

Slender women like Sheila tend to be at higher than average risk for osteoporosis. (Fat cells produce estrogen, which moderates the hormonal drop-off usually seen with menopause.) Other risk predictors include early menopause (especially before age 45), a family history of osteoporosis, a personal history of several bone fractures, drinking too much alcohol, physical inactivity, low nutritional calcium intake, heavy cigarette smoking, the prolonged use of cortisone-type hormones, and possibly, chronic use of thyroid hormone supplements.

Women who are identified through bone density tests as particularly vulnerable to osteoporosis can not only rely on estrogen, but also take other measures to build up their bones. These include quitting smoking, taking calcium and other mineral supplements, and engaging in weight-bearing exercises. Also, if the problem is severe, they may take medically supervised doses of vitamin D or other medications.

WHAT TO DO: If you have one or more risk factors for osteoporosis then you should definitely obtain a bone density measurement at the time of your menopause, with a repeat measurement about 18 months later to plot your rate of bone loss.

Those charged with balancing the health care budget would probably not endorse the recommendation that all women without osteoporosis risk factors also have a bone density measurement at menopause. Nevertheless, I personally believe that your individual interests would be best served by doing exactly that.

If your bone density measurement indicates an above-average risk you should review all your options, both hygienic and medical, with a doctor who has a special interest in osteoporosis. Usually this will be an arthritis specialist (rheumatologist) or an endocrinologist. However, many orthopedists and gynecologists and some family physicians and internists are also well qualified.

ERROR:

Your Doctor Uses the Right Drug—Estrogen—Along with a Wrong Drug to Treat Osteoporosis

Anna suffered from a severely curved spine and a tendency toward frequent fractures, both signs of her advanced osteoporosis. She regularly experienced pain from the compression fractures of her spine. Her doctor treated her with several drugs, including estrogen therapy, etidronate (Didronel), and a fluoride solution. Yet her pain worsened.

Was he giving her the wrong treatment?

FACTS: The estrogen therapy was appropriate and should be used for advanced cases of osteoporosis. The etidronate is able to reduce bone loss in the immediate postmenopausal years but may lose its effectiveness later on. In the longer term it may even promote bony fractures by building poor-quality bone. Some of the same problems accompany high-dose fluoride treatments, especially the stimulation of new but poor-quality bone.

A better approach may be to use estrogen therapy along with a new medicine called calcitonin. This drug is actually a natural hormone that actively prevents bone loss. It can quickly relieve bone pain in patients like Anna, who suffer from osteoporosis-caused compression fractures of the spine. Calcitonin is expensive, but except for potential allergic reactions, it appears to be safe. It's now used only as an injection, but a nasal spray form should be available eventually.

Another promising drug is calcitriol, a vitamin D derivative sold as a medication. It probably reduces the progression of osteoporosis, but more research will be needed before it gains Food and Drug Administration support. Recent results using lower doses of fluoride have also been encouraging.

WHAT TO DO: Estrogen plus calcitonin make sense if you are suffering from a severe case of osteoporosis. Also, calcitriol, though not yet approved by the Food and Drug Administration, may be a good idea if your osteoporosis is far advanced. But if you take this drug, you should see your doctor often enough to keep very close tabs on your blood calcium level—which can become elevated to toxic levels. For now, I would steer away from Didronel, fluoride medications, or anabolic steroids, which are sometimes used for osteoporosis.

ERROR:

Your Doctor Has Been Too Quick to Recommend Surgery for Your Carpal Tunnel Syndrome

Maggie, a 32-year-old cashier at a grocery store, developed a chronic pain in her right hand, which was diagnosed as carpal tunnel syndrome. Her doctor immediately suggested that the best treatment would be surgery.

Was this the correct recommendation?

FACTS: Carpal tunnel syndrome, a pain in the hands due to damage to a nerve passing through the wrist, is the best known of several important injuries that result from small, repeated stresses and strains to a particular part of the body. (See the accompanying box, Common Work Injuries.)

Most carpal tunnel cases improve with conservative treatment—especially among younger people—rather than with the more aggressive, surgical approach recommended by Maggie's doctor. For example, the doctor might try splinting the wrists and also using a nonsteroidal, antiinflammatory type of medicine. He might also identify the cause of the problem (in Maggie's case, repetitive use of the cash register with one hand) and then suggest ways to change the patient's habits so as to relieve the stress. In Maggie's situation, the doctor might have suggested that she try using her left hand more.

Surgery for carpal tunnel syndrome is relatively simple to perform and usually effective. Surgery is more likely to be needed for older people, where the tissues within the wrist may be unhealthily thickened. In older patients with carpal tunnel, delaying surgery too long, may, unfortunately, reduce the chances of an excellent result.

There have also been a few reasonably well designed studies that suggest there may be benefits from modest doses of vitamin B_6. But other studies have failed to confirm these results and most carpal tunnel experts remain skeptical of these claims.

WHAT TO DO: If you have carpal tunnel syndrome or symptoms suggestive of other overuse syndromes, such as those listed in the

Common Work Injuries: Their Symptoms and Likely Victims		
Name	*Symptoms*	*Who's Vulnerable*
Tension neck syndrome	Stiff, aching neck often with headache	Typists, key-punch operators, cashiers, bicyclists, small-parts assemblers, packers and others who work with their forearms while bracing at shoulder
Cervical syndrome	As in tension neck symptoms but may have pain radiating to one or both arms or numbness or tingling in hands	People who must flex or extend neck repeatedly or assume awkward positions, e.g., painters, cash register operators, data entry operators, dental surgeons
Thoracic outlet syndrome	Numbness, pain in arm especially when shoulder thrown back and hand raised	People who reach above shoulder level; carry heavy loads, e.g., suitcases; or wear knapsacks, e.g., letter carriers; auto mechanics; cashiers; musicians; operating room personnel; truck drivers
Rotator cuff tendinitis	Pain on elevating arm above 70 degrees at shoulder	Welders, painters, riveters, construction workers, installers of aluminum siding and awnings
Bicipital tendinitis	Pain, tenderness in upper arm near shoulder	Workers who must reach overhead, e.g., assembly workers, cleaners, window washers, construction workers, stock room employees

	Common Work Injuries: Their Symptoms and Likely Victims (*Continued*)	
Name	*Symptoms*	*Who's Vulnerable*
Frozen shoulder (more often with trauma but also with repetitive strain injury)	Reduced range of motion in shoulder	When arm or shoulder injury has caused decreased use, frozen shoulder may set in as a complication
Acromioclavicular syndrome	Pain, tenderness where shoulder and collarbone meet	People who carry heavy weights at waist level
Epicondylitis (tennis elbow on the thumb side, golfer's elbow on the little-finger side)	Pain at elbow when try to move hand against pressure	From repeated forceful rotation of forearm with wrist bent, e.g., small-parts assemblers, musicians, construction workers, woodworkers, tennis players, golfers
Carpal tunnel syndrome	Pain, tingling, or numbness in hand, often disturbs sleep; affects middle and thumb side of hand	Repeated forced hand movements, e.g., cashiers, assembly line workers, grinders, typists, keypunch operators, seamstresses and cutters, musicians, packers, bricklayers, drill operators
Ulnar nerve entrapment near the elbow from minor trauma	Like carpal tunnel syndrome but mainly toward fifth-finger side of hand	Work where inner aspect of elbow is strained or injured
De Quervain's tenosynovitis	Tenderness toward base of thumb, popping sensation when extend thumb backward	Hand tools that require repeated twisting motion

accompanying box, you should certainly raise the issue with your orthopedist, your company physician, or physiatrist (a specialist in physical training and therapy). But, especially if you are in your twenties or thirties, *don't* book an operation for carpal tunnel syndrome until you've tried more conservative treatments, such as splinting or identifying and eliminating repetitive injury patterns at work or home. Of *course*, if your symptoms progress despite conservative treatments, then the surgical option should be considered.

A good source of help for workers with carpal tunnel problems is the Job Accommodation Network, a federal program designed to advise citizens about work place modifications that can reduce the risk of injury. Call 1-800-526-7234.

ERROR:

Your Doctor Wrongly Diagnoses Your Backache as a Simple Muscle Spasm

Anyone who has had a long-lasting backache knows how frustrating it can be to bounce from doctor to doctor and diagnosis to diagnosis without finding an answer—or any relief from the pain. When I confronted this situation while writing this book, I became much more sympathetic to the plight of these patients.

My problem started when I simply turned over in bed, an act that caused my back to throb and pain to radiate down the back of my left leg. The first physician I consulted was a well-qualified specialist, but he was in a hurry that day. After a brief exam, he decided that the problem was a muscle spasm. He provided great relief by rolling me over onto a table to apply electrical stimulation to my back muscles for about 20 minutes. After two days of bed rest, I was back at work and also doing regular muscle-strengthening exercises with a physical therapist. But two weeks later, the backache worsened again.

Frustrated, I called an orthopedist, who tapped and tugged for what seemed like forever before pronouncing that I most likely had a herniated disk, which was causing damage to my sciatic nerve. A magnetic resonance imaging (MRI) exam confirmed that a protruding disk was pressing on two of my nerves. Two weeks of absolute bed rest accompanied by pain medication and muscle relaxants relieved the pain. When I was 95 percent better, I tried physical therapy again.

FACTS: The first doctor was too quick to assume that my back problem was a simple muscle spasm. He didn't look carefully enough for subtle signs of neurological damage. We both became overconfident when his treatment for spasm gave me temporary relief, and so I wrongly embarked too soon on a physical therapy program.

WHAT TO DO: Good family doctors and internists should be able to evaluate most routine back problems—if they give your case the full time and attention it deserves. But whether you first see your primary physician or you go directly to a specialist (usually an orthopedist or a neurologist), you must always insist that a thorough neurological and orthopedic exam be conducted. The doctor should evaluate your pain, strength, and flexibility as they relate to the nerves, muscles, and joints throughout the back, hips, and legs.

Be biased toward *resting* through the acute phase of your illness. Stay in touch with your doctor so she'll know if you're getting better on schedule.

If you find you're not doing well, go back to the doctor so that she can repeat her physical exam and look for subtle changes in your condition. If you have not yet seen a specialist, this would be a good time to obtain such a consultation. Ask your primary physician to refer you to a specialist she respects.

At this stage, despite the expense, an MRI or a computed tomography scan of the spine may be money well spent. These tests are better than plain spinal X rays because they can outline your disks and also pick up other causes of back pain, such as narrowing of the spine (spinal stenosis).

What about chiropractors? That's a "seeing-red" issue for most of my orthopedist friends, who are quick to point to patients they have seen who have had their problems made worse by overaggressive manipulation by a chiropractor. Still, there is fairly strong research evidence to show that chiropractic manipulation *does* help certain low back pains more quickly than does conventional medical therapy. I am very skeptical of chiropractors who claim to treat problems outside their realm of expertise, such as asthma or heart disease. I also want you to recognize that overzealous manipulation of an unstable low back (or far worse, a fragile neck!) could cause irreversible harm. But where low back problems are involved, my personal experience with and feelings about chiropractic are basically positive.

ERROR:

Your Doctor Thinks Your Back or Leg Pain Is Caused by a Disk or Muscle Spasm When the Real Problem Is an Artery Blockage

Kent experienced a pain and then numbness in his right leg, which his doctor attributed to a long-standing disk problem. But the pain increased, and Kent's leg turned a sickly pale color. He was admitted to the hospital, where the diagnosis was a clogged artery in the leg.

FACTS: Blockage of an artery in the pelvis or leg can cause leg pain or numbness that can mimic a disk problem. Usually, the blockage symptoms come and go; typically, they worsen with walking or running (a condition known as *intermittent claudication*). Sometimes, though, the condition progresses rapidly, as happened with Kent. In this situation, the patient may confront a true emergency in a matter of days or hours. A typical symptom is a leg that turns pale or even blue.

Arterial blockage is probably not your problem if the doctor can feel pounding pulses in your foot, behind your knee, and in your groin. But these beats can be difficult to feel if you retain fluid, are heavy, or already have arteriosclerosis to a degree. An ultrasound sonar-type exam of your arteries may be necessary to be sure arterial blockage isn't the problem.

WHAT TO DO: If you have serious leg or lower back pains, be sure your doctor examines the pulses in your feet and tells you the result. If the pulses aren't strong, ask whether arterial blockage is a possibility.

Physicians who deal with many back complaints should be able to avoid the confusion between back and vascular problems. But even orthopedists or neurology specialists can fall into the trap of focusing on just one formulation of a diagnosis and not thinking through alternatives.

I'd be especially concerned that non-physicians, e.g., physical therapists or chiropractors, might be apt to overlook the key question, *Is this really a bone-muscle problem or could it be vascular?*

ERROR:

Missing a Change in Back Symptoms That Can Signal a Dangerous Emergency

Benny, a 70-year-old former accountant, was told by his orthopedist to go to bed whenever his chronic back condition, a slipped disk, flared up. He did so faithfully every time the pain hit, and usually, he recovered within a few days to a week.

But then he noticed on one occasion that even though the pain had improved after about three days, his leg seemed weaker. In fact, he could barely walk on it to the bathroom. He didn't make the connection that something different might be going on in his body, and in a brief conversation on the phone with his doctor, he just said, "I felt a little weak today." The doctor, apparently assuming the weakness arose from his having been in bed for an extended period, didn't probe to find out exactly what Benny meant by "weak."

Weeks later, when Benny's son-in-law realized what was happening and frantically persuaded the orthopedist to make a house call, Benny's right leg had shriveled to two-thirds the size of the left. Only an emergency operation prevented further damage. Though Benny lived another six years, he never fully recovered the strength in that leg.

FACTS: Pressure on a nerve from a protruding disk, arthritis, a tumor, or inflamed muscles can cause pain through the area touched by that nerve. For the back that means pain anywhere along the low back, buttock, hip, thigh, knee, leg, or ankle. As pressure increases, reversible and later irreversible damage to the nerve may result. Approximately 1 to 3 percent of disk operations are due to emergencies to relieve this type of increased pressure on the nerves, and fast action is absolutely essential.

WHAT TO DO: Call your doctor immediately if you develop

- Numbness or weakness in one or both legs. For example, you can't rise up on your toes or your heels, not because of the pain but because you're weak.
- Difficulty moving your bowels or urinating. These problems might be due to the side effects of medication or to your disease. In either case, you should have the situation dealt with promptly.

Your Orthopedist Is Too Quick to Recommend Back Surgery

Jack had a steady but relatively moderate lower back pain. He knew that the problem stemmed from a big, bulging disk, which could be seen on an MRI machine. Because Jack complained regularly about his back, his surgeon decided to recommend an operation.

Was he right?

FACTS: Many experts believe that 40 percent or more of the 200,000 or so disk operations (laminectomies) done each year should not have been performed. A University of Wisconsin study found that the rate of back surgery varies as much as 700 percent from one county to another! Since these operations do carry a small but significant risk of doing harm to the back, it's best to view all proposals for disk surgery with some wariness.

One common misconception is that a big, bulging disk of the type that Jack saw on his MRI means that surgery is required. Quite a few people have only modest low back pain, only occasional symptoms, or even *no* symptoms despite an impressive abnormal MRI picture.

The people most likely to benefit from back surgery are in these categories:

- Their spinal disks have actually broken down or ruptured.

- The disk is pressing on a nerve—the same nerve that is linked to the site of their symptoms.

- Pain radiates down the leg, past the knee.

- The leg pain worsens when they lie on the back and raise the leg straight into the air.

- They have some objective loss of neurological function, such as diminished reflexes, weakness, difficulty rising on their toes or heels, or an abnormal nerve conduction study (a test that measures the health of individual nerves).

- Their back problem has recurred or progressed despite bed rest, antiinflammatory medicines, and physical therapy.

Surgery is much less likely to help even if you have severe or prolonged back pain, if your pain is confined to the back (that is, it doesn't radiate down the leg), and there is no neurological damage. Of course, life isn't always so simple. My orthopedist consultants insist that some back operations should be done even when there is not yet objective evidence of neurological damage. In certain situations, objective findings may appear only relatively late as the problem progresses, and to delay the operation might decrease the chances of full recovery.

The point of these guidelines, of course, is not to supersede your doctor's judgment, but to help you decide when to be more aggressive about seeking additional opinions.

WHAT TO DO: Except in emergency cases, such as when your leg turns numb or your bladder or bowel stops working, a second opinion should be routine before any surgery, including back surgery. Your questions to the physician giving the second opinion should include these:

1. What are the odds that the proposed surgery will help me and for how long?

2. What are the odds that nonsurgical alternatives might help?

3. Is the doctor who is proposing to operate on me well qualified?

Your second opinion doctor as well as your surgeon should be board-certified orthopedists or neurosurgeons. Both of these specialists are qualified to operate on backs. They should also do 100 to 150 back operations each year, though all don't necessarily have to be disk surgery. In addition, they should be respected as "conservative" surgeons among doctors in the community, in the sense that they don't do surgery at the drop of a hat but often rely on nonsurgical procedures to treat back problems. (Your family physician may be able to help you check on this point.)

$$\boxed{\text{E R R O R :}}$$

Your Doctor Is Ignorant About Identifying and Treating Fibromyalgia

Ellen, who was in her late fifties, complained to her doctor on several occasions of general muscle aches, an inability to sleep well, stiffness in various joints every morning, and tenderness over many parts of her body. The doctor had a variety of responses during the visits when Ellen brought up her symptoms:

"It must be arthritis. What do you expect at your age? I'll give you a painkiller to make you feel better."

"You need to find a comfortable sleeping position. Try a firmer mattress."

"It's probably because you're anxious or depressed. I can refer you to a psychotherapist."

"There's nothing else to be done. You'll just have to live with it."

What had the doctor missed?

FACTS: The doctor had missed the fact that Ellen had fibromyalgia, a condition of muscle soreness and tenderness that affects an estimated one American in twenty. This disease wasn't even in the medical books 20 years ago when I was a medical resident. Now fibromyalgia has established itself as a physical disorder, which involves a large array of symptoms, including muscle aches and tenderness, fatigue, headache, irritable bowel, stiffness in the morning, and poor sleep.

Because this problem is such a newly defined syndrome, many doctors aren't up to speed on its symptoms and diagnosis. Yet the key to diagnosing fibromyalgia is the presence of the symptoms listed above as well as tenderness to the touch of certain key points on the body. These include the following sites: midway along the firm muscle that connects the base of the neck and the shoulder; the upper, inner border of the scapula (shoulder blade); the base of the side of the neck; the spot where the second rib connects to the sternum; the inner side of the knee; an area just off the midline near the lowest part of the back; the outer side of the elbow; and the upper, outer part of the buttocks.

Before your doctor concludes that fibromyalgia is the difficulty, he must exclude various other inflammatory diseases, such as rheumatoid arthritis, Lyme disease, polymyalgia rheumatica, low thyroid production, and any localized injury or trauma.

How should fibromyalgia be treated? The best drugs are certain antidepressants but in doses much lower than those used for depression. Most experts now think that fibromyalgia results from a brain chemistry imbalance. Another helpful medicine that's often used is cyclobenzaprine (Flexeril). Gentle physical therapy, moderately paced exercise, good-quality sleep, and, possibly, certain nutritional supplements are also important aids for this problem.

Drugs such as aspirin, Advil, or other nonsteroidal antiinflammatory medicines, though good for arthritis, get only mixed reviews for fibromyalgia. Many rheumatologists prescribe them in combination with antidepressants, but most find that they provide only modest benefit. Also, even though narcotic pain medicines may provide some relief, you should avoid them because they are likely to be habit-forming when used for a chronic condition like fibromyalgia.

Tranquilizers and sleeping pills, like Valium and Dalmane, can relax the muscles and sometimes help fibromyalgia. But again, the risk of addiction is too great to justify more than occasional use.

WHAT TO DO: If your doctor, like Ellen's, can't seem to identify the source of your aches and pains, ask him about fibromyalgia. If he seems to know something about this disease, talks knowledgeably about the symptoms, and indicates he has had other cases of this type, that's encouraging. But be cautious if your doctor proposes that you use habit-forming medicines or cortisone-type drugs.

If you draw a blank stare from your doctor when you mention this disease or if he seems at all nonresponsive, seek a consultation with an arthritis specialist, an orthopedist, a physiatrist (a rehabilitation specialist), or a sleep specialist. They will all have seen many patients with fibromyalgia and should know how to diagnose and treat it.

ERROR:

Your Doctor Fails to Educate You About the Early Symptoms of Lyme Disease

Tim, who lived on Long Island, New York, developed a flulike illness and rash. The rash involved a small, reddish area on his arm, which expanded a couple of inches into a red ring with a pale skin-colored interior, like a kind of bull's-eye. But then the symptoms disappeared, and Tim forgot about them—until he awoke one morning about six months later with excruciating pain in both knees and one ankle. He immediately made an appointment with his doctor.

The complaint sounded to the doctor like arthritis. But because Tim lived in an area that has a high incidence of Lyme disease, he added a Lyme antibody test to a standard arthritis blood test. The result was strongly positive.

The doctor placed Tim on a three-week course of doxycycline, and he now feels fairly well. But like many patients with Lyme disease, he still doesn't feel 100 percent. His muscles ache and feel sore, and mild fatigue and restless sleep have become an annoying fact of life.

Did Tim's doctor make any mistakes?

FACTS: The only mistake this physician seems to have made was not educating Tim about the symptoms of Lyme disease, which was a prevalent threat in his area. Due to a lack of time, most physicians allow the media to educate their patients about Lyme disease—and this is a major mistake.

Doctors who see patients regularly have a responsibility not only to check for standard conditions they learn about in medical school, but also to keep in mind special health threats in their locality. When those threats involve initial symptoms that are subtle and may go unnoticed—as is the case with Lyme disease—ideally the doctor *must* take steps to educate patients about what to look for.

More and more Americans are finding Lyme disease intruding on their lives. The disease has appeared in almost every state, though 90 percent of the cases remain clustered in the Northeast, the mid-Atlantic region, the north central states, and the Pacific Coast.

Lyme disease is a bacterial infection, actually, a close cousin of syphilis. But it's transmitted by the bite of an infected tick, primarily deer ticks, which are tiny, black-legged, hard-to-see creatures.

The typical initial symptoms are a flulike illness and rash that often turns into a bull's-eye shape. You may notice the bite of a tiny deer tick, and a few days or weeks later, a small red flat or slightly raised rash will form near the site of the bite. The rash doesn't hurt or itch, but it expands over the next weeks to a circle that is one to seven inches or more in diameter, with a bright red outer ring and a paler center. Unfortunately, however, many Lyme victims don't develop or don't notice this typical rash. At this early stage, the flu-related symptoms may include fatigue, achiness, fever, swollen glands, and a headache.

The initial symptoms typically disappear after a few weeks, and the disease goes underground. But Lyme then tends to resurface months or years later with more serious complications, including arthritis, brain and nerve inflammation, or even damage to the heart.

Early recognition and treatment with antibiotics will usually cure the problem. But a few patients mysteriously go on to late-stage symptoms even after a vigorous round of early antibiotics. Many others, like Tim, may seem to be cured but then continue to carry strange aches and pains or suffer from a general malaise.

WHAT TO DO: If the above-described classic Lyme disease sequence occurs, with the bull's-eye rash and perhaps flu symptoms, see your doctor immediately. He may give you the Lyme disease blood antibody test but shouldn't wait to begin treatment. First of all, if the Lyme test is taken at a very early stage, say, within the first four weeks of infection, the result is often still negative. (See the accompanying box, Is the Lyme Disease Test Reliable?)

In any case, for your best chance of a complete cure, it's probably best to treat the condition early. So if your doctor has a strong suspicion that you have Lyme disease, there's no need to wait until the blood test turns positive.

Unfortunately, most people with Lyme disease don't recall being bitten by a tick, and 30 to 40 percent don't see a rash. Their only early symptoms may resemble a viral infection. As a practical matter, this type of Lyme disease can't be detected until a blood antibody test is done. So if there's a fair chance that you've been exposed—and especially if you have an accompanying flulike illness—it's best to follow up with a blood test for Lyme, perhaps six to eight weeks later.

Most specialists don't treat low-probability situations such as an imbedded deer tick, especially if it has been attached less than 24 hours. If they did, they might have almost everyone on antibiotics throughout the summer. However, a few physicians in areas with a

---

Is the Lyme Disease Test Reliable?

The current standard Lyme disease test requires that the infection be in the body four to eight weeks before it turns positive. An early negative means nothing. So there's little reason to take one immediately after a tick bite.

Even a Lyme test that is done at a later stage may come back falsely negative. So if the circumstances and symptoms you're experiencing strongly suggest Lyme, antibiotic treatment should be given.

Some Lyme disease tests may come back positive, but the reason may be the presence of *other* diseases. For example, you may get a positive Lyme result if you have autoimmune disease, neurological disease, syphilis, or Rocky Mountain spotted fever.

In one 1992 study of laboratories that test for Lyme, 4 to 21 percent of the labs failed to detect the disease in a sample known to have high levels of the Lyme antibody. Furthermore, 55 percent couldn't detect a low level of the antibody.

Many Lyme disease experts have much more confidence in the results at certain laboratories that have a special interest in the issue. These include the school of medicine at the State University of New York, Stony Brook; Yale University, New Haven, Connecticut; New England Medical Center, Boston; and the University of Connecticut, Hartford.

---

high occurrence of Lyme disease are more aggressive, preferring to err on the side of unnecessary antibiotics rather than risk the ravages of Lyme.

I feel that both viewpoints are defensible. The key is that you and your doctor should discuss the pros and cons of treating versus observing for your particular case, so that your values and preferences are weighed in making the decision.

ERROR:

Your Doctor Treats You with the Right Antibiotics for Lyme Disease but for Too Short a Period of Time

Winston was diagnosed as having an early stage of Lyme disease and was placed on ten days of oral doxycycline.

What was wrong with this treatment?

FACTS: Unlike most infections, where seven to ten days of antibiotics is enough, most experts treat Lyme for twenty to thirty days with high doses of the drugs. The most commonly used antibiotics are oral doxycycline, tetracycline, amoxicillin, penicillin, Ceftin, or Suprax.

Erythromycin has been used, but it's not effective enough. Also, children, pregnant women, or nursing women shouldn't use tetracycline and doxycycline, because these drugs can stain growing teeth.

For long-lasting Lyme disease or where symptoms affect the brain or heart or cause arthritis, intravenous antibiotics are in order, usually for about a four-week period. If this course doesn't work or if you improve but then relapse, there is considerable controversy about what to do next.

Many Lyme disease specialists believe that Lyme is grossly overdiagnosed, especially by certain physicians who diagnose almost all mysterious ailments as probably due to Lyme. On the other hand, other specialists argue that Lyme is also *under*diagnosed because of the insensitivity of current antibody tests.

A growing minority of specialists also take issue with the standard view that four weeks of intravenous antibiotics is always enough to treat even the most difficult cases of Lyme.

My opinion: There is no doubt that some so-called Lyme specialists are too quick to assume that every patient they see needs treatment. At the same time, however, recent research also makes it likely that some patients with active Lyme are probably missed by current antibody tests. There is also evidence that some patients with Lyme continue to have active disease even after four weeks of antibiotics.

Most academic specialists in infectious disease are conservative about diagnosing Lyme unless the evidence is strong. You can find such a specialist on referral from your family physician or from a local infectious disease doctor. Lyme specialists who are more aggressive in diagnosing Lyme and in treating it are on the referral list of this consumer advocate organization: the Lyme Borreliosis Foundation, P.O. Box 462, Tolland, CT 06084-0462, phone 203-871-2900.

WHAT TO DO: If your doctor places you on a course of antibiotics for less than twenty days for any stage of Lyme disease, tell her you understand that's not long enough to knock out the infection. If she insists on this course of treatment, seek a second opinion from a physician who has had considerable experience treating Lyme disease patients.

With ambiguous cases, most infectious disease specialists will take a conservative position in diagnosing Lyme and prescribing treatment. That is, they will be more likely to take a wait-and-see attitude. Physicians referred through the Lyme Borreliosis Foundation will tend to be more aggressive prescribing antibiotics and using them for longer courses of treatment. If your consultants can't agree on what to do, you may find a resolution by seeking an opinion from a medical school department that has access to new Lyme diagnostic tests that may not yet be available to community physicians.

For patients with chronic symptoms, where Lyme is suspected but not proven to be the cause, I've found that certain experimental tests on spinal fluid can be useful. These are done at centers like the department of neurology at the State University of New York, Stony Brook, Long Island.

PART SIX

Some Anti-error Strategies for Women Only

Special Alerts: For Women Only

- You're treated for vaginitis even though you're in the early stage of pregnancy. (See error, p. 321.)

- Your pelvic, rectal, or back pain is caused by endometriosis, but your physician thinks the problem is an irritable bowel. (See error, p. 324.)

- You are diagnosed as having the flu when you really have the deadly toxic shock syndrome. (See error, p. 325.)

- You're not warned that you can get pregnant during the first phase of menopause. (See error, p. 330.)

Your Doctor Gives You Medication Without Taking into Account Your Birth Control Pills

Barbara, a young mother in her midthirties, was taking birth control pills regularly when she came down with a bacterial infection. Her doctor prescribed penicillin, which knocked out the infection. Two months later, she found that she was pregnant.

What had happened?

FACTS: So many women take the Pill these days that doctors sometimes forget to take it into account when they review potential drug interactions with new medications.

Certain antibiotics may decrease the effectiveness of oral contraceptives. These include penicillin, tetracycline, griseofulvin, and rifampin. A similar problem exists with barbiturates and hydantoins (such as Dilantin). So it's wise for those women on these drugs to rely on a backup form of birth control, such as the diaphragm or condom, during the period when they are taking these medications.

Also, birth control pills tend to slow the metabolism and increase the risk of side effects for a number of drugs, such as the benzodiazepines (Valium, Librium); caffeine; cortisonelike medications; the beta-blocker metoprolol (Lopressor); tricyclic antidepressants; and theophyllines.

Furthermore, birth control pills may increase the risk of liver damage from acetaminophen (Tylenol) in women who have liver disease. And they can increase *or* decrease the effect of warfarin (Coumadin) and other anticoagulants.

WHAT TO DO: Whenever you plan to take any medication, prescribed or over-the-counter, check with your doctor and pharmacist to see if there might be any interactions with your birth control pills. Always remember: Oral contraceptives are a drug, and they can react explosively with many medications.

E R R O R :

Your Doctor Prescribes an Intrauterine Device, Even Though You Have a Past History of Pelvic Infections

Jane had become dissatisfied with her normal method of birth control, a diaphragm. After evaluating her situation, including that she was involved in a monogamous relationship and did not plan to have more children, her doctor chose the intrauterine device (IUD). But he overlooked that before she had come under his care, she had experienced two pelvic infections, which the doctor had managed to clear up with a round of antibiotics.

A few months after the IUD was inserted, Jane came down with another quite severe pelvic infection.

Should the doctor have anticipated this?

FACTS: Although the IUD is an extremely convenient form of contraception, its downside risks are severe, including increased risk for pelvic infections; ectopic pregnancy (a potentially fatal complication, where the fertilized egg implants itself outside the uterus); and irregular bleeding and menstrual cramps.

The IUD only makes sense for women who value convenience above all else; who have already had all the children they want; and who are in a monogamous relationship, which puts them at low risk for contracting a sexually transmitted disease. Obviously, Jane fit into these categories.

But her doctor failed to note that she was also in a high-risk situation for complications from an IUD because she had a past history of pelvic infections. Other women who should not be fitted with an IUD include those who have had a sexually transmitted disease; an infection of the cervix or uterus; unexplained vaginal bleeding; cancer of the reproductive area; previous major pelvic surgery; a small or distorted uterus; or a history of ectopic pregnancy. In addition, those who are pregnant or think they may be should stay away from an IUD.

WHAT TO DO: Although all forms of contraception have their drawbacks, for most women the risks from an IUD outweigh the advantages. My advice is to stay away from them unless you have no realistic alternative. If you feel you must have one, be absolutely *sure* you aren't in any of the high-risk groups I've described under Facts. Contact your doctor *immediately* if you experience any of these symptoms: a late or missed period; abdominal pain; fever; chills; four-smelling or unusually heavy vaginal discharge; spotting; heavy periods; or clotting.

ERROR:

Your Doctor Fails to Check How You Insert Your Diaphragm

Joanne's doctor recommended birth control pills or the IUD for contraception, and he pointed out, quite correctly, that unwanted pregnancies came about more often with devices like the diaphragm. But she wanted a diaphragm because she felt, also correctly, that it was the least likely to be dangerous to her health.

Reluctantly, the doctor prescribed the diaphragm, and he described how she should insert it, but he didn't actually have her insert it to check its placement while she was still in the office. Six months later, Joanne became pregnant.

What is wrong about this interaction with her doctor?

FACTS: It is instructive to understand, as Joanne's doctor indicated, that the odds of becoming pregnant do vary according to the method of contraception that is used. (See the accompanying box, Your Chances of Becoming Pregnant with Different Methods of Contraception.) On average, many more women using the diaphragm become pregnant than do those using the Pill or the IUD.

On the other hand, the diaphragm can be an excellent method if your doctor has experience fitting it on patients *and* shows you *exactly* how to use it *and* watches you insert it to be sure that you're following the correct procedure.

WHAT TO DO: As effective as the diaphragm usually is, it requires active, conscientious attention each and every time you insert it, or there will be a high risk of pregnancy. (See the accompanying box, Rules for Proper Diaphragm Use.) So if you decide on the diaphragm, choose a doctor who is enthusiastic about the device, not one who tries to talk you out of it. The enthusiasts are much more likely to be experienced and competent in fitting you properly.

	Your Chances of Becoming Pregnant with Different Methods of Contraception	

The table below lists the number of women out of 100 who become pregnant in the first year of using different methods of birth control. The column Lowest Pregnancy Rate shows the rate when people use the method without any mistakes. The column Typical Pregnancy Rate lists the results with the use by the average person, who periodically makes mistakes.

Method	Lowest Pregnancy Rate	Typical Pregnancy Rate
Birth control pills	0.1	3
Rhythm method		20
Calendar	9	
Cervical mucus method	3	
Cervical mucus plus temperature method	1	
Withdrawal (coitus interruptus)	4	18
Diaphragm with spermicide	2–6	18
Cervical cap with spermicide	6	18
Vaginal sponge		
Women with children	9	28
Women without children	6	18
Condom (without spermicide)	2	12
Intrauterine device (IUD)		3
Progesterone T	2	
Copper T 380 A	0.8	
Norplant (progesterone) placed under skin	0.04	0.04
Depoprovera (progesterone) injections every 3 months	0.3	0.3
Male sterilization (vasectomy)	0.1	0.15
Female sterilization	0.2	0.4

Once you've been fitted, you should practice inserting the diaphragm in your doctor's office—that means the entire device, not just the fitting ring. This way, the doctor can check you on the spot to see if you've put it in correctly.

If you still lack confidence in your ability to put the diaphragm in correctly even after you've done it right once or if you feel nervous

Rules for Proper Diaphragm Use

1. Urinate before insertion. Check diaphragm for any leaks or cracks. Never use petroleum jelly (e.g., Vaseline). It can harm the rubber. Do use spermicidal cream.

2. After you insert the diaphragm, check to be sure the cervix is covered by feeling for its firm, knoblike projection behind the rubber of the diaphragm. Also, the top part of the diaphragm's ring should fit snugly against the pubic bone.

3. Insert the diaphragm within two hours of intercourse. (Some doctors feel that within six hours is okay.)

4. Apply more spermicide vaginally after first ejaculation, if further intercourse is expected. Do not remove diaphragm! (Some doctors feel repeat spermicide is necessary only if several hours have elapsed.)

5. Leave diaphragm in for at least six to eight hours after intercourse. Then remove and wash with mild soap such as Ivory. Dry and store. Do not use talc. You may use cornstarch.

6. Ask your doctor to recheck the diaphragm fit every 3 years, or if you gain or lose 10 percent of your body weight, or after a pregnancy.

when you're inserting it, have your doctor recheck your ability to insert it at a later visit. When your nervousness subsides, your vaginal muscles tend to relax, and that can change the fit of the diaphragm. Ask your doctor to recheck your diaphragm if you have gained or lost considerable weight because this might alter your fit.

If you are a virgin, it may be best to use foam and condoms for a while before fitting the diaphragm, since your vaginal cavity may enlarge as a result of intercourse.

Warning: A diaphragm is an extremely safe device—with one exception. The diaphragm and also the cervical cap and the vaginal sponge should *not be used by women who have a history of toxic shock syndrome.* This is an often fatal infection that occurs with a certain strain of staphylococcal (staph) bacteria. Though rare, this condition may be encouraged by the use of these three types of contraception.

E R R O R :

Your Doctor Treats You for Vaginitis Without Checking Whether You Are Pregnant

Ruth went off the Pill because she and her husband were trying to have another child. A few weeks later, she began to experience a vaginal discharge, which her doctor diagnosed as vaginitis, an inflammation of the vagina that she had encountered several times in the past. He immediately prescribed an oral antibiotic. A month later, Ruth announced that she was two months pregnant.

What are the implications of the doctor's treatment?

FACTS: If possible, drugs should never be prescribed during pregnancy—and especially during the first three to four months—because of possible negative effects on the fetus.

In this case, the doctor should have checked to see if Ruth was pregnant or trying to get pregnant before he prescribed a treatment for vaginitis. Pregnant women are quite vulnerable to vaginitis, especially candida. But a noninfectious vaginal discharge, which requires no treatment, is also common in pregnancy.

If a pregnant woman does develop vaginitis during pregnancy, a doctor must choose carefully the drugs that are least likely to have a negative effect on the baby. Those that are often recommended are class B-rated drugs, such as clotrimazole, miconazole, ampicillin, and first-generation cephalosporins.

"Class B" means that no problems with pregnancy have been reported in humans or in animal experiments. Relatively few drugs are class B. Most are class C, meaning no problems reported in humans, but harm to the fetus was seen when high doses of the drug were given to pregnant animals. Another class B-related oral antibiotic, flagyl, is often used to treat certain types of vaginal discharge. But I recommend that it be avoided during pregnancy because of lingering concern about the medication's possible mutational or cancer-causing effects.

WHAT TO DO: If you think there's any chance you may be pregnant, you should make sure about your condition before you take medications for vaginitis or any other condition. *Remember:* You want to do everything reasonable to minimize your exposure to medicines, especially during the first three to four months of pregnancy, in order to protect the health of your child.

ERROR:

Your Doctor Doesn't Take Your Premenstrual Syndrome Symptoms Seriously

Every time Arlene's menstrual period approached, she began to feel depressed; she cried easily, and she felt bloated. She mentioned this to her doctor, but he just replied, "There are some things you have to live with."

Was he right?

FACTS: No, he was dead wrong. He represents a still significant group of doctors, mostly male, who downplay the impact of premenstrual syndrome (PMS). The standard medical position now is that PMS is indeed a real condition, partly physical, partly psychological, and definitely related to the monthly hormonal cycle. But too many doctors don't take it seriously enough to treat it as an illness.

There are four main patterns of PMS symptoms that have been identified:

Type A: Anxiety, irritability, nervousness, mood swings.
Type C: Food cravings (especially chocolate or sugar), headache, palpitations, dizziness.
Type H: Fluid retention, abdominal swelling, feeling bloated, breast congestion and tenderness, anxiety.
Type D: Depression, crying easily, insomnia, confusion.

PMS can also bring out other symptoms, such as acne, digestive disturbances, and worsening of preexisting illnesses, including arthritis, asthma, and migraine.

WHAT TO DO: If you have any of the above symptoms and your doctor doesn't pay much attention to your complaints, find another doctor who is sympathetic. An understanding internist or gynecologist will be the most likely candidate. Endocrinologists, with some exceptions, are not the best choice. Their routine lab tests, other than the one for basic thyroid conditions, are likely to be expensive and are almost never helpful in explaining or treating the symptoms of PMS.

In any event, getting the right doctor is the first step. Then, expect to be introduced to a number of guidelines and techniques that have been advocated (but not proved 100 percent effective) for reducing your PMS symptoms. These include

- Relaxation techniques, such as visual imagery, self-hypnosis, yoga, and biofeedback.

- Physical exercise.

- More adequate sleep.

- More frequent sex.

- A hypoglycemia-type diet, with small, frequent meals that are *low* in caffeine, alcohol, sugars, and simple carbohydrates.

- Restriction of your salt intake.

- The use of nutritional supplements, especially vitamin B_6 (in doses of 50 to 100 milligrams), vitamin E, magnesium, and oil of evening primrose plant (a source of the essential fatty acid gamma linolenic acid—GLA).

Your doctor may also prescribe a medicine like fluoxetine (Prozac), an antidepressant that has been shown to be able to prevent or reduce PMS symptoms. Diuretics may also help if fluid retention is a prominent factor in your PMS. Aches, pains, and other specific problems may be decreased with such drugs as aspirin, Advil, tricyclic antidepressant medicines, or antianxiety agents (such as Valium and BuSpar). Also, some doctors advocate the use of birth control pills or other hormonal manipulations.

Many PMS specialists advocate treatment with natural progesterone hormones. (Natural progesterone is said to have different effects from the synthetic progesterones physicians usually prescribe.) However, this approach remains controversial. Most gynecologists, and most research studies, indicate the the benefit claimed for natural progesterone is mainly due to coincidental improvement or to a "placebo effect."

ERROR:

Your Doctor Overlooks the Possibility That Your Pelvic, Rectal, or Back Pain May Be Caused by Endometriosis

Ida, who was in her early thirties, had been experiencing discomfort in her pelvic area. Also, even though she and her husband had been trying to have a child for about a year, they had been unsuccessful.

Her doctor decided that her problem was probably an irritable bowel that she had complained about several times in the past, and he began to treat her for that. But the pain increased, and a gynecologist determined that she actually had endometriosis, the spread of functioning uterine tissue to surrounding organs from their usual location inside the cavity of the uterus.

FACTS: Endometriosis affects about 5 percent of women who are fertile and approximately 25 percent of women who can't have children. The condition, which involves the presence of functioning uterine tissue outside the uterus, has been identified in almost every organ of the body except, oddly enough, in the spleen. As these endometrial cells first swell and then shrink with the ebb and flow of the monthly menstrual cycle, they trigger pelvic, back, or rectal pain; pain with intercourse; and very painful menstrual cramps.

When pelvic pain is cyclical and severe, doctors routinely suspect endometriosis. But sometimes, more subtle discomforts, such as those experienced by Ida, can be confused with irritable bowel syndrome or chronic pelvic infections. Or there may be no pain at all; infertility may be the only complaint.

Diagnosis can sometimes be made by ultrasound images of the pelvis, a computed tomography (CT) scan, or magnetic resonance imaging (MRI). But the gold standard for identifying this problem remains actually observing the site in the body and taking a piece of tissue from the abnormal site. Usually this procedure is done with an instrument such as a laparoscope or culdoscope, which is employed through small incisions in the pelvic region.

WHAT TO DO: If you are infertile or have distress in your pelvis— or, for that matter, elsewhere in your body—and the distress grows worse with your period, consult a gynecologist about endometriosis.

If the problem is endometriosis, hormone treatments may be ordered. These include the use of such medications as progesterone, Danazol, and Lupron, which prevent sex hormone production. All of these have potential side effects and should be used only by experienced physicians. Lupron is one of a new group of medicines that have been used; they are called "gonadotropin-releasing hormone agonists." They block the action of certain pituitary hormones that would normally stimulate the ovaries. In effect, these blocking drugs put the body into a temporary menopause.

Nonsteroidal antiinflammatory painkillers, like aspirin or Advil, are often less effective for endometriosis than they are for standard menstrual cramps.

Various surgical techniques are available for removing endometrial implants while preserving the functioning of the uterus and ovaries. But the most serious cases may have to be treated by complete hysterectomy, or removal of the uterus and ovaries—a step that eliminates the possibility of childbearing and induces premature menopause. You should always seek a second opinion by an independent specialist to confirm the necessity of this sort of surgery.

ERROR:

Your Doctor Overlooks That Flulike Symptoms with a Peeling, Red Rash May Actually Be Toxic Shock Syndrome

Nan, who was in her late thirties, began to suffer from fever, diarrhea, and vomiting. She also noticed the appearance of a red rash on her abdomen, which peeled like a sunburn. Her doctor gave her a prescription to quell the nausea and reduce the fever, but he just told her to "keep an eye on" the rash and inform him about its progress.

What was his mistake?

FACTS: This doctor slipped up by not thinking of toxic shock syndrome (TSS) as a possibility when Nan came in with her symptoms. This deadly illness, which is a complication of an infection involving a particular strain of staphylococcus bacteria, isn't too common. But menstruating women—usually those who use tampons—are the most frequent victims. When treatment is delayed, the illness can become quite severe, with fatalities in about 5 percent of the cases.

Initial symptoms often include fever, vomiting, and diarrhea, often accompanied by headache, sore throat, aching muscles, or feeling faint. Any of these symptoms may also signal possible viral illness, food poisoning, or an intestinal infection. But with TSS, blood pressure may drop and trigger mental confusion, shock, and breakdown of vital organs, such as the kidney, blood, or lungs. A tip-off clue that sets TSS apart from other illnesses is a red rash that peels like sunburn. That's what the doctor missed in his diagnosis.

Some first cases of this disease may resolve by themselves. But there's a tendency for TSS to reappear a second or third time, and when this happens, the condition is more likely to be fatal.

Early treatment of TSS with intravenous fluids and intensive medical care can make all the difference. But too often, the doctor will continue to treat the condition as a bad flu until it's too late. The biggest obstacle to care is getting the doctor himself to ask the question, "Could this be TSS?"

WHAT TO DO: If you're menstruating and especially if you use tampons, be alert if you develop a sudden fever (usually over 102 degrees Fahrenheit), especially if it is accompanied by vomiting or diarrhea and a red, peeling rash. With such symptoms, you should contact your doctor immediately. And don't be shy: Suggest the possibility of TSS and demand to be seen or taken to the emergency room. If you are wearing a tampon, remove it.

To prevent TSS, you should avoid tampons or use those that have a lower absorbency. Also, if you do use tampons, change them frequently—at least four times a day. If you develop TSS once, *never* use tampons again.

ERROR:

Your Doctor Tries to Make the Estrogen Decision for You

Margaret, who was 51 years old, had been placed on estrogen-progesterone therapy because she was going through menopause. She had a family history of breast cancer; her mother and a sister had been stricken with malignancies. With this background and after reading that there might be a link between taking estrogen and progesterone and breast cancer, she worried that she might be increasing her risk.

When she raised this issue with her doctor, he said, "The benefits of taking estrogen, such as maintaining your bone mass and reducing your likelihood of having a heart attack, far outweigh any risks. Besides, you haven't had any indication of breast cancer. So don't worry about it."

Was he right?

FACTS: The issue of whether or not to take estrogen and progesterone is a complex matter—more complex than Margaret's doctor indicated.

What we know for sure is that giving women estrogen reduces their risk of broken bones from osteoporosis but at the same time increases their risk for cancer of the uterus. Fortunately, adding progesterone to the estrogen drastically reduces the uterine cancer risk.

Breast cancer, which affects about 10 percent of women, is another factor to consider when taking estrogen and progesterone. Those who have had breast cancer or who have a strong family history of the disease are best advised to stay away from estrogen, and so Margaret's doctor possibly did increase his patient's risk.

The current consensus (which has changed before and might change again) is that estrogen, when taken during menopause and thereafter for a period of no more than five years, probably doesn't increase the risk of breast cancer. But the risk of breast cancer may increase by about 25 percent for women who take estrogen for ten to twenty years, and adding progesterone may worsen those risks still further.

Estrogen supplements definitely improve the cholesterol profile in many women, but taking progesterone largely nullifies this advantage. Overall, experts estimate that taking estrogen may decrease heart disease risk by about one-third, with the adding of progesterone reducing the possible benefits below that level. (See the accompanying box, The Benefits and Risks of Estrogen and Progesterone Therapy.)

WHAT TO DO: If you are going through menopause and are considering estrogen therapy, here are some issues to keep in mind as you discuss the situation with your doctor:

- If you've had a hysterectomy, the main risks of taking estrogen—uterine cancer or uterine bleeding—have been eliminated. So the chances are that you'll be placed on estrogen supplements *without* additional progesterone.

The Benefits and Risks of Estrogen and Progesterone Therapy		
Postmenopausal Estrogen Treatment	*Confidence Level*	*Comments*
POTENTIAL BENEFITS		
Cholesterol profile improved	Certain	Adding progesterone reduces benefit
Coronary heart disease risk decreases	Moderate	Adding progesterone probably reduces benefit
Risk of hip and other fractures due to osteoporosis decreased	Certain	Benefit probably persists with added progesterone
POTENTIAL RISKS		
Cancer of the uterus increased by about 800% for 10 to 20 years of estrogen alone	Certain	Adding progesterone largely eliminates this risk
Cancer of the breast increased by about 25% among women taking estrogen for 10 to 20 years, risk may not be increased for women taking for less than 5 years	Moderate	We are not sure, but some experts are concerned that adding progesterone might further increase risk
Side effects: 5%–10% get (usually mild) headache, bloating, or breast tenderness; 35%–40% get vaginal bleeding; increased gallstone risk	Certain	Progesterone may cause bloating, weight gain, irritability, depression (usually mild)
Increased probability (20%) of hysterectomy because of uterine changes	High	Adding progesterone largely avoids this risk

SOME ANTI-ERROR STRATEGIES FOR WOMEN ONLY 329

The Benefits and Risks of Estrogen and Progesterone Therapy
continued

Postmenopausal Estrogen Treatment	Confidence Level	Comments
Increased need for regular medical exam of uterus	Certain	Adding progesterone reduces this need except if bleeding occurs at time other than expected or if heavy, prolonged, or frequent bleeding persists beyond first 6 months

- If you've had breast cancer or have a strong family history of breast cancer, the situation in which Margaret found herself, you should probably avoid any hormone supplements.

- If you have strong coronary heart disease risk factors (such as high cholesterol or a parent who had a heart attack before age 55), you should probably take hormone supplements.

- If you have a low bone-density measurement, which places you at risk for osteoporosis, you should probably take the hormone supplements.

- If your menopause was premature, say, before age 40, you should probably take estrogen because of its probable protection against heart problems. Similarly, if you've had an early menopause due to a total hysterectomy, you should be on estrogen.

If none of the above scenarios or risk profiles describes you, then the best course will most likely be for you to use estrogen plus progesterone for only the first five years of menopause. The reason for this limited period of hormone treatment is that the risk of uterus and breast cancer seems to increase the longer you use the hormones. Also, the most critical period for rapid bone loss is in the first years after menopause.

ERROR:

Your Doctor Fails to Tell You That You Can Get Pregnant During Menopause

Connie, a 47-year-old, had just started going through menopause, and she was showing some of the symptoms of this condition, including irregular periods, hot flashes, headaches, and vaginal drying. Her doctor prescribed estrogen supplements for this problem, and he tried to reassure her by saying, "Well, at least you won't have to worry about having any more children!"

In fact, she became pregnant a few months later. What happened?

FACTS: As women approach menopause, periods often become irregular, with the bleeding stopping and starting intermittently. But most experts don't consider menopause to be firmly in place until there have been no periods at all for at least six months. During this transition time, you can become pregnant, as Connie did, though the risk is certainly lower than it is among more fertile younger women.

WHAT TO DO: As you enter menopause, continue using contraception until your doctor tells you specifically that you can stop it. Usually that will be after six months to one year with no periods.

To determine if you're actually entering menopause, your doctor should check your blood level of a pituitary hormone called follicle-stimulating hormone (FSH). If you are indeed entering menopause, blood FSH levels should rise, and that means that before long, your fertility will cease. But again, the main signal that contraception is no longer necessary is the complete ending of menstrual periods for at least six months.

ERROR:

Your Doctor Attributes Too Little Significance to Your Pattern of Menstrual Bleeding During Menopause

Jeanne experienced the normal spotting and irregular bleeding as she entered menopause, and when menopause seemed to be over, all bleeding stopped for several months. But then, Jeanne had another discharge, similar to her periods before menopause. When she told her doctor, he said, "You're probably still at the end of menopause. Just keep me posted."

Was this the right response?

FACTS: No, her doctor should have conducted a standard pelvic exam and Pap smear. Then, he should have considered whether she needed a uterine biopsy in his office or a full-scale uterine scraping (a dilatation and curettage, also known as a *D and C*).

Most spotting and irregular bleeding during the transition into menopause (or perimenopause) is due to changing hormone levels. But sometimes the problem is cancer of the uterus, cancer of the cervix, or other difficulties with internal organs. In particular, when bleeding stops and then resumes after the lapse of many months, as happened with Jeanne, the doctor should be alert to the need for an extensive examination.

WHAT TO DO: Despite the probability of a negative result from a thorough examination, you must keep checking with your doctor about abnormal bleeding during the transition into menopause. Keep precise records about when and how much you experience bleeding during menopause. Be especially alert if you seem to have finished menopause and all bleeding has stopped, but then the bleeding resumes months later.

I usually ask patients to call if there is any bleeding between their periods; if menstrual flow lasts 10 days or more; or if periods come every 2 weeks or sooner.

E R R O R :

Your Doctor Recommends an Unnecessary Hysterectomy

Darlene was diagnosed as having endometriosis (a spreading of functioning uterine tissue to organs outside the uterus) and also a small fibroid tumor (a benign growth on the uterus). The doctor said, "I think you should have a hysterectomy [removal of the uterus] just to eliminate any chance of cancer."

Was he right?

FACTS: In a situation like the one facing Darlene, a hysterectomy shouldn't be an automatic procedure. In fact, further investigation might very well show that a hysterectomy isn't necessary at all.

About one American woman in three will have a hysterectomy by age 60, but most researchers say that between 25 and 50 percent of hysterectomies are unnecessary and inappropriate. Furthermore, the incidence of these operations varies widely, depending on the part of the country where you and your doctor live. For example, the procedure is done twice as often in the South as in the Northeast. Yet it's not likely that there's that much difference in medical need from one geographical location to another.

So it's important to forget the surgical fashion of the moment or the area where you're living and look at the facts. Everyone seems to agree that a hysterectomy is proper if you have these conditions:

- Cancer or a precancerous condition affecting the uterus or nearby pelvic structures.

- Severe, painful damage to the pelvic organs due to infections from pelvic inflammatory disease, childbirth, or abortion.

- Severe endometriosis (the eccentric growth of uterine tissue outside the uterus) that is not responding to medical treatment. (In Darlene's case described above, the doctor apparently didn't even consider confining his operation to the areas of endometriosis.)

- Prolapse of the uterus, where the organ drops down into the vagina, causing pressure, pain, or loss of bladder control.

- A large, though benign fibroid tumor that causes excessive pain or bleeding, especially if severe anemia becomes a problem.

- Excessive bleeding from the uterus that can't be controlled with hormonal treatments or a simple D and C procedure.

Hysterectomy should never be done lightly. It's serious surgery, with all the potential risks that the procedure implies, including pelvic infection and accidental damage to the bladder, the ureter (tube running from the kidney to the bladder), and the bowel. In addition, there are always risks from the application of anesthesia during an operation and about a 10 percent chance of the need for a blood transfusion.

Some feminist and patient advocate groups believe that a hysterectomy, in addition to preventing a woman from having children, may also cause long-standing problems such as an inability to enjoy sex fully or a tendency toward depression.

One colleague put this controversy in a more positive light: "I think that most women who had a bad experience after hysterectomy are those who had their hysterectomy for the wrong reason in the first place. If the justification for the hysterectomy is secure, such as *severe* pain or *heavy* bleeding, then most women will be satisfied with the outcome."

WHAT TO DO: Have a direct, complete discussion with your doctor about all the reasons she feels you should have a hysterectomy. If the reasons are not completely compelling, of course a second opinion is in order.

Here are a few alternatives to surgery:

- *A large, painful, or bleeding uterine fibroid tumor.* You can take a hormone called gonadotropin-releasing hormone analog (GnRH), which can be prescribed under the brand name Lupron. This helps shrink the fibroid. Or you can have less extensive surgery to cut out only the tumor.

- *Vaginal bleeding.* A progesterone hormone supplement often reduces the bleeding. Or a gynecologist can cauterize the inner lining of the uterus.

- *Endometriosis.* You can take any of a number of hormones or drugs, including progesterone, testosterone, danazol (Danocrine), or Lupron. Or a skilled surgeon can remove the critical patches of endometriosis tissue without removing the entire uterus.

- *A dropped or prolapsed uterus.* Estrogen supplements can improve muscle tone. Or you can try the pelvic muscle strengtheners called Kegel exercises.

In any event, if the hysterectomy is being proposed for nonurgent reasons, such as those described for Darlene, be sure to get a second opinion before you agree. Also, if you feel you might want to have more children, you should secure a second, third, or even fourth opinion before you act.

Always be suspicious of proposals to remove your uterus to treat a small fibroid, vague pelvic area symptoms, pain from an unidentified source, vaginal discharge, or backache. Also, avoid this procedure when it's to be used solely as a cancer preventative, a means to correct a hormonal imbalance or an abnormally tipped uterus, or a method of permanent contraception.

PART SEVEN

Eliminating Errors Involving Your Eyes, Endocrine System, and Urinary Tract

Special Alerts:
The Eyes, Endocrine
System, and Urinary Tract

- Your doctor has done cataract surgery on one of your eyes and suggests operating on the other eye before the first one has healed. (See error, p. 339.)

- Your physician fails to recognize that you have thyroid cancer. (See error, p. 342.)

- Your doctor orders a urine culture, kidney X ray, or cystoscopy instead of a simple, inexpensive urinalysis after you're diagnosed with a urinary tract infection. (See error, p. 345.)

- The hospital staff misses the fact that your elderly father's malaise and loss of appetite are caused by a urinary tract infection. (See error, p. 348.)

- Your doctor has prescribed oral medications for your diabetes without telling you that you are increasing your risk of heart disease. (See error, p. 350.)

ERROR:

Your Doctor Recommends Operating on Your Cataracts Just Because They Are There

Wayne, who was 70 years old, began to have difficulty reading in less than optimal light, though he could read quite well under a bright lamp. He called this problem to the attention of his doctor, who determined that he had cataracts (a clouding of the lens of the eye) and recommended that he have surgery.

Should Wayne have questioned this recommendation?

FACTS: Often a cataract is first detected by a doctor during a routine eye exam. But this doesn't mean that the cataract must come out. Many cataracts never deteriorate to the point where they interfere seriously with vision. If eyeglasses, contact lenses, bifocals, or better lighting allow you to see well enough to do your daily activities without great distress, you don't need a cataract operation.

Still, those who depend heavily on their eyes for work or other activities may need a cataract operation earlier than those with ordinary vision needs.

In fact, American eye doctors perform more than 1.7 million cataract operations each year—a rate that makes cataract surgery about the most popular form of operation in the United States. Cataracts are mainly a problem for people over age 65. Fifty percent of those over this age have this problem to some degree. Because this age group is covered by Medicare, it's highly likely that pressure from the federal government will increase on ophthalmologists to avoid unnecessary cataract surgery.

Most people who need cataract surgery score 20/50 or worse on the traditional eye chart exam. Those with 20/40 vision or even better may also qualify for surgery if their visual function fluctuates because of glare or low lighting, they have double vision, or their vision ability differs substantially between their two eyes.

In general, cataract surgery is very safe, but like any kind of operation, there may be complications. For example, there is a small risk of infection or bleeding during the operation, which could lead to blindness.

WHAT TO DO: If you are diagnosed as having cataracts, use this checklist to help you decide with your doctor whether or not you should have surgery. In general, you should consider an operation if any of the following apply to you:

- The glare from the sun or headlights interferes significantly with your driving.
- You don't see well enough to do your best at work, in your hobbies, or working around the home.
- You can't enjoy TV, sewing, playing cards, or otherwise being independent.
- Glasses or contact lenses don't do a good enough job to satisfy your needs.

If an eye surgeon suggests you should have a cataract operation even though you think you're doing all right visually, definitely seek a second opinion from another ophthalmologist.

ERROR:

Your Doctor Suggests You May Want to Have an Operation for Cataracts in Your Second Eye Before Vision Has Been Fully Restored in the First Eye

Dave had cataracts in both his eyes but underwent surgery for only one. He had more difficulty seeing after the operation than before, but his doctor assured him that the eye was recovering nicely and that his vision would be better than ever in a few weeks. In the meantime, the physician said he had an immediate opening in his surgical schedule and would be willing to go ahead with the second eye.

What should Dave's response have been?

FACTS: Dave should have said, "Thanks, but I'll wait until my first eye has recovered completely."

Since cataract operations pose a small risk of harm, you should never, ever allow an operation on both your eyes at once or on a second eye before the first has fully recovered. Instead, enough time must pass for you to gain the full benefits from the first operation. Then you are ready to consider a second.

WHAT TO DO: Take one eye at a time. If vision in the first eye doesn't recover satisfactorily, consider carefully the pros and cons of a second operation, including the possibility that a second failure could leave you mostly blind.

If you feel that because of the demands of your work or some other good reason you must seriously consider an operation on the second eye when the first operation wasn't completely successful, always seek a second opinion.

ERROR:

Failing to Do a Blood Test for Thyroid Function on Every Person Who Feels Unwell When the Source of the Problem Can't Otherwise Be Identified

I think of thyroid disorders as the great masqueraders. In particular, I remember the following cases:

- Sharon, a 38-year-old housewife, had developed the habit of drinking bourbon every night and most of each day to keep herself calm. Her physician focused on dealing with the alcohol consumption when, in reality, her agitation was due to an overactive thyroid. When this was finally treated, her drinking problem vanished.

- Henry, a 70-year-old retired factory foreman, became forgetful, tired, and withdrawn. At the suggestion of a doctor, his family began plans to move him into a nursing home. Then, a blood test revealed the real cause of the problem: Henry's thyroid was failing. When this was corrected with medication, he rapidly resumed his old way of life with alertness and vigor.

Why do mistakes like these occur?

FACTS: The main mistake that doctors make is not doing a blood test to screen for thyroid function on every person who complains of hard-to-pin-down symptoms.

Thyroid disorders affect millions of Americans. The symptoms can mimic many other diseases and affect any organ of the body. (See the accompanying box, Common Symptoms of Overactive and Underactive Thyroids.)

It's also easy for thyroid symptoms to be misinterpreted as being due to psychiatric disorders, such as anxiety or depression, stress, aging, or a variety of other conditions.

WHAT TO DO: If you haven't been feeling well for some time, regardless of the symptoms, insist that your thyroid be checked. Even if you've had another diagnosis that makes sense, ask for a thyroid test when the symptoms don't seem to be clearing up with treatment.

Your doctor can test your thyroid with blood tests such as the thyroxine (T_4) test, which measures thyroid hormone, and the thyrotropin (TSH) test, which measures a pituitary gland hormone involved in regulating the thyroid.

ERROR:

Your Doctor Overlooks Potential Interactions Between Thyroid Hormone Supplements and Other Drugs

Earlene had been on medications for an underactive thyroid for several years when she decided to switch her contraception method from an intrauterine device to birth control pills. About eight weeks after she began the Pill, however, she began to feel fatigued and weak, and she also experienced a lower heart rate. A subsequent diagnosis revealed that her thyroid medicine wasn't working as well.

What had happened?

FACTS: Her doctor failed to take into account the fact that birth control pills can lower the effectiveness of thyroid hormone medication.

Also, iron taken at the same time as a thyroid hormone supplement may reduce significantly the absorption of the thyroid hormone. Thyroid medications may alter the dosing requirements for insulin or other diabetes medication.

WHAT TO DO: Take your thyroid and iron pills at separate meals. Ask your doctor to recheck your thyroid levels if you start or stop estrogen. If you are a diabetic, recheck your blood sugar if you start or change your thyroid dose.

Common Symptoms of Overactive and Underactive Thyroid
Common Symptoms of an Overactive Thyroid (Hyperthyroidism)
Nervousness or emotional instability. Difficulty concentrating. Fatigue. Muscle weakness or tremor. Rapid or irregular heartbeat. Perspiration or heat intolerance. Increased bowel movements. Weight loss. Menstrual irregularities. Eye irritation or protruding eyes. Thyroid swelling or tenderness in neck. Decreased exercise tolerance.
Common Symptoms of an Underactive Thyroid (Hypothyroidism)
Fatigue or lethargy. Difficulty concentrating. Depression or mood changes. Constipation. Weakness. Dry or rough skin or brittle hair. Intolerance to cold. Husky voice. Puffy hands or face. Weight gain. Joint or muscle aches. Slow heart rate. Decreased exercise tolerance.

ERROR:

Your Doctor Fails to Recognize Thyroid Cancer

Kyle, a 22-year-old, had a nodule near the thyroid area on his neck. Over a two-month period, the lump seemed to grow harder and slightly larger. His doctor said, "This bears watching," but didn't order any tests.

Was this a mistake?

FACTS: In this case, the doctor should probably have done a *fine-needle aspiration test,* an office procedure that involves placing a needle into the nodule and applying suction to pull out a small sample of thyroid tissue. The tissue is then analyzed for malignancy. The signals that should have alerted the doctor to the need for action were first that Kyle was young. Thyroid lumps in young people are relatively more likely to be due to cancer. Also, the nodule had changed in a relatively short period of time, and such a change may mean malignancy.

But it's understandable that a doctor might overlook the importance of performing this procedure. Tens of millions of American adults have lumps or nodules on their thyroids, which their doctors can feel on a routine exam. Among those over age 50, nodules can be felt on almost half. Most of these nodules are harmless. But lurking within this group are about 11,000 people a year who actually have cancer of the thyroid.

Radioactive iodine scanning of the thyroid can correctly classify most thyroid nodules as not being cancer. But this procedure does miss some malignancies. For those lumps that seem particularly suspicious, like Kyle's, a fine-needle aspiration is in order.

It's not hard for a physician to learn the mechanics of this procedure, but it does take a fair degree of experience. Most experts recommend that you have the procedure done only by someone who has done at least fifty of these tests. Otherwise, there's a fairly high chance of an inaccurate result.

A second issue involves the expert who will evaluate the tissue. It's best to have a specialist, a cytopathologist, perform this task. An ordinary hospital pathologist may be able to do an adequate job, but you're usually better off with a specialist who has extensive experience in doing this type of analysis.

WHAT TO DO: If your doctor detects a thyroid nodule that is not changing rapidly, it may be all right to observe it for a while. Or you might have it ranked high or low risk for cancer with a radioactive thyroid-imaging test.

At the same time, your doctor should evaluate your risk for thyroid cancer. Any of these factors will raise your risk:

- A history of X-ray treatments to the neck area—a common treatment for acne, tonsillitis, and other health problems until about 1960.

- A family history of thyroid cancer, especially if there is also a family history of other endocrine cancers or abnormalities.

These may include hyperparathyroidism, which causes high blood calcium, or pheochromocytoma, which causes high blood pressure, flushing, and headache.

- A young age. A higher proportion of nodules are malignant in young versus older adults. Thyroid nodules in children must be *assumed* to be cancer.

- A hoarse voice.

- A lump or nodule that changes noticeably.

If there is serious concern or suspicion about the lump, you should have a fine-needle aspiration biopsy done. A few family doctors who have taken special training can handle this test all right, but be sure that the one you pick has done at least fifty of the procedures. If he hasn't, I would ask to be referred to a specialist, an endocrinologist, for the procedure. Also, you should ask that the specialist who will read the slide be a cytopathologist who has substantial experience.

<hr>

ERROR:

You Are Sexually Active, but Your Doctor Resists Giving You Preventive Antibiotics to Counter Possible Urinary Tract Infections

A young single woman came into my office with bitter criticism for her previous two doctors, who had refused to give her antibiotics to prevent urinary tract infections that occurred almost invariably after she had sex.

Was her criticism justified?

FACTS: Most sexually active women don't always get urinary tract infections after sex. But one study, which checked the urine of women volunteers before and after they had sexual relations, showed a sixty-fold increase in urinary infection rates in the twenty-four hours after intercourse! The typical signs of these infections include a burning sensation upon urination, an increase in urinary frequency, and, in some cases, cloudy urine.

With many women, urinary infections can be prevented if they take a very brief course of antibiotics shortly before or after sexual intercourse or at the first sign of urinary tract symptoms. Another way to prevent such infections is to clear the bladder by urinating within five to ten minutes after intercourse. Also, when you choose a contraceptive, it helps to pick an alternative to the diaphragm or spermicide because these two can increase your vulnerability to urinary infections. Menopausal women might benefit from a vaginal estrogen cream, which may increase resistance to infection.

WHAT TO DO: If sex often triggers urinary infections, be sure your doctor knows about this tendency. Discuss changing your contraceptives away from a diaphragm or spermicide. Discuss the option of your doctor giving you an open or standing prescription, which you can refill and use at the time of intercourse or when any symptoms of a urinary tract infection appear.

Note: This practice of multiple drug refills is *not* recommended in most situations. But in the unusual case where a woman gets a urinary infection after almost every act of intercourse (typically in circumstances where she is involved in intermittent but intense sexual activity), the practice may be justified if the patient stays in close touch with her doctor as she treats herself.

ERROR:

At the First Sign of a Urinary Tract Infection, Your Doctor Immediately Orders a Sophisticated Urine Culture or Other Expensive Test Instead of a Simple Urinalysis

Eloise typically had one or two urinary tract infections a year. At first her doctor checked her routinely with a simple urinalysis, where he provided a urine sample to be looked at under the microscope or tested with a quick "dip" stick. But then he began to order more expensive urine culture tests.

Was this change in his approach warranted?

FACTS: Most women who get one or two urine infections a year and whose infections respond well to standard antibiotics need only a simple urinalysis. They don't require an expensive urine culture, which currently may cost about $75, or other more extensive tests.

Urine cultures seek to grow the bacteria that are infecting your urine so that the doctor can identify the type and determine which antibiotics to use for treatment. Complicated or hard-to-cure urinary infections may require this approach, but not simple infections.

If your doctor is a urologist or if you are referred to a urologist for recurring infections, you're likely to be subjected to more invasive (and expensive) procedures. These may include a kidney X ray with an intravenous injection or a cystoscopy, which involves looking into the bladder with a fiber-optic light. Women with occasional urinary tract infections—and even those who have them moderately frequently—usually don't need these procedures unless there is suspicion of serious complicating factors, such as an anatomical abnormality in the urinary tract.

WHAT TO DO: Question your need for a urine culture if you are a woman who has only a rare urinary infection. Usually, the initial antibiotic choice will work fine. If it doesn't, then a culture will make sense. Also, you should agree to a culture in these situations:

- You have three or more urinary tract infections a year.

- You have structural abnormalities of the urinary tract, such as an abnormal kidney or scarring of the urethral tube, which leads from the bladder to the outside.

- Your urinary infections began in childhood.

- You have had a previous urinary infection within the last six weeks.

- You're pregnant, have diabetes, or suffer from immune system disorders.

If you're referred to a urologist, don't automatically assume that when she recommends a sophisticated test, she is looking for an additional fee. But this is an area of medicine that's vulnerable to overuse. So demand a full justification for each procedure that is suggested.

By the way, a good reason to seek out a urologist is the situation where you've had previous urinary tract infections and you're concerned that the simpler tests your doctor is using aren't picking up a new outbreak. Sometimes, standard tests like urinalysis, urine dip sticks, or even urine cultures register negative even when you are infected. Research studies show that these tests might miss 10 to 25 percent of urinary tract infections. A urologist will be in the best position to be certain whether or not you have a problem.

E R R O R :

Your Doctor Mistakes Your Urinary Tract Infection for a Prostate Problem

Garth's doctor had been monitoring his moderately enlarged prostate very closely. So when Garth, who was 47, complained that his urine stream was decreasing and he had to get up more often during the night to urinate, the doctor immediately concluded, "The prostate is getting worse!"

What was his mistake?

FACTS: Although young and middle-aged men don't get urinary tract infections very often, they do sometimes develop this condition with symptoms that may suggest another problem, like prostate infection (prostatitis). Sometimes, there are the classic urinary tract infection symptoms of burning or urgency during urination. But with some patients, the diagnosis becomes more difficult because their urinary infections display other kinds of signals.

For example, a man may have obstructive symptoms, like slow urine stream, dribbling, increased urination at night, and a delay before he can begin urination. Such symptoms, of course, are similar to those with an enlarged or diseased prostate, and they may confuse an otherwise alert physician.

Also, sexually transmitted diseases, such as gonorrhea and non-gonococcal urethritis (an inflammation of the urethral tube, which leads from the urinary bladder to the outside), can mimic a urinary tract infection.

WHAT TO DO: If you are a man with either irritation or obstruction in the urinary tract and the cause isn't clear, insist on a urinalysis and urine culture. You should also undergo a prostate exam and an evaluation for sexually transmitted diseases.

ERROR:

The Hospital Staff Has Missed That an Elderly Father's Malaise and Loss of Appetite Are Caused by a Urinary Tract Infection

The condition of an elderly gentleman had been deteriorating during the two weeks that he had been in the hospital. He was suffering from a complete lack of energy, loss of appetite, and apparently worsening mental status, with an increased tendency to be depressed and forgetful. Members of the hospital staff recommended that he be considered a candidate for a nursing home.

But the family insisted on another complete round of tests, and a urinary tract infection was found. After being treated for a couple of weeks with antibiotics, the elderly man experienced a "miraculous" recovery.

FACTS: Urinary tract infections, usually without symptoms, are extremely common in the elderly, especially in those who are hospitalized, who live in nursing homes, or who have needed catheterization of the bladder. This procedure involves placing a plastic tube into the bladder to drain out the urine. Infection rates are estimated to range from 16 to 30 percent among those undergoing this procedure.

Urinary infections in the elderly can emerge with irritation or obstructive symptoms, as they do in younger people. But often, the symptoms are minimal and may not be recognized for what they are. Instead, elderly people with urine infections have symptoms that seem unrelated to the urinary tract, such as malaise, loss of appetite, or worsening mental status.

WHAT TO DO: If an elderly person deteriorates physically or mentally, the medical work-up to search for causes of the problem should include a urinalysis and probably a urine culture even if there are no obvious complaints of urinary symptoms.

ERROR:

You Have Juvenile-Onset Diabetes, and Your Doctor Fails to Inform You That a High Blood Pressure Drug Can Slow the Onset of Kidney Disease

Beth, who is in her early twenties, had been treated for juvenile-onset diabetes since she was a child. Her doctor either didn't know or had neglected to tell her that the ACE-inhibitor class of high blood pressure drugs (such as Vasotec, captopril, and Monopril) can slow the development of kidney disease in her type of diabetes.

Was this a significant oversight?

FACTS: Kidney disease is a major killer of diabetics, especially those with the juvenile-onset variety of the disease. So many specialists in diabetes are beginning to offer ACE-inhibitor medicines to their juvenile diabetics. In addition to benefiting the kidneys, these drugs also help lower blood pressure. For diabetics, even mildly high blood pressure seems to be more hazardous than it is for people without diabetes.

On the other hand, adult-onset diabetes is in many ways quite different from juvenile diabetes. For one thing, most adult diabetics never face severe kidney disease, and so there is not yet any justification for giving ACE inhibitors to those with the adult type of condition, unless, of course, these patients also have high blood pressure.

WHAT TO DO: If you have juvenile-onset diabetes, ask your doctor about the effects of ACE inhibitors in delaying kidney disease. If your doctor seems uninformed about this issue, you should seek another opinion.

ERROR:

Your Doctor Doesn't Tell You That Your Oral Diabetic Medicine May Increase Your Risk of Heart Disease

At his doctor's suggestion, Peter decided to begin taking an oral medicine for his diabetes, primarily because of the convenience. But his doctor neglected to inform him about the possibility that these drugs may increase the risk of heart disease.

FACTS: Of ten patients I recently spoke to who were taking pills to control their diabetes, only two had been told about the warning on the drug package, which reads in part: "the administration of oral hypoglycemic drugs has been associated with increased cardiovascular mortality as compared to treatment with diet alone or diet plus insulin. . . ."

Oral diabetic medicines are great for day-by-day control of blood sugar for those with mild to moderately severe diabetes. But these superconvenient medicines might also increase the risk for heart and other blood vessel diseases, which are the main causes of death and disability for diabetics. The admittedly incomplete studies done up to this point suggest that oral diabetes medicines might not be as great a bargain as they once seemed to be.

Some experts argue against too much concern, citing flaws in the key study that showed oral diabetic pills to be harmful. My feeling and that of most diabetes specialists is that many, and perhaps most, diabetics who are now taking diabetes pills could achieve good blood sugar control without taking medicines if they could maintain a commitment to aggressive diet control and a regular exercise program. Ideally, therefore, exercise and diet control would be the path to take.

Realistically, though, many patients, even those who try to motivate themselves, will not be able to keep themselves on the ideal diet they require. While insulin shots are an alternative, few patients would choose them unless they absolutely had to. Therefore, despite possible adverse effects, oral diabetic pills often remain the best choice.

WHAT TO DO: Think of oral diabetic medicines as a stopgap while you work seriously on weight and diet control. Discuss their potential long-term risks frankly with your doctor, along with your key alternatives: diet control and insulin shots.

ERROR:

Your Doctor Fails to Recognize That High Blood Sugar in the Morning May Result from Too Much Insulin

Martin, a diabetic, started having trouble sleeping, and he noticed that his heartbeats were irregular. His doctor first identified the problem as stress. Then, he suggested that the problem might be in Martin's heart, but an electrocardiogram showed that everything was normal.

Special Alert for Those with Juvenile-Onset Diabetes

Typically, diabetics check their blood sugar and give themselves insulin injections about twice a day. But diabetes specialists have long debated whether much tighter blood sugar control might reduce the risk for diabetes complications, such as heart attacks, stroke, blindness, kidney failure, and infections. Specifically, they have wondered if it might not be better to measure blood sugar and give finely calibrated insulin doses three or four times a day.

Recent research is beginning to support this more intensive approach, at least for some diabetics. People who have developed diabetes as children or teenagers have been shown to have a decreased rate of eye and nerve damage with ultratight blood sugar control.

But questions still remain about whether the heart, brain, and kidneys will be helped by the same approach. Also, it's unclear if patients with adult-onset diabetes will be protected in the same way as those with the juvenile-onset variety.

Although this issue is still being studied, it does seem that those with juvenile-onset diabetes should seriously consider the new, intensive regimen if they are motivated enough to handle this demanding approach. On the other hand, there is as yet no strong scientific support for recommending that those with adult-onset diabetes take the intensive self-care route.

Noticing that Martin's blood sugar levels were quite high in the morning, he decided to increase his dose of insulin at night (a step designed to lower the blood sugar). But then, Martin's blood sugar levels registered even higher in the morning.

What was the doctor missing?

FACTS: Doctors are usually quite adept at recognizing the signs of severe low blood sugar (hypoglycemia). These include feeling sweaty, cold, tense, shaky, irritable, mentally confused, or hungry. The diagnosis can be clinched if the blood sugar level is checked or if there is quick improvement after eating a sugary food or having an injection of the sugar-raising hormone glucagon.

But sometimes, as in Martin's case, the symptoms of low blood sugar can be masked, particularly during sleep. Taking too much insulin at night can cause disturbed sleep, heartbeat irregularities, or, rarely, a stroke or seizures. The cause may go unrecognized, or the doctor may assume another condition is involved, because blood sugar levels may rebound up to very high levels by morning.

A classic trap that some doctors, such as Martin's, fall into is to look at the morning blood sugar reading and to prescribe *larger* doses of insulin or oral diabetic medications at night. This causes even lower blood sugar levels in the early morning hours and an even higher blood sugar rebound later in the morning. Then, the doctor may raise the night time insulin even more. The vicious cycle only ends when the doctor (or patient!) finally recognizes the rebound pattern—a mistake that is common enough to be given a name, the *Somogyi phenomenon.*

Beta-blocker drugs may mask low blood sugar symptoms—making its presence difficult to recognize.

WHAT TO DO: Become proficient at testing your blood sugar at home. Check it immediately if you have odd symptoms. Or if you are not up to testing it yourself because you're not feeling well, have a family member or co-worker trained so that he or she can do it.

If your blood sugar level keeps rising in the morning despite increased insulin at night, bring this fact to your doctor's attention. Ask if you could be experiencing a rebound effect due to low blood sugar during the night.

ERROR:

Receiving the Wrong Diabetes Drug at the Pharmacy

One patient received a $4 million malpractice award from a pharmacy because the pharmacist misunderstood the doctor's prescription and handed out a pain medicine instead of the diabetic drug, which had a similar name. The result for the patient in this case was out-of-control blood sugar and catastrophic health complications.

FACTS: Gross errors of this type aren't common, but they happen often enough that every patient should examine closely all drugs received at the pharmacy or in the doctor's office. For example, you might be given an incorrect dose of a diabetes pill because of a pharmacist's error or a slip of the doctor's pen.

You can usually recognize that a switch has occurred because the pill may look different. But the only certain method is to read the label and the package insert, if there is one, in addition to examining closely the appearance of the pill.

WHAT TO DO: When you go to the pharmacy, always read the label on your prescription very carefully. If you're getting a pill, look at the pill to be sure it has the same size, color, and markings as the ones you've been taking. If you see any variations, ask the pharmacist, and don't leave until he gives you some satisfactory answers.

Drug reference books such as the *PDR* and *The Pill Book* have pictures of many "brand name" medications, but they do not provide pictures for their many generic non-brand-name substitutes.

ERROR:

Your Doctor Prescribes Medicine That Will Interact with Your Diabetes Medicine

Liz, who was taking glyburide, an oral medicine for diabetes, was placed on fluconazole (Diflucan), a powerful antibiotic used to treat yeast infections. Shortly afterward, she suffered a low blood sugar reaction (hypoglycemia), with clamminess, chills, and mental confusion.

What had happened to her?

FACTS: The problem with Liz was one of the most common mistakes that occur with a wide variety of illnesses: Her doctor forgot one or more of the medicines that Liz was taking and gave one that interacted dangerously with another. Specifically, he forgot that her glyburide could interact with Diflucan to produce a low blood sugar reaction.

The following medicines may *increase* the tendency of insulin or oral diabetic medicines to lower blood sugar and produce a hypoglycemic reaction:

Alcohol.
Aspirin and nonsteroidal antiinflammatory medicines (e.g., ibuprofen and indomethacin).
Beta-blockers (these drugs may also block recognition of hypoglycemic symptoms).
Coumadin (anticoagulant).
Fluconazole (Diflucan), an antifungal medicine.
MAO inhibitor antidepressants (e.g., Parnate)
Sulfa-type antibiotics (e.g., Bactrim and Gantrisin), though a rare side effect.
Tricyclic antidepressants.

The following medicines may *reduce* the ability of insulin or oral diabetic medicines to lower blood sugar. This may make blood sugar more difficult to control or lead to unanticipated lowering of blood sugar if the medicine is stopped:

Calcium channel blockers.
Cholestyramine (Questran), a cholesterol-lowering drug.
Certain contraceptives, female hormones.
Cortisone-type medicines (prednisone, Medrol).
Diazoxide, a blood pressure medicine.
Nasal decongestants (e.g., pseudophedrine).
Rifampin, an antibiotic.
Thiazide diuretics.
Thyroid hormones.

WHAT TO DO: Check with your doctor before any medication changes are made to see if any negative drug interactions are likely.

The interactions listed above are only a rough guide. Some of these are quite predictable and affect both insulin and oral diabetic medicines. Others are less certain or may apply only to one diabetic medicine.

The moral with any drugs is to stay on your toes! Pay special attention to measuring your blood sugar for the week or two after you add, subtract, or change doses on any medicine. If you notice changes in your blood sugar or experience any unusual symptoms, notify your doctor immediately.

PART EIGHT

Is It Your Body or Your Mind?

Special Alerts: Body or Mind

- You have an alcohol problem, but your doctor fails to warn you about the danger of ending your drinking too abruptly. (See error, p. 361.)

- Your doctor is unable or unwilling to try psychotherapy without drugs. (See error, p. 367.)

- Your doctor doesn't realize that your headache relief medicine is causing your headaches (See error, p. 381.)

- Your physician misses the possibility that your worsening headache could be signaling a medical emergency—and may result in blindness or worse. (See error, 382.)

$$\boxed{\text{E R R O R :}}$$

Your Doctor Fails to Identify You as an Abuser of Alcohol

Tim had been going to the same doctor for fifteen years, yet the doctor never recognized the fact that Tim was an alcoholic until he came down with gastritis, an inflammation of the stomach resulting from the overuse of alcohol. The symptoms were abdominal pain and a black-colored stool.

How was this possible?

FACTS: Many people with alcohol problems cannot or will not recognize that fact, and the same limitation often applies to their physicians. On average, doctors recognize less than half of the problem drinkers in their practices.

To avoid this mistake, every doctor should use a remarkably simple questionnaire, which does an excellent job of identifying those who have serious problems with alcohol. Called the *CAGE questionnaire*, this tool is meant to be asked by physicians of the patients. I'm including it here for readers whose doctors may have overlooked this helpful device:

Answer the following questions. Over the past twelve months:

1. Have you ever felt you should cut down on your drinking?

2. Have people annoyed you by criticizing your drinking?

3. Have you ever felt bad or guilty about your drinking?

4. Have you ever had a drink the first thing in the morning to steady your nerves or get rid of a hangover?

A score of two or more yes answers indicates a high probability that the patient has a significant drinking problem. Even one positive reply is a reason for looking further into the matter.

WHAT TO DO: If you think you have a drinking problem or know someone who does, the best course is to involve an expert who can at least *begin* the process of recovery. This may be a physician, a substance abuse counselor at a hospital or outpatient alcohol treatment program, a psychologist, a clergy person, or a self-help group, such as Alcoholics Anonymous (AA) or Al-Anon.

You should also take the CAGE test and discuss it with your doctor. When you see her, have a periodic SMA blood test, which will measure your liver functions. Even mild elevations of liver function tests can be a sign of an alcohol problem.

ERROR:

You Have an Alcohol Problem, and Your Doctor Fails to Warn You About Ending the Drinking Too Abruptly

I once reasoned with a patient about his problem drinking without expecting much result, but he took me very seriously. Two weeks later, he cleaned out his liquor cabinet and turned over a completely new leaf by going "cold turkey." Twenty-four hours later, he was hospitalized with an epileptic seizure and early symptoms of the DTs (delirium tremens).

Was I wrong to advise him to quit drinking?

FACTS: I should have monitored his decision to stop drinking more closely. Because alcohol is addicting, if you drink regularly and then stop or cut back suddenly without active medical monitoring and treatment, you can be subjecting yourself to extreme danger.

A common situation is the heavy drinker who develops pneumonia, diarrhea, or any other illness, which makes continued drinking impossible. The abrupt cessation of drinking can lead to withdrawal symptoms, such as anxiety, shakiness, sweating, muscle aches, hallucinations, seizures, or full-scale DTs. These reactions may occur within twelve to thirty-six hours.

Ironically, these physical problems are unnecessary *if*, with your quitting the bottle, you use simple medication such as chlordiazepoxide (Librium) to help you taper off the addiction.

WHAT TO DO: If you drink alcohol daily and want to drink less often, let your doctor know about your plans immediately. Set up a schedule with your doctor to get you off of alcohol. Specifically discuss whether you should take a medicine such as Librium while you withdraw.

Notify the doctor immediately if you have any of the withdrawal symptoms listed above. Discuss whether you should do your withdrawal as an outpatient, or as part of an inpatient hospital program.

Join Alcoholics Anonymous (AA) or another alcohol treatment program—and stick with it. In the long run, committing yourself to an AA-type program is often the most important step to recovery.

E R R O R :

Your Doctor Is Too Quick to Diagnose Alzheimer's Disease

Walter began to display signs of mental deterioration, including increased forgetfulness and confusion. His doctor first attributed these symptoms to possible senility or Alzheimer's disease, given his advanced age of 88. But finally, after a lengthy battery of tests, the doctor determined that the real problem was congestive heart failure.

FACTS: People suffering from the common Alzheimer-type senility usually get worse slowly and subtly. Some other factor is probably at work when the deterioration occurs quickly or dramatically.

The most frequent causes of mental deterioration other than senility or Alzheimer's are the following:

- *Depression.* This should be suspected if there is loss of enthusiasm for activities a person used to enjoy. Depressed people haven't really lost their mental powers, but they may feel and act as if they have.

- *Any physical illness.* For example, mental problems may arise with a urinary infection, slow internal bleeding, pneumonia, low blood pressure, congestive heart failure, or a stroke.

- *Side effects of many medicines or toxic substances, including alcohol.*

WHAT TO DO: If a friend or loved one deteriorates mentally, insist that the doctor obtain a thorough evaluation for physical and mental illness. This step is necessary even if the patient is already suffering from a lesser degree of senility.

Be sure the doctor thinks through systematically the possibility of alternative causes of senility. This requires at least thirty to sixty minutes devoted entirely to this problem. A geriatrics specialist or a neurologist will be the most skilled for this evaluation, though some family physicians, internists, and psychiatrists are excellent.

A minimum evaluation should include the following:

- A review of medicines and alcohol and drug use.

- Various blood tests, including a complete blood cell count (CBC), SMA panel, thyroid, vitamin B_{12}, VDRL (a syphilis test), sedimentation rate, and a human immunodeficiency virus (HIV) test, if indicated.

- A chest X ray and electrocardiogram.

- A neurological exam.

Although many cost-conscious experts will disagree, I believe strongly that if no other cause can be found, a magnetic resonance imaging (MRI) or computed tomography (CT) examination of the brain should also be done. I would certainly insist on this with one of my relatives!

As a preliminary step, you can give your companion the accompanying Mini–Mental Status Exam, which has been used widely as a preliminary test for senility, but don't assume that this can take the place of a medical checkup by a qualified physician.

ERROR:

Your Doctor Is Unable or Unwilling to Recognize Physical Symptoms of Stress

Katey, who was constantly under deadline pressure at her job, frequently complained of headaches, fatigue, and dizziness. Her doctor conducted a variety of blood tests and other evaluations but couldn't isolate the source of the problem. He never questioned her about the nature of her job or family life and whether any pressures she was under might be contributing to her symptoms.

FACTS: Both doctors and patients often turn a blind eye to the symptoms of anxiety. Yet small stressors challenge our bodies many times each day, with the result that we face chronic overstimulation

Mini–Mental Status Exam

The following exam, which can be an indicator of possible senility, has been given to more than 18,000 people. The scores for the top and bottom 25 percent are listed at the end of the test and are broken down by the number of years of formal education the test taker has had. As a rough guide, it's reasonable to seek further evaluation for scores in the bottom quarter. But a few people with early senility might score higher, especially if their basic intellectual skill started out at a high level. Be reassured by scores in the top 25 percent.

1. What is the year ____ , season ____ , date ____ , day ___ , month ____ ? (Score one point for each correct answer.)
   Total (5)____

2. Where are we? State ____ , Country ____ , Town/city ____ , Address ____ , Floor ____ .   Total (5)____

3. Name three objects, taking one second to name each. Then ask the subject to repeat all three. (Score 1 for each correct answer.) Then keep repeating names until subject learns all three (see question 5).   Total (3)____

4. Ask subject to subtract 7 from 100, then to keep subtracting for a total of five subtractions. (Correct: 93, 86, 79, 72, 65. Score 1 point for each correct answer.)   Total (5)____
   As an alternative, ask subject to spell *world* backward.

5. Ask for the names of the three objects from question 3. (Score 1 point for each correct answer.)   Total (3)____

6. Point to a pencil and a watch. Have the subject name them as you point.   Total (2)____

7. Have subject repeat "No ifs, ands, or buts."
   Total (1)____

8. Have subject follow a three-stage command: "Take the paper in your right hand. Fold the paper in half. Put the paper on the floor." (Score 1 point for each correct action.)
   Total (3)____

9. Have the patient read and obey the following: "Close your eyes."   Total (1)____

10. Have the subject write a sentence of his or her own choosing. (It should contain a subject and object and make sense. Ignore spelling errors.)   Total (1)____

11. Enlarge the design printed below to ½ inch to 2 inches on each side and have subject copy it. (Give 1 point if all sides and angles are preserved and if the overlapping sides form a four-sided figure.   Total (1)____

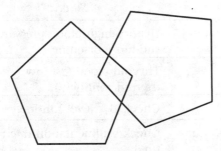

Total (30)____

Reprinted from JAMA, 5/93, with the permission of Marshall Folstein, M.D., Dept. of Psychiatry, Johns Hopkins University School of Medicine.

Scores on the Mini–Mental Status Exam (30 = perfect), all ages combined

Years of Education	0–4	5–8	9–12	12+
Bottom 25%	19	21	23	25
Top 25%	25	27	28	29

Reprinted with permission.

of the adrenal gland hormones and its neural network. This response leads to a perpetual high-alert state of mind and an outcropping of a host of physical and mental ailments.

Common physical responses to excessive stress include headache, fatigue, irritable bowel, heart palpitations, dizziness, and ulcer symptoms. Also, those experiencing too much stress and anxiety may be taking in too much tobacco, caffeine, alcohol, or drugs.

WHAT TO DO: Don't assume or allow your doctor to assume that your stress-related symptoms are illegitimate or "all in your head." Stress reactions are frequently physical. And if you remove the source of the stress or at least learn to handle it better, the physical symptoms, such as those listed under Facts, will disappear.

One way to see if stress may be the cause of the symptoms you're having is to take the accompanying short test, Do You Have Stress-

Causes of Senility Other Than Alzheimer's Disease	
Although Alzheimer's disease is currently incurable, other causes of senility symptoms may to some extent be treatable or even reversible. The following table lists some of these other problems with their telltale medical signals.	
Problem	*Suspect If*
Multiinfarct dementia (many small strokes)	History high blood pressure or sudden worsening
Low thyroid	Thryoid blood test low (check thyroid routinely)
Low vitamin B_{12}	Check B_{12} level routinely
Polymyalgia rheumatica (an inflammatory disease)	Check sedimentation rate routinely
Alcoholic dementia	History of alcohol abuse
Subdural hematoma (blood clot pressing on brain)	History of head trauma in previous weeks or months or rapid progression of symptoms even if no history of trauma
HIV dementia	High risk for acquired immunodeficiency syndrome
Parkinson's disease	Hand tremors, shuffling gait, "cogwheel" type arm stiffness
Syphilis, late stage	Check VDRL syphilis test routinely
Depression masquerading as senility	Loss of enthusiasm, reasoning skills and personality intact
Sleep-related disorders	Long pauses in breathing or struggling for breath during sleep
Low blood oxygen or high blood carbon dioxide	History of chronic lung problems, e.g., emphysema, bronchitis
Normal pressure hydrocephalus (pressure increase within the brain)	Unsteadiness on walking, loss of urine or bowel control

Related Symptoms? This test can be used as a screening tool; so after you've finished the evaluation, sit back for a moment and look at your answers. If you see a pattern of checkmarks all over—say, 5 or more checks—then there's good reason to suspect a problem. If so, bring this to your doctor's attention, and if he can't help you, ask him to refer you to a psychiatrist or psychotherapist who can.

ERROR:

Your Psychiatrist Is Unwilling to Try Psychotherapy Without Drugs

Joan often experienced extreme nervousness as she tried to juggle her many career and family responsibilities. Consequently, her psy-

---

Do You Have Stress-Related Symptoms?

1. Symptoms related to physical muscle tension or activity:
___ Jitteriness   ___ Furrowed brow
___ Tooth grinding   ___ Jaw tension
___ Restlessness   ___ Easily tired out
___ Trembling   ___ Fidgeting
___ Muscle heaviness or aches

2. Symptoms related to overactivation or hyperalertness:
___ Pounding heart   ___ Lump in throat
___ Cold or clammy hands   ___ Impatience
___ Upset stomach   ___ Sleep problems
___ Diarrhea   ___ Dry mouth
___ Rapid breathing or breath-   ___ Numb or tingling hands or feet
    lessness   ___ Frequent urination
___ Rapid heart   ___ Flushing
___ Light-headedness or dizzi-   ___ Poor concentration
    ness
___ Hot or cold spells

3. Apprehension or fearful expectations:
___ Worried about the future
___ Worried that something bad might happen to you or to a loved
    one

chiatrist, deciding that nondrug psychotherapy sessions either would not work or would take too long to have an effect, prescribed a benzodiazepine drug, Valium, for her symptoms. Furthermore, "to make it convenient," as he put it, he gave her the right to have multiple refills without checking back with him (a practice that is allowed in a number of state jurisdictions).

Joan began to take the pills at first three to four times a week, then nightly. After a while, she increased her intake to twice daily, since it did help her relax. Her sleep also improved, but she still felt tired in the morning, and developed difficulty concentrating. Then she began to feel depressed. When she tried to skip her Valium, she felt worse.

What were the doctor's mistakes?

FACTS: I usually prefer that my patients with chronic anxiety try every nondrug means at their disposal before they turn to drugs as a regular treatment for their anxiety. Benzodiazepine drugs, such as Valium, Librium, Xanax, and Klonopin, often provide prompt dramatic relief from anxiety symptoms. That's why they are so popular with both patients and doctors.

But because they work so well, patients tend to ask for more, and doctors, trying to please, often give more without establishing adequate controls. Before the patient knows it, he can become hooked, and reducing the dosage actually makes the anxiety get worse.

On the other hand, benzodiazepines are actually safer than the barbiturates and other antianxiety medicines that came before them, and I myself prescribe them for my patients when appropriate. But the trick is to keep the dose low and the duration of treatment limited. This is one point where Joan's doctor slipped up.

Although most ordinary anxiety problems can be treated successfully without routine use of drugs, there are other, special forms of anxiety where aggressive use of medicine usually does make sense. These include panic disorder (where there are episodes of extreme fear or anxiety, verging on panic), obsessive-compulsive disorder (where people find it difficult to ignore certain thoughts or resist certain actions), or post-traumatic stress disorder (where a traumatic physical or emotional event triggers recurring dreams, memories, or symptoms).

Like anxiety, depression can often be treated without using medicines. However, medicines can be extremely helpful: when depression is severe, long-standing, or recurring they are often a wise choice—done together with "talk" therapy. Fortunately, antidepressant medicines do not have the high habit-forming potential that we see with the benzodiazepine antianxiety drugs.

WHAT TO DO: If you are taking Valium, Librium, Xanax, or another antianxiety medicine more than three times a week, for either sleep or anxiety, you should seek a second opinion from a psychiatrist.

Also, before you go on one of these drugs, go over the possible negative side effects, such as memory loss, depression, and difficulty in concentrating.

Be skeptical if your doctor prescribes you a multimonth supply of benzodiazepine at a time or if she gives you the right to multiple refills. If this approach is chosen, there should be agreement among you, your family doctor, and a psychiatrist.

Be sure to ask your doctor about the various antianxiety drugs that have no or minimal addictive or dependence-producing qualities, such as the antidepressants Prozac, Zoloft, Elavil, and doxepin. These medications often can help both anxiety and depression. BuSpar is also an effective antianxiety agent without an addictive potential.

If you need antianxiety medicines on a regular basis, you probably also should be involved with "talk" psychotherapy or psychological counseling.

Finally, you might explore with your doctor nondrug strategies for dealing with stress, such as relaxation techniques, self-hypnosis, biofeedback, guided visual imagery, and religious disciplines such as prayer. *Remember:* In managing your emotional life, it's essential to get adequate sleep, good nutrition, and regular exercise and to limit your caffeine and alcohol intake.

ERROR:

Your Doctor Doesn't Sufficiently Explore Whether You Are Depressed

One of my patients, whom I'll call Dan, was a 60-year-old whose son had died in an auto accident. He came in to see me for an exam three years after this tragedy and claimed to feel just fine. His only problem, he said, was that he had gained some weight and was experiencing bouts of constipation. I thought about asking him about his child's death and whether the loss was still weighing heavily on him. But I chose not to, because, I told myself, I didn't want to upset him. Besides, on the surface, he seemed all right.

I learned of my error a few days later when I called back to convey the results of his lab tests. As I spoke to his wife, she told me how depressed Dan had become and how this emotional problem seemed to be sapping his energy.

FACTS: Strange as it may seem, many, perhaps most, people who are depressed don't consciously recognize feelings of sadness, guilt, or lack of hope that we often associate with depression. Or if they do have these feelings, they may downgrade their importance.

Instead, these depressed patients may complain of physical symptoms, such as fatigue, headache, backache, diarrhea, constipation, muscle soreness, weakness, craving for sugar, a tendency to gain or lose weight, difficulty sleeping, or a propensity to sleep too much. These physical symptoms, some of which Dan had mentioned, are caused by the same biochemical imbalances in the brain that also create the emotional pain of depression.

When the main complaints are physical, doctors tend to focus on the physical problem and may overlook the underlying emotional trigger. Medical researchers have shown again and again that unrecognized depression is a component of 10 to 30 percent of all symptoms that bring people to the doctor's office.

WHAT TO DO: You can best help your doctor help you with your depression if you understand what the symptoms of depression are. The accompanying box contains a simple screening test for depression. I also find one "quick and dirty" question to be extremely helpful in raising a warning flag: Have you lost enthusiasm for many or most things that you used to enjoy? If the answer is yes, there's a good likelihood that you are depressed.

If you determine that you probably are depressed, bring this fact up with your doctor. If he doesn't seem to know how to help you, ask for a referral to a therapist or psychiatrist.

ERROR:

Not Recognizing When You and Your Therapist Make a Poor Match

Ken mentioned that he was feeling tremendous anxiety about his job, and his doctor suspected that some of the physical problems he was experiencing, like headaches and insomnia, were related to

A Screening Test for Depression

A yes answer to five or more of these statements, including questions 1 and 2 suggests that you might be depressed, and professional evaluation is strongly recommended. If you answer yes to question 3, you should seek help immediately.
  For at least two weeks, have you

1. Felt blue, sad, or downhearted?

2. Not enjoyed the things you used to?

3. Felt that others would be better off if you were dead?

4. Felt that you were not useful or needed?

5. Noticed that you were losing weight without trying to?

6. Had trouble sleeping through the night?

7. Been sleeping much longer than you usually do and often felt you didn't want to get out of bed?

8. Been restless and unable to keep still?

9. Sensed your mind hasn't been as clear as it used to be?

10. Tended to become tired for no good reason?

11. Felt hopeless about the future?

stress. So the doctor referred Ken to a psychiatrist who rarely talked or gave advice during the therapy sessions.

Ken soon decided that the psychiatrist was giving him no help and costing far too much money. He felt disconnected, as if he were talking to himself. But when he complained to his internist, the response was, "These things take a while, and believe me, this man is well qualified. He was at the top of our medical school class. I think if you stick with it, he'll take good care of you."

Should Ken have been told to switch therapists?

FACTS: One critical factor predicting the success of psychotherapy turns out to be "chemistry"—a feeling between the patient and therapist that they are well connected. You don't have to like the therapist to do well, but it's important to feel involved and believe you can make progress.

Obviously, Ken didn't relate well to the psychiatrist to whom his doctor had referred him. He should have discussed this directly with the therapist to identify possible reasons. Sometimes a frank discussion—even including your sense of disappointment—helps treatment go forward. At other times it does not. In any event, not matching well with a particular therapist or style of therapy doesn't mean you won't be helped by a different therapist or style of treatment.

To communicate well with the therapist, you want to feel that he or she is interested in you as a person. You might also need to feel that you are on the same wavelength as far as personal or religious values are concerned. Although that's not always necessary, it might make it easier for you to trust the advice you're getting.

How important are a psychotherapist's professional credentials? Many studies make clear that successful "talk therapy" has relatively little to do with the degree held by the therapist. A psychiatric social worker with a master's degree may be as effective a partner for your personal therapy as, or more effective than, an esteemed M.D. or professor of psychiatry. Again, the key factor predicting success is chemistry or a sense of connection between patient and therapist.

Of course, it's also important that your therapist be well trained. The best chemistry in the world won't do you much good if your therapist's judgment leads you in the wrong direction. Psychiatrists and Ph.D. psychologists undergo longer and more intensive training than do therapists with a master's degree. So all else being equal, they should have clearer insight into your needs. That's why I strongly recommend that if you do choose a therapist with a master's degree or less, prefer one who purchases regular supervision of his cases from a psychiatrist or a Ph.D. psychologist.

A psychiatrist is the best option in certain situations, especially where the reason for emotional turmoil is unclear: Is the problem mainly depression, mainly anxiety, or some different psychiatric disorder? Is the cause mainly psychological, or is there a physical disease at work? Psychiatrists usually have the best developed skills to do an initial complete evaluation of just what is wrong and what sorts of treatment are most likely to help.

The other critical time to prefer a psychiatrist is when symptoms are so severe, urgent, or nonresponsive to treatment that treating with medicines should be considered. Psychiatrists, who are physicians, are entitled to prescribe drugs. Psychologists cannot.

WHAT TO DO: If after a session or two, you, like Ken, don't feel connected with your therapist, discuss the issue frankly with him or her and also with your doctor who made the referral. You may be able to talk through the block you're feeling and actually stimulate some chemistry in the relationship. But if your sense of uninvolvement persists, you should seek a different therapist, or an alternative style of treatment.

ERROR:

Your Doctor Lacks an Organized Approach to Dealing with Your Chronic Fatigue

Nancy had severe chronic fatigue along with a number of other symptoms. After nearly two years of feeling tired, having headaches, loose bowel movements, and various other aches and pains, she demanded a complete medical work-up from as many specialists as it took to get to the root of her problem.

So her family doctor referred her to a gastroenterologist, who passed a long tube into her rectum and told her she had spastic colitis. A cardiologist then listened to her heart, did an echocardiogram, and told her she had mitral valve prolapse syndrome. A neurologist did an MRI scan of her brain and told her she had tension headaches. An arthritis specialist did some blood tests and concluded that her muscle aches were from fibromyalgia. An infectious disease specialist checked her for Lyme disease. A nonphysician nutritionist told her she had hypoglycemia and was infected with candida yeast. Finally, a psychologist said that the root of her problem was chronic depression.

Why all the confusion?

FACTS: As it turned out, the psychologist was the one who came closest to the truth, though there was some truth in what several of the other specialists concluded. The problem for Nancy, as for many other patients whose main symptom is fatigue, was that no single doctor took a systematic, organized approach to sorting through her symptoms. Her experience reflects the problem with the narrow training that specialists receive: If the only tool you have is a hammer, then pretty soon, everything you look at begins to resemble a nail.

In fact, there are fifteen to twenty or so common causes of chronic fatigue, and each of Nancy's experts hit on at least one. But a better approach would have been for one doctor to go through all of the possibilities, prioritize them, and evaluate them in order until the real cause or causes of the fatigue were found.

WHAT TO DO: While there are many exceptions to this rule, it's my experience that your odds of curing your fatigue increase if you *begin* your evaluation not with a specialist, but with your family physician or internist. You should spend at least one hour with her, during which she gets a complete up-to-date medical history and gives you a complete physical exam.

In addition, you should expect your family doctor to do basic laboratory tests. Everyone with fatigue should get a CBC count, SMA panel, thyroid test, and urinalysis. Some should also receive a chest X ray, a sedimentation rate (a measure of inflammation in the body), an antinuclear antibody test (another sign of inflammation), an HIV test, a Lyme test, an exercise stress test, or psychological testing.

Your personal physician is likely to be the most broadly trained and open-minded doctor you encounter. She's also more likely to treat your complaint with respect. On the other hand, if she is stumped, as Nancy's doctor was, the next logical step may be to seek a second opinion from another physician, who may be more organized and analytical than your own.

If these attempts to get to the root of your fatigue don't work, then you should schedule two or three sessions with a psychiatrist or psychologist. You're not going to this therapist for regular psychotherapy at this point. You just want an initial evaluation to answer a specific question: Do you believe I have psychological issues that are sufficiently important to be the cause of my fatigue?

Only after this basic evaluation is completed does it make sense to begin to consult with subspecialists for subtle, missed diagnoses. Your last stop should be the alternative medicine crowd, who specialize in diagnoses that regular physicians may reject.

ERROR:

Your Doctor Misses an Elusive Physical Cause of Your Chronic Fatigue

Harry had been feeling well when a bad respiratory infection put him in bed for more than a week. Although his nose remained somewhat stuffy, his main respiratory symptoms cleared. After he recovered from this illness, he continued to feel frequent fatigue over the next four months. He saw four doctors, who were unable to help him.

Finally, an astute internist took a long shot. He figured that since Harry's problems began with a respiratory infection, he should order a CT scan of Harry's sinuses. The test revealed that the patient had a low-grade sinus infection that had gone undetected and was probably left over from his original illness. A long course of antibiotics allowed Harry to recover his previous sense of vitality.

FACTS: A variety of physical conditions can cause chronic fatigue. If you have appropriate, telltale signs or symptoms of any of these conditions, it's important for them to be checked out before a definite diagnosis is rendered of excessive stress or a psychological disorder. See the accompanying box, Easily Missed Physical Conditions That Can Cause Fatigue. The first column lists the conditions; the second, the signs and symptoms that should make you suspect the condition; and the third, techniques that you can expect your doctor to use to check whether you really have a particular condition.

WHAT TO DO: Reflect on all the changes you have experienced in your health since you began to feel fatigued. Also, list all symptoms you've noticed; use the accompanying box. Take your notes to your doctor's office when you go in for your next visit, and be sure that he answers all your questions satisfactorily. If you feel dissatisfied with any of his responses, seek a second opinion.

ERROR:

When You Complain of Chronic Fatigue, Your Doctor Fails to Check for Sleep Apnea

Lenny, a 55-year-old department store manager, developed congestive heart failure so severe that his cardiologist listed him as a heart transplant candidate. But Lenny also suffered from sleep apnea, a condition involving long, frequent spells of not taking a breath during sleep. He was constantly tired and had to deal with frequent periods of depression. As a result, he was referred to me for treat-

Easily Missed Physical Conditions That Can Cause Fatigue		
Condition That Can Cause Fatigue	*Suspect If*	*How to Check*
Nasal or sinus congestion or allergies	Stuffy nose, postnasal drip, especially if you have sinus headache and non-restorative sleep	Trial of antibiotics, nasal decongestants or nasal cortisone, CT scan of sinuses, allergy tests
Too little sleep	Need an alarm clock, sleep longer on weekends, sleep <6 hours, sleep 45 minutes less than you did when you felt well, fall asleep during the day	3-week trial of an extra 45 minutes of sleep each night
Poor-quality sleep	Not feeling rested in morning, wake often at night, toss and turn, snore badly, stop breathing or struggle for breath while asleep, muscle twitching while asleep or restless legs during the day	Someone should observe your sleep, see a sleep specialist
Fibromyalgia	Muscles sore or tender, sleep not refreshing	Consult an arthritis, sleep, pulmonary, or rehabilitation specialist
Lyme disease	Typical bull's-eye rash, tick bites even if Lyme tests are negative, see pp. 309–310	Lyme blood tests, see infectious disease specialist (Caution: some Lyme specialists overdiagnose Lyme)
Polymyalgia rheumatica, temporal arthritis	Muscle aches, headaches, especially if age >60	Sedimentation rate, see arthritis specialist

Easily Missed Physical Conditions That Can Cause Fatigue *(Continued)*

Condition That Can Cause Fatigue	Suspect If	How to Check
Autoimmune disease (e.g., rheumatoid arthritis, lupus)	Swollen, painful joints	Antinuclear antibody test, sedimentation rate, see an arthritis specialist
Chronic urine or prostate infections	Frequent or burning urine, slow urine stream	Urinalysis, prostate exam
Subtle heart and lung disease	Shortness of breath with mild physical exertion, cough, swollen ankles	Chest X ray, echocardiogram, electrocardiogram, lung function tests, lung scan
Vitamin and mineral deficiencies	Poor diet, alcohol excess, diuretic medicines	See a registered dietitian to review diet, blood potassium
Irritable bowel syndrome (50% of these patients also have fatigue)	Constipation, diarrhea, gas	Trial of high-fiber diet, elimination diet, gastroenterologist versus nutritionally oriented physician
Adrenal gland deficiency (rare)	Dizziness on standing up, poor stamina	See an endocrinologist
Physical deconditioning	Increased heart rate or shortness of breath on mild physical exertion	Exercise stress test, supervised exercise training program
Dizziness syndrome	Spinning or off-balance feeling, fatigue	See an ear, nose, and throat specialist or neurologist
Low blood pressure	Feel worse standing up	Measure blood pressure lying, sitting, and standing
Extreme obesity or recent weight gain	Gained weight recently or >50 pounds overweight	Trial of diet and exercise

Easily Missed Physical Conditions That Can Cause Fatigue *(Continued)*		
Condition That Can Cause Fatigue	*Suspect If*	*How to Check*
Thyroid problems, low or high	Double-check to be 100% sure thyroid tests were done with standard blood work	Triiodothyronine (T_3), thyroxine (T_4), and thyrotropin (TSH)
Hidden cancer	Weight loss, changed bowel habits, especially if age >60	Complete physical including attention to colon and pancreatic cancer
Low vitamin B_{12} (can occur without anemia)	Age >60, strict vegetarian, a long history of gastritis	Blood vitamin B_{12} level
Low iron (can occur without anemia)	You are a woman who menstruates, red blood cells on CBC are small	Check blood iron or ferritin
Chronic fatigue syndrome	Fatigue persisting for 24 hours after exertion, often begins with a flu	An infectious disease versus a chronic fatigue specialist

ment because I have developed some expertise with sleep disturbances.

I treated his sleep apnea with a device that forces pressured air into the nose during sleep, and he quickly showed improvement. Now, he can walk three miles at a stretch and is on much less medication than before. Most important, he's been taken off the heart transplant list.

FACTS: Sleep apnea affects about 1 adult in 100 and is most common among overweight men, people who snore, and those above age 65. It can cause daytime fatigue, depression, high blood pressure, and congestive heart failure. Yet only a small proportion of sleep apnea victims are recognized and treated.

Part of the problem is that most doctors haven't been alerted to look for sleep apnea as a possible cause of fatigue or other symptoms. In my first fifteen years of practice, I recognized only one case of sleep apnea. But since I've started looking for the condition routinely among all my patients who complain of fatigue, I now find about ten cases each year.

WHAT TO DO: If you regularly feel tired and sleepy and no good reason has been found, ask your doctor to check out the possibility of sleep apnea. One preliminary test you can do is to ask someone you trust to watch you while you sleep, preferably for one full ninety-minute dream cycle. If you snore, sleep apnea is a distinct possibility. But even if you don't snore, the condition may be signaled by pauses in breathing of ten seconds or longer that occur more than about ten times an hour. Snorting or struggling for breath is also an abnormal sign.

If this amateur observation raises suspicions of sleep apnea, ask your doctor about a referral to a sleep center so that you can undergo a home sleep apnea monitor test. This is done by strapping electrodes to your chest so that your chest movements can be measured during breathing.

Also, ask your observer whether you often have small kicks or muscle twitches when you sleep or if you toss and turn excessively. Any of these habits can be clues to a different specific and treatable sleep disorder.

ERROR:

Your Doctor Prescribes Sleeping Pills Unwisely

Lydia couldn't sleep for weeks after she hurt her back in an auto accident. The painkiller Advil helped some, but she also needed a sleeping pill, the benzodiazepine Restoril, to help her sleep through the night.

Her pain diminished over the next few weeks, and her doctor reduced the dosage of Restoril, but Lydia began to sleep fitfully again, waking several times at night and waking unrefreshed in the morning.

When she was referred to me, I persuaded her to switch from Restoril to a low dose of the antidepressant Elavil. She protested at first: "But I'm not depressed!" But when I explained that I was using the Elavil to get her off the stronger, habit-forming benzodiazepine, she agreed.

Within a few weeks, we tapered off the Elavil, and Lydia's sleep pattern remained healthy. Now she takes the Elavil for sleep at most only once or twice a month. She's also found that Benadryl, an allergy medicine, can help her on those infrequent occasions when she can't get to sleep.

FACTS: Too many doctors are too quick on the draw in continuing to prescribe habit-forming sleeping medicines. There's a saying among sleep specialists: Sleeping pills don't increase your sleep time, they just borrow it from tomorrow.

The currently popular benzodiazepine-type sleeping pills have fewer side effects and are less addictive than the older barbiturates (such as Seconal) or chloral hydrate. But still, the benzodiazepines have a significant tendency to lose their effectiveness when you take them regularly. Also, they can depress breathing, a particularly dangerous effect with those who have lung disease or mix alcohol with sleeping pills. They may also cause decreased memory, depression, hallucinations, agitation, mental confusion, and dizziness. Stopping these drugs suddenly can cause anxiety or even epileptic seizures.

For most people, these benzodiazepine medicines are safe when used occasionally. When taken more than three times a week, however, the risk of side effects or addiction increases dramatically. Various research reports have suggested that many physicians, especially nonpsychiatrists, make it too easy for their patients to get hooked on these sleeping pills.

The shorter-acting benzodiazepine sleeping pills like triazolam (Halcion) don't leave you tired the next day. Also, because it wears off in five or six hours, Halcion—when taken as a sleeping pill—is less likely to induce addiction than are longer-acting forms of benzodiazepine sleeping pills. But Halcion sometimes causes people to be anxious the morning after they take it.

Medium-duration sleeping pills, like temazepam (Restoril) and estazolam (Pro Som), may become less effective with more frequent use. They also have a moderate potential for addiction if they are used too often. A minority of users find these drugs still keep them sleepy the next day.

Long-acting benzodiazepines, such as flurazepam (Dalmane), quazepam (Doral), and diazepam (Valium), are more likely to cause addiction and daytime fatigue. But their long sedating action can be a helpful side effect for people who suffer from daytime anxiety.

Often the best approach to treatment is to begin with the stronger sleeping medications if necessary but to be careful to taper them off within a few weeks by using less habit-forming sedating drugs, such as the antidepressant Elavil or an over-the-counter antihistamine, e.g., diphenhydramine (Benadryl).

WHAT TO DO: For most people with poor sleep—with the exception of alcoholics and lung disease victims—there is no harm and often some good from occasionally using a benzodiazepine-type sleeping pill. You should definitely prefer them to the former favorites, the barbiturates.

However, insist that your doctor also explain the down side of any sleeping medicine she gives you. Especially go over the risks of developing an addiction. Resist the temptation to push your doctor to prescribe more than fifteen or so pills at a time. That's a good way to get yourself addicted.

Ask your physician about the sedating antidepressants or antihistamines as alternatives to traditional sleeping pills. They aren't as potent in knocking you out, but they may work even better to improve the quality of your sleep. The important thing is that their addictive potential is much less than that for standard sleeping potions.

ERROR:

Your Doctor Doesn't Recognize That Your Headache Relief Medicine Is Actually Causing Your Headaches

Frank was taking Cafergot, an ergot-type medicine, which had been prescribed by his doctor, for his migraine headaches. The drug worked for several months, but then the migraines returned in greater intensity than before.

What had happened?

FACTS: Most headache relief medicines can have an addictive effect if they are taken every day or nearly every day. The body gets used to the drug and needs it more and more, so that any delay in taking a dose can actually bring on a headache. Patients with migraines may take these drugs more often to reduce the pain, but then they may begin to suffer from a less intensive but chronic daily headache between migraines. Also, if they ever cut back on their medicine, an acute migraine can result.

Pain medicines that can trigger headaches include ergot-type drugs (Cafergot, ergostat), sedatives (Fiorinal, Esgic), narcotics (codeine, Percodan, Demerol), caffeine-containing drugs (Excedrin, coffee), and perhaps even aspirin.

Headache experts now agree that many people with daily or almost-daily headaches actually feel better after they are supervised to taper off their headache medicines—at least once they get past their painful "withdrawal headaches." The most qualified physicians in this area are neurologists or others who make headache the major focus of their practice. Most belong to the American Association for the Study of Headache, 875 Kings Highway, Suite 200, West Deptford, N.J. 08096, phone 1-800-255-ACHE.

WHAT TO DO: If you have problems with headaches, and your medication doesn't seem to be working or even appears to be making the condition worse, pose these questions to your doctor:

- Could the overuse of acute-relief headache medicines be making my headaches worse? (If you take them daily, chances are the answer could be yes.)
- Should I be taking nonaddictive, preventive medicines instead of or in addition to my acute-relief medicines? (These may include beta-blockers, tricyclic antidepressants, and calcium channel blockers.)
- Should I be referred to a specialist who can supervise my withdrawal from potentially addictive medication for headache?

If you have headaches that continue to require pain relief medicines almost daily, you should consult a neurologist or a medical specialist in headaches. If your physician doesn't know of such an expert call the American Association for the Study of Headache at the above phone number and ask for a referral.

ERROR:

Your Doctor Misses the Possibility That Your Worsening Headache Could Signal a Medical Emergency

Sol, who was 75 years old and apparently in good health, began to experience pain around his temples. He had experienced occasional migraines in the past, and his doctor assumed that this was another instance of that problem even when the pain began to intensify. The next day, Sol was admitted to the hospital with a condition that was diagnosed as temporal arteritis, an inflammation of the temporal artery, which feeds the temple area.

FACTS: Although headache emergencies aren't common, it's crucial to recognize them when they occur. Here are some possible causes of headache emergencies:

- Temporal arteritis (an inflammation of the arteries near the temple). If not detected and treated promptly, blindness can result. This problem is most common in those over the age of 60.
- Severe high blood pressure.
- Meningitis (infection of the spinal column).
- Encephalitis (infection of the brain).
- Brain tumor.
- A rapidly expanding or leaking blood vessel in the brain (an aneurysm or cerebral hemorrhage).
- Strokes.
- Acute glaucoma (high pressure in the eye).

WHAT TO DO: If you suspect an emergency headache or your headache grows steadily worse, contact your doctor immediately. Don't delay if your doctor is slow to answer. Call the emergency squad, or if you are a family member or friend, bring the patient to the nearest emergency room.

If your problem is thought to be temporal arteritis, as happened with Sol, your doctor should check with a blood test called the *sedimentation rate*. Temporal arteritis responds dramatically well to cortisone-type medicines.

Other signs that you may be dealing with an emergency are situations where the headache is unusual in any way; is very painful; or is accompanied by other symptoms, such as fever, stiff neck, vomiting, confusion, slurred speech, weakness of any part of the body, impaired vision, or the enlargement of one of your pupils. Also, you should look on the headache as an emergency if you've suffered a blow to the head recently, especially if you were knocked out, even briefly.

Conclusion

Making the Health Care System Work for You

Being an activist on behalf of your own health is not easy.

As we've already seen, you first have to gain a basic understanding of the specific medical conditions you're facing. Then, you have to know some of the danger signals that may warn "Possible error!" when you're in your doctor's office or in the hospital.

In the turmoil and crisis atmosphere surrounding today's medical scene, you must also be aware of another important factor that may trigger error: the inherent flaws and weaknesses of the particular health plan that you've chosen.

There are several basic types of health care programs that are now available, and these will almost certainly continue in some similar form in the foreseeable future. Each has its own peculiar strengths and weaknesses—weaknesses that may trigger error. So in addition to understanding the specific diseases and patient responses described in the foregoing text, it's important to keep in mind the characteristics of the particular form of health care you're using.

You Have Four Choices

I like to divide the main programs into four different categories:

1. Fee-for-service private practice.
2. Health maintenance organizations (HMOs), where physicians are salaried employees of the plan.

3. Individual practice associations (IPAs), where privately practicing physicians contract to see patients who are referred by a managed care insurance plan. A variation on this is the preferred provider organization (PPO), where patients pay less for member doctors than they would for physicians outside the organization.

4. Hospital- or government-run clinics.

Current estimates suggest that of Americans who see doctors with some regularity, about 50 percent now depend on private fee-for-service doctors, 40 percent rely on an HMO or IPA, and 10 percent use a walk-in clinic plan.

What are the main strengths and weaknesses of each of these types of medical programs and the issues that should cause you to stay on the alert for error? In the introduction to this book, I mentioned a couple of considerations, but briefly, here is a summary of some other points to ponder.

The fee-for-service private practice plan. This approach usually provides the most personal attention and maximum freedom to chart your medical course, including the hiring and firing of your physician. But as we've seen time and time again throughout this book, private practice is expensive and vulnerable to the triple errors of overdiagnosing, overtreating, and overcharging.

The HMO. These organizations, which include programs like Kaiser Permanente, are the most cost-effective model of health care. They try to assure adequate care for everyone through incentives and controls that discourage their employee-doctors and patients from consuming medical resources beyond what the HMO considers to be reasonable and efficient. The problem is that when a patient feels strongly that he should have a particular test or procedure and the HMO disagrees, the HMO will almost always win out.

The IPA. The IPA model is a cross between the HMO and private practice. In an IPA, privately practicing physicians contract with managed care plans, such as Aetna, U.S. Health Care, or PruCare. The doctors accept lower fees and agree to various controls on their work as a trade-off for higher patient volume. The IPAs provide more flexibility in choosing a physician than do the HMOs. But like the HMOs, they strictly monitor each physician and restrict his or her ability to recommend expensive procedures, even if the patient feels she needs the procedure, and even if the physician agrees.

Both HMOs and IPAs suffer from a number of inherent flaws, which can lead to error or to a limitation on the patient's right to correct or redress error:

- They limit the ability of doctors to order diagnostic tests or prescribe treatments because they are deemed too costly for the probable benefits involved.

- They often require patients to sign a document that in effect forfeits the individual's right to sue for medical malpractice. The patient must rely on compulsory arbitration rather than a formal law court.

- Many of these plans selectively avoid taking on high-risk or high-cost patients. They may either try to raise premium rates or reject prospective subscribers if the patients seem at risk to develop a costly illness such as cancer, mental disease, or acquired immunodeficiency syndrome. This selective bias is known in the industry as *cherry picking*.

Clinic care. Many patients use walk-in clinics at hospitals or government facilities because they are cheap or the only available program in their area. Many clinic workers, who tend to be paid relatively low wages and who are often overworked, are concerned about the welfare of their patients. A few are genuine idealists. But the sheer volume of their practice works against individual attention and tends to foster fatigue and mistakes.

On the whole, this type of plan tends to be inflexible, inefficient, and relatively unresponsive to patient's desires. So if you can afford to, avoid using most clinics.

As I've said, it's likely that each of these types of plans will continue in some form in the coming years. But in light of the pressure to make low-cost care available to more people, there will certainly be some changes, and I expect those changes will favor a movement toward the HMO-IPA model.

The Future Directions of Health Care and How You Can Best Protect Yourself

Medical care seems to be moving strongly in the direction of some form of the HMO and IPA, where the doctors are either employees or under the strict control of cost-conscious managers. You may be tempted to switch from a private fee-for-service situation to an HMO because the reduction in costs can be quite attractive. But take care! Before you jump, ask the managers of the plan some of the following pointed questions.

Note: Of course, if your company has a contract with a particular managed care plan, you won't have a choice about your program. Still, it will be helpful to ask these questions upon your first contact with the plan to learn what to expect when you have to go in for a checkup, diagnosis, or treatment.

- What is their policy on coronary heart disease? You want to know what the policy is concerning angioplasty and heart surgery. If the plan you're considering consistently comes down on the less expensive side, or refers its procedures to a less desirable hospital, you may want to shop around if you have that option.

- What types of cancer treatments does the organization approve? Some of the more advanced cancer treatments used at the great cancer treatment centers aren't available in most hospitals, and they are also very expensive. You should inquire: If the standard treatments fail, will the plan send me where I need to go to get extra care, or will I be left to fend for myself? (Try to get this answer in writing, if you can.)

- What is their policy on mental health care? How many mental health visits are covered each year? What are the credentials of their therapists? What choice do you have in selecting a therapist? If depression, schizophrenia, or a drug abuse problem doesn't respond to standard treatment, does the plan have a backup facility on call? If you are wrestling with a neurosis, a common condition where long-term counseling may be the best choice, will the plan help you pay?

- Check into the care for stroke, Alzheimer's disease, and dementia. How good is the physical therapy program offered by the plan? Also, look into the home care services and the training and emotional support for family caregivers.

- How does the plan respond to chronic headache? Ask if there is a comprehensive, holistic approach to treatment, including the use of relaxation techniques. Or are headache victims passed off with quick prescriptions or with vague explanations that they may be "just dealing with some excessive stress"?

- Does the plan provide nutrition counseling or support groups to deal with overweight problems?

- What is the policy in dealing with kidney failure due to diabetes or other conditions? It's possible you or a family member may require dialysis or a kidney transplant. How will these measures be handled by your HMO?

- Ask about how the plan handles health conditions with "mysterious" symptoms, including fibromyalgia, sleep disorders, chronic fatigue syndrome, or chronic Lyme disease. Check the descriptions of errors related to these conditions (refer to the index), then see how the plan representative responds when you raise a few pertinent questions. Ask for a few examples of how these problems were handled by the plan. If the representative seems evasive, you should consider placing your health care business with another program.

- Find out if there is provision for a hospice program for those with a late-stage terminal illness. If there's not, your care choices will be limited if you or a loved one is dying from cancer or some other serious disease.

Those who are satisfied with the answers to the above questions and decide to go with an HMO or IPA will still have to be on the alert to avoid error when they go in for a checkup or treatment. Here are some tactics that will enable you to protect yourself.

Tactic 1: Make friends with your doctors, nurses, lab technicians, appointment clerks, and administrators, even the telephone operators, whose names you should learn. Remember, even the most rule-bound of systems is usually run by normal people much like you or me. You should do all you can to get your caregivers to see you as a *person*, not just as a package to be processed. When you become a friend, most people are willing to bend rigid rules in order to give you the best service.

Tactic 2: When you go in for a visit, know in advance what you want, make sure your desires are reasonable, and then be persistent in asserting your demands. Suppose you have bronchitis and want to see the doctor today or tomorrow, but the first available opening isn't for a week. A doctor can almost always see one more patient today if the need is urgent. Your responsibility is to get across the emergency nature of your situation, such as by telling them, "The last time I had bronchitis, it turned into pneumonia."

The real issue here is your ability to communicate clearly. If the receptionist hears you asking for a nonemergency visit, you won't get quick service. But if you say unequivocally that your need *is* an emergency and that you're sure your health will suffer if you're not seen immediately, you're quite likely to get action.

If this approach doesn't work, don't give up. Ask to speak to a nurse or doctor. Or call back an hour later to report that your condition is worse. Appeal to the person's sympathy. Rely on the friendships you've been cultivating. Be assertive and persistent, but don't get nasty. Always remember that your ultimate objective when you meet a roadblock to immediate treatment is to become an exception to the plan's rules.

Tactic 3: Understand how your program works politically. As quickly as possible you should learn the buzz words that get action. For example, terms like *medical necessity, irreparable damage,* or *human concern* will often make a plan representative take notice.

Also, identify the major sources of authority in the plan. You may learn that the word or opinion of a particular doctor carries great weight. Or the buck may stop with a senior nurse, the medical director, or a middle level administrator. Get to know by name the individuals who wield the power, and don't hesitate to appeal to them if you reach an impasse.

Most managed care plans have a formal grievance procedure for patients who are dissatisfied. But I would exhaust every informal, personal avenue of appeal before I entered the formal grievance process. You're more likely to be labeled a "complainer" if you frequently use the grievance procedures.

Another way to put pressure on a resistant HMO or IPA is to enlist the aid of your personnel director at work. This is the individual who decides which program will be sponsored by your company. Too many complaints from workers like you could motivate the company to withdraw its account.

Tactic 4: If the stakes are high enough, that is, if your health or that of a family member is in real jeopardy, be prepared to litigate or use the power of the press.

The ability of HMOs and IPAs to survive and prosper depends on their ability to maintain the trust and confidence of politicians who write the laws, the employers who pay the bills, and the general public, who must remain satisfied. Just one *Wall Street Journal* article describing a malpractice horror in an HMO is not what a plan wants or needs to maintain a rosy profit picture.

This tactic should be your last resort after all else has failed. But just the threat of such action will often be enough to get the health plan to give you what you want.

The more controls the government or others place on our health care system, the more adept the patient must become at dealing with bureaucracy. Many mistakes—through medical oversight, or outright refusal to pay for an important but expensive procedure—can arise from health plans that are overorganized and overcontrolled. But by learning to operate within the particular system that you've chosen or that has been imposed on you, you can minimize your exposure to these errors.

Although we are in the midst of a health care crisis—and confusion and uncertainty are, unfortunately, the order of the day—there is no need to despair. The need may have intensified for you to stay on the alert in guarding your family's health care. But at the same time, plenty of powerful, effective tools are now at your disposal to reduce or even eliminate the threat posed by any health care challenge you may face.

Acknowledgments

Our deepest and warmest thanks go to our literary agents, Herb and Nancy Katz, and to our editor at Simon & Schuster, Fred Hills. Laureen Rowland, Fred's assistant, has been unfailingly helpful.

Our greatest debt is to the many patients, friends, physicians, and nurses who shared their life experiences with us to form the basis for the case studies that illustrate this book.

My partner, David Brown, M.D., and his wonderful wife, Melissa Brown, M.D., have my special gratitude for their support and encouragement, as do the members of my office staff: Jodi Geller, R.N.; Nancy Carter, R.N.; Peggy Stiner; Betty Giordano; Felicia Carter; Nora Cielo, M.A.; and Lorri Katz, R.D.

Many physicians and health care administrators have made special contributions as critics or teachers. These include Douglas Ashendorf, M.D.; David Befeler, M.D.; Howard Blank, M.D.; Richard Blum, M.D.; Johanna Burani, R.D.; Paul Carniol, M.D.; Joel Duberstein, M.D.; James Espinosa, M.D.; Stuart Fischer, M.D.; Jeff Fisher, M.D.; Tom Foley; Fred Goldberg, Ph.D.; Joan Goldberg, M.D.; Larry Goldfarb, D.C.; Michael Gutkin, M.D.; Mitchell Jablons, M.D.; Ben Josephson, M.D.; Joyce Jukofsky, R.N.; Donald Kent, M.D.; Michael Kerner, M.D.; Michael Kreitzer, M.D.; Gerald Lazar, M.D.; Beverly Licata, R.N.; Lynn Lind, R.N.; Marvin Lipsky, M.D.; Dennis Lowenthal, M.D.; Paul Marcus; Arthur Millman, M.D.; Robert Morrison, M.D.; Jeffrey Nahmias, M.D.; John Penek, M.D.; Mark Peppercorn, M.D.; Dolores Phillips; Fred Pine, D.C.; Robert Restifo, M.D.; Kenneth Ring, M.D.; Tom Robertson, M.D.; William Rea, M.D.; Steven Rosenthal, M.D.; David P. Saur, M.D.; Jack Scharf; Sharon Selinger, M.D.; Garry Sherman, D.P.M.; Bennett Silver, M.D.; Fred Silverberg, M.D.; Michael Sniffen; Ronald Sorvino, M.D.; Steven Stanzione, M.D.; Elliot Stein, M.D.; Kenneth

Storch, M.D.; Michael Suhl, M.D.; David Swee, M.D.; Mark Van
Cooy, M.D.; Harris Vernick, M.D.; Melvin Vigman, M.D.; John
Weinstein, M.D.; H.H. Wittmann, M.D.; David Worth, M.D.

Special thanks to these good friends and editorial critics: Louis
Gary, Joel Nisenbaum, Andrew Kaldor, Sandra Kaldor, Avi Yos-
kowitz, Reggie Yoskowitz, Renie Carniol, Ellen Gilbertson, Robert
Hirschfeld, Bennet Tittler, Andrew Weiss, Ph.D., Bonnie Weiss,
Arthur Chotin, Betsy Chotin, Shelly Pilberg, Howard Useem, and, of
course, Patricia, Carrie, Lisa, and Tracy Podell.

And most critically at times of crisis, the unfailing support of Mark
Bara and Bob Blidner from The Gentle Computer, Summit, New
Jersey.

Index